PROCEEDINGS

WORKSHOP ON NEEDLE EXCHANGE AND BLEACH DISTRIBUTION PROGRAMS

Panel on Needle Exchange and Bleach Distribution Programs

Commission on Behavioral and Social Sciences and Education

National Research Council

and

Institute of Medicine

NATIONAL ACADEMY PRESS
Washington, D.C. 1994

NOTICE: The project that is the subject of this report was approved by the Governing Board of the National Research Council, whose members are drawn from the councils of the National Academy of Sciences, the National Academy of Engineering, and the Institute of Medicine. The members of the committee responsible for the report were chosen for their special competences and with regard for appropriate balance.

This report has been reviewed by a group other than the authors according to procedures approved by a Report Review Committee consisting of members of the National Academy of Sciences, the National Academy of Engineering, and the Institute of Medicine.

The National Academy of Sciences is a private, nonprofit, self-perpetuating society of distinguished scholars engaged in scientific and engineering research, dedicated to the furtherance of science and technology and to their use for the general welfare. Upon the authority of the charter granted to it by the Congress in 1863, the Academy has a mandate that require it to advise the federal government on scientific and technical matters. Dr. Bruce M. Alberts is president of the National Academy of Sciences.

The National Academy of Engineering was established in 1964, under the charter of the National Academy of Sciences, as a parallel organization of outstanding engineers. It is autonomous in its administration and in the selection of its members, sharing with the National Academy of Sciences the responsibility for advising the federal government. The National Academy of Engineering also sponsors engineering programs aimed at meeting national needs, encourages education and research, and recognizes the superior achievement of engineers. Dr. Robert M. White is president of the National Academy of Engineering.

The Institute of Medicine was established in 1970 by the National Academy of Sciences to secure the services of eminent members of appropriate professions in the examination of policy matters pertaining to the health of the public. The Institute acts under the responsibility given to the National Academy of Sciences by its congressional charter to be an adviser to the federal government and, upon its own initiative, to identify issues of medical care, research, and education. Dr. Kenneth I. Shine is president of the Institute of Medicine.

The National Research Council was organized by the National Academy of Sciences in 1916 to associate the broad community of science and technology with the Academy's purposes of furthering knowledge and advising the federal government. Functioning in accordance with general policies determined by the Academy, the Council has become the principal operating agency of both the National Academy of Sciences and the National Academy of Engineering in providing services to the government, the public, and the scientific and engineering communities. The Council is administered jointly by both Academies and the Institute of Medicine. Dr. Bruce M. Alberts and Dr. Robert M. White are chairman and vice chairman, respectively, of the National Research Council.

This project was sponsored by the National Institute on Drug Abuse.

Library of Congress Catalog Card No. 94-67632
International Standard Book Number 0-309-05084-7

Additional copies of this report are available from:
National Academy Press
2101 Constitution Avenue N.W.
Washington, D.C. 20418

Call 800-624-6242 or 202-334-3313 (in the Washington Metropolitan Area).

B349
Printed in the United States of America

PANEL ON NEEDLE EXCHANGE AND BLEACH DISTRIBUTION PROGRAMS

LINCOLN MOSES (*Chair*), Department of Statistics, Stanford University
RONALD S. BROOKMEYER, Department of Biostatistics, School of Hygiene and Public Health, The Johns Hopkins University
LAWRENCE S. BROWN, Jr., Department of Medicine, Harlem Hospital, College of Physicians and Surgeons, Columbia University *and* Division of Medical Services Evaluation and Research, Addiction Research and Treatment Corporation, Brooklyn
RICHARD F. CATALANO, Social Development Research Group, Seattle
DAVID S. CORDRAY, Vanderbilt Institute for Public Policy Studies *and* Department of Human Resources, Peabody College, Vanderbilt University
DON C. DES JARLAIS, Chemical Dependency Institute, National Development and Research Institutes, Inc., Beth Israel Medical Center, New York
CASWELL A. EVANS, Jr., Public Health Programs and Services, County of Los Angeles Department of Health Services
MARK B. FEINBERG, Gladstone Institute of Virology and Immunology, San Francisco
HERBERT D. KLEBER, Department of Psychiatry, College of Physicians and Surgeons, *and* Center on Addiction and Substance Abuse, Columbia University
PATRICK M. O'MALLEY, Institute for Social Research, University of Michigan, Ann Arbor
NANCY S. PADIAN, Department of Obstetrics, Gynecology, and Reproductive Sciences, University of California, San Francisco General Hospital
MARIAN GRAY SECUNDY, College of Medicine, Department of Community Health and Family Practice, Howard University
DAVID VLAHOV, School of Hygiene and Public Health, The Johns Hopkins University
W. WAYNE WIEBEL, AIDS Outreach Intervention Project *and* School of Public Health, Epidemiology and Biostatistics, University of Chicago at Illinois
DAVID R. WILLIAMS, Institute for Social Research, University of Michigan, Ann Arbor

National Research Council Staff

SUSANNE M. STOIBER, *Division Director* (through January 1994)
ALEXANDRA K. WIGDOR, *Division Director* (from February 1994)
JACQUES L. NORMAND, *Study Director*
SAHR J. KPUNDEH, *Staff Officer*
ELAINE McGARRAUGH, *Research Associate*
SUSAN R. McCUTCHEN, *Senior Project Assistant*

Institute of Medicine Staff

MICHAEL A. STOTO, *Division Director*
LESLIE M. HARDY, *Program Officer*

CONTENTS

PREFACE

The July 1992 ADAMHA Reorganization Act mandated that the Secretary of Health and Human Services, acting through the Director of the National Institute on Drug Abuse, request the National Academy of Sciences to conduct a study on the impact of needle exchange and bleach distribution programs on drug use behavior and the spread of the human immunodeficiency virus. In response to that legislative directive, the National Research Council and the Institute of Medicine of the National Academy of Sciences organized the Panel on Needle Exchange and Bleach Distribution Programs in May 1993, under the auspices of the Committee on AIDS Research and the Behavioral, Social, and Statistical Sciences. Specifically, the panel was asked to: (1) examine the scientific evidence pertaining to the effects of needle exchange and bleach programs on rates of drug use and the behavior of drug users in the United States; (2) evaluate the efficacy of needle exchange and bleach programs in reducing the spread of HIV and other infectious diseases among injecting drug users and their partners, and (3) evaluate the potential risks and benefits associated with the implementation of such programs. The panel is examining related issues of importance to the research and service communities (e.g., characteristics associated with successful programs, community issues, and service delivery issues) and will make recommendations regarding future research directions and appropriate methods for evaluating needle exchange and bleach programs.

In its effort to gather and analyze the relevant scientific evidence, the panel invited both U.S. and foreign experts to participate in a two-day workshop September 27-28, 1993, devoted to the presentation and discussion of recent research on and experience with needle exchange and bleach distribution programs. (A second workshop, held in January 1994, elicited the views of the many communities with a stake in the outcome of the ongoing needle exchange and bleach distribution debate.) The agenda for the workshop was designed to inform the further work of the panel by focusing on particular salient issues to be considered in the establishment of needle exchanges and bleach distribution programs. Because substantial public interest in data on the efficacy of needle exchange and bleach distribution programs has been expressed and most of the presentations made at this workshop summarize ongoing research projects, panel members decided it would be beneficial to publish the papers.

This proceedings is organized to follow the five sessions that constituted the workshop: U.S. needle exchange data, international evaluations of needle exchange programs, legal issues and drug paraphernalia laws, evaluation methods, and bleach distribution programs. Each section consists of the papers that were presented, followed by a brief summary of the presentations by the designated discussant.

Panel members are indebted to the presenters and discussants who participated in this workshop and to the workshop participants who volunteered time to share their insights and expertise. We note with sadness the recent death of Noreen Harris, one of the presenters, and offer our sympathy to her family and colleagues. Noreen's research has contributed greatly to enhancing the knowledge and understanding of critical issues in the areas of HIV/AIDS and drug abuse.

The panel extends its sincere thanks and appreciation to Sander Genser and Peter Hartsock of the National Institute on Drug Abuse and T. Stephen Jones of the Centers for Disease Control and Prevention for their valuable assistance in organizing the workshop.

The panel also benefited from the work of the staffs of the National Research Council and the Institute of Medicine, including Susanne Stoiber, Michael Stoto, and Leslie Hardy, who provided valuable suggestions for this panel activity. Special thanks are due to the panel staff: Jacques Normand, study director; Sahr John Kpundeh, staff officer; Elaine McGarraugh, research associate; and Susan McCutchen, senior project assistant, for their many hours of work expended in bringing this workshop to fruition and producing this proceedings.

Lincoln E. Moses, *Chair*
Panel on Needle Exchange and Bleach
Distribution Programs

INTRODUCTION

Between 1.1 and 1.5 million people in the United States are injection drug users (Turner, Miller, and Moses, 1989), and over 3.2 million people have injected drugs at some point in their lives (National Institute on Drug Abuse, 1991). The sharing of injection equipment among drug users is the second most common risk behavior (Turner, Miller, and Moses, 1989), after male homosexual contact, among people with acquired immune deficiency syndrome (AIDS). It is also the major risk factor associated with heterosexual and perinatal transmission of the human immunodeficiency virus (HIV) in the United States (Centers for Disease Control and Prevention, 1993). By early 1993, according to the Centers for Disease Control and Prevention (1993), a third of the more than 280,000 people in the United States who had been diagnosed with AIDS were drug injectors (29 percent), people who had heterosexual contact with such a drug user (3 percent), or children born to injecting drug users or their sex partners (1 percent).

African-American and Latino communities have been particularly affected by drug-related transmission of HIV. In 1991, AIDS cases related to injection drug use accounted for 52 percent of African-American and 45 percent of Latino AIDS cases in the United States, compared with 19 percent for whites (Jones et al., 1991). Moreover, the proportion of AIDS cases occurring among people whose primary risk factor is injection drug use has been steadily increasing since the beginning of the epidemic (Krepcho et al., 1993).

Needle exchange programs, in which used needles and syringes are exchanged for new, sterile ones, are widely used in Europe and Australia as part of public health efforts to reduce the spread of HIV and other needle-borne infections among drug users and their sexual partners. Programs that distribute household bleach to injecting drug users so they can disinfect shared injection equipment have also been established abroad. In the United States, although needle exchange programs have been initiated in a number of cities, they are generally small and frequently operate illegally. In addition, health outreach workers in many U.S. communities distribute bleach as part of their work among drug users. In the U.S. Congress, an intense debate about whether needle exchange programs encourage either continued injection behavior or initiation of injection drug or other drug use has blocked any federal funding of needle exchanges. Prior to the passage of the ADAMHA Reorganization Act of 1992 (P.L. 102-321), the use of federal funds to evaluate needle exchange programs was also prohibited.

This proceedings presents original papers and the discussants' summaries from the Workshop on Needle Exchange and Bleach Distribution Programs. The workshop was structured to address, in five sessions, topics considered important to the panel's inquiry: (1) U.S. needle exchange data, (2) international evaluations of needle exchange programs, (3) legal issues and drug paraphernalia, (4) evaluation methods, and (5) bleach distribution programs. Following this brief introduction, these five areas also structure this report. In each area, the complete text of the workshop presentation is followed by a summary by the designated discussant for the session. The agenda and list of participants are included at the end of the report.

The first workshop session on U.S. needle exchange data focused on what has been learned about the impact of needle exchange on HIV transmission and drug use behaviors in this country. Data were presented from evaluations of needle exchange programs in four cities: New York, New York; Portland, Oregon; San Francisco, California; and Tacoma, Washington. In addition, researchers from the University of California (Berkeley and San Francisco) presented highlights of their recent study on the impact of needle exchange programs in the United States and abroad, which involved an intensive review of the research literature and site visits to needle exchange programs in 10 U.S. and 5 foreign cities.

The second session continued the theme of what has been learned about the impact of needle exchange programs on HIV transmission and drug use behaviors--but from programs outside the United States. Data were presented from evaluations of programs in the Netherlands, Canada, and Australia. In addition, findings were presented from a U.S. General Accounting Office evaluation of research results from nine needle exchange study projects, all but one of which involved needle exchange programs outside the United States.

The focus of the third workshop session was the legal perspective on needle exchange programs, and three presentations were made. The first provided a description of drug paraphernalia and needle prescription laws in the United States and the obstacles they pose to needle exchange programs. The second reported on an evaluation of whether changes in Connecticut's drug laws had an impact on pharmacy practice, in regard to the sale of needles and the needle purchasing and usage behavior of injectors of illegal drugs. The third presentation described the results of a national survey of Canadian pharmacies in their response to HIV prevention and harm reduction strategies.

The presentations in the fourth workshop session dealt with research methods and designs strategies used in studies of the impact of needle exchange and bleach distribution programs, as well as methodological issues that can arise in such studies. Four presentations were made: the first three discussed epidemiologic and qualitative methods of evaluating the impact of HIV prevention programs and related methodological issues. The fourth provided a detailed description of two mathematical models that were derived to assist researchers in estimating the impact of needle exchange programs.

In the final workshop session, three presentations were made: the first reported on a series of investigations into the efficacy of bleach as an inactivation-disinfectant agent and the compliance of drug users with bleach protocols. The second provided a review of HIV inactivation and disinfection methods as background for an examination of why cleaning needles with bleach in the field may not work even though it has been shown to work in the laboratory. The third presentation described the results of a study of the compliance of injecting drug users with bleach protocols.

REFERENCES

Center for Substance Abuse Treatment
1993 *HIV/AIDS Prevention Bulletin* April 19. Substance Abuse and Mental Health Services Administration, Public Health Service, U.S. Department of Health and Human Services.

Centers for Disease Control and Prevention
1993 U.S. AIDS cases reported through March 1993. *HIV/AIDS Surveillance Report* 5(1) January. Public Health Service, U.S. Department of Health and Human Services.

Jones, T., L. Slutsker, B. Frey, and B. Ward
1991 AIDS cases associated with injection drug use, United States 1991. In Final Program and Abstracts of the VIII International Conference on AIDS, 1992. Amsterdam.

Krepcho, M., M. Fernandez-Esquer, A. Freeman, E. Magee, and A. McAlister
1993 Predictors of bleach use among current African-American injecting drug users: A community study. *Journal of Psychoactive Drugs* 25(2):135-141.

National Institute on Drug Abuse
1991 National Household Survey on Drug Abuse: Population Estimates 1991. Rockville, MD: National Institute on Drug Abuse.

Turner, C. F., H. G. Miller, and L. E. Moses, eds.
1989 *AIDS: Sexual Behavior and Intravenous Drug Use*. Washington, D.C.: National Academy Press.

U.S. NEEDLE EXCHANGE DATA

THE UNIVERSITY OF CALIFORNIA NEEDLE EXCHANGE PROGRAM EVALUATION PROJECT: METHODS, CONCLUSIONS, AND RECOMMENDATIONS

PETER LURIE, JAMES G. KAHN, BENJAMIN BOWSER,
and DONNA CHEN, JILL FOLEY, JOSEPH GUYDISH,
T. STEPHEN JONES (Centers for Disease Control and Prevention),
SANDRA LANE, ARTHUR L. REINGOLD, and JAMES SORENSEN,
Needle Exchange Program Evaluation Project,
The University of California

In this paper we describe the multidisciplinary methods used in our report on needle exchange programs (NEPs) in the US and abroad[1, 2, 3 *] and list our conclusions and recommendations. The project was funded through a cooperative agreement between the Centers for Disease Control and Prevention (CDC) and the Association of Schools of Public Health, which contracted with the University of California, Berkeley to conduct the study. A significant amount of the work was subcontracted to the Institute for Health Policy Studies at the University of California, San Francisco. The project began in April 1992 and was funded through October 1993. Draft/Interim Reports were completed and submitted to the CDC on April 1 and July 16, 1993.

METHODS

Project Personnel

We assembled a 12-person research team in which no investigator was identified in his or her writing as either in favor of or opposed to NEPs. In order to better understand the diverse epidemiological, social, and policy aspects of NEPs, and to design a research methodology appropriate to their evaluation, investigators representing a variety of disciplines were involved in the project. The research team included members with training in clinical medicine, nursing, psychology, anthropology, sociology, cost-benefit modeling, and epidemiology. In addition, project investigators were accompanied on site visits to seven cities by one of four CDC staff, including the Project Officer.

---

* Copies of the 2-volume, 700-page full report are available through the National AIDS Clearinghouse at 1-800-458-5231.

Goal and Research Questions

The goal of the project was: "To assess the public health impact of needle exchange programs." The central research questions surrounding NEPs were identified by team members. Revisions to the list of research questions were made based on comments solicited from members of the project Advisory Committee (see below), public health officials, NEP staff members, researchers and experts in drug treatment and injection drug use, and community leaders either favoring or opposing the programs. Three team members also made two trips to CDC headquarters in Atlanta, GA early in the project to seek further input on the research questions and to delineate methods for answering them.

This process yielded a list of 14 research questions, grouped into seven categories: (1) NEP Descriptions; (2) Populations Reached by NEPs; (3) Community Responses to NEPs; (4) NEP Effect on HIV Risk Behavior; (5) Studies of Syringes; (6) NEP Effect on Disease Rates; and (7) NEP Cost-effectiveness (see Appendix 1). Project members were aware that in several cases available data might prove insufficient to answer the research question definitively. In each such case we intended to review available data, indicate gaps in existing information, and suggest research methods that might prove fruitful in answering that research question.

Ensuring Community and Expert Input

Due to the strong community reactions to NEPs in some settings, it was crucial to ensure adequate community and expert input. This was sought in three distinct manners: (1) Advisory Committee; (2) expert reviewers; and (3) Kaiser Family Foundation Forum.

Advisory Committee

A 13-member Advisory Committee based in the San Francisco Bay Area was formed. Members included injection drug use researchers, staff of the San Francisco NEP, a representative of the San Francisco Department of Public Health, and members of ethnic minority and religious groups. Care was taken to include members who supported and opposed NEPs.

Two Advisory Committee meetings were held: shortly after the initiation of the project (June 26, 1992) and prior to submission of the first Draft/Interim Report (March 5, 1993). At each meeting, project investigators reported on progress made to date and sought input from the Advisory Committee.

Expert Reviewers

Letters describing the project's research questions and proposed methods were sent to 31 leading researchers, public health officials, and community members, and comments from 10 respondents were received and integrated into the project approach.

We also solicited comments from the staff of the approximately 20 NEPs known to the project investigators at the beginning of the project; five responses were obtained. To promote accuracy in the descriptions of individual NEPs, staff at all sites visited were sent copies of sections of the report describing their NEP and given the opportunity to suggest corrections. Finally, five expert reviewers were contracted to review the full report and submit their comments. Two mathematical modeling experts also reviewed the chapter on cost-effectiveness.** Several additional chapters were reviewed by individuals at CDC and the National Institute on Drug Abuse who had specific expertise in the material covered in that chapter.

Kaiser Family Foundation Forum

On December 10 and 11, 1992 the Kaiser Family Foundation sponsored a forum entitled "Needle and Syringe Availability and Exchange for HIV Prevention" at the Foundation headquarters in Menlo Park, California. The approximately 60 attendees included researchers, NEP staff, law enforcement and public health officials, injection drug users (IDUs), and community members. Project members assisted in designing the Forum program, identifying speakers, developing a bibliography on NEPs, and producing a list of active NEPs for dissemination to Forum attendees. At the Forum, project members described the project methods, summarized the history of NEPs in North America, and offered preliminary descriptions of the NEPs visited.[4, 5] Feedback obtained was integrated into the Draft/Interim and Final Reports.

Consent and Confidentiality

The research protocol was submitted to and approved by the Committee for Protection of Human Subjects at the University of California, Berkeley. Focus groups with IDUs were conducted anonymously, while other key informants were offered the opportunity to remain anonymous in the Final Report; only one accepted. IDUs participating in the focus groups were provided with a participant information sheet. NEPs were only listed in the Final Report if they provided permission.

Formal Review of Existing Research

Data analysis in this portion of the report included published and unpublished materials from the US and foreign countries.

** The expert reviewers were Don Des Jarlais, Mindy Fullilove, Edward Kaplan, Herbert Kleber, Douglas Owens, Beny Primm, and Beth Weinstein.

Assessment of Data Needs

In order to assess the data necessary to answer the research questions, a Data Collection Outline was drawn up. For each research question, the outcome variables of interest were listed and likely data sources identified. This document formed the basis for interview protocols (see below) and the chapters in the Final Report addressing each research question.

Data Collection

To assemble a data file on NEPs, AIDSline and Medline computer searches were undertaken. In the articles identified by these searches, references were examined for additional articles related to the research questions. Abstracts from the annual International AIDS Conferences from 1988 to 1993 were examined. Authors of abstracts on NEPs were contacted by mail for original poster or oral presentation materials as well as any published articles based on the abstract or otherwise germane to NEPs. Conference abstracts from the annual American Public Health Association conferences (1987–1992) were also obtained and the authors similarly contacted.

To identify additional unpublished materials, NEP staff were contacted and asked about internal program reports or other unpublished materials they were willing to share. Newspaper clippings, magazine articles, government and institutional reports, and book chapters dealing with NEPs were also collected. The American Public Opinion Index (1985–1991) and Gallup Index (1987–1991) were searched to identify local and national public opinion poll questions addressing NEPs.

Per capita city AIDS case rates and selected HIV seroprevalence data were obtained from the CDC and demographic information on the cities visited came from the Bureau of the Census[6] and Statistics Canada.[7] Information on drug treatment availability in the US cities where site visits were conducted was obtained from the National Drug and Alcoholism Treatment Unit Survey (NDATUS).[8] Data sources used in an effort to track drug use trends over time were the Drug Abuse Warning Network (DAWN),[9] Drug Use Forecasting (DUF),[10-19] and the Uniformed Crime Reports (UCR).[20]

Data Synthesis

All materials assembled were reviewed by the Project Director or the Research Assistants. Documents were coded according to which research question(s) they could help answer and filed with each NEP site to which they referred. All data sources were entered into a bibliography software program called EndNote Plus[21] and coded according to research question and NEP site. Table 1 describes the data sources reviewed.

Project members were assigned responsibility for synthesizing information on one or more of the 14 research questions. This process included data collected in the manner described above as well as the interview and observational information collected during the site visits (see below).

Table 1

Data Sources Reviewed

Newspaper and magazine articles	499
Journal articles	475
Conference abstracts	381
Reports	236
Unpublished materials	159
Personal communications	106
Books and book sections	94
Other sources	22
Total	1,972

Drafts of all chapters were circulated within the group and modified accordingly. Six of the chapters addressing the research questions and seven additional chapters on the site visits were part of the first Draft/Interim Report. The second Draft/Interim Report contained the remaining chapters. Both Draft/Interim Reports were reviewed by both paid and unpaid outside reviewers, whose comments were then integrated into the Final Report.

Site Visits

Between May and September 1992, site visits to 15 cities were conducted: 10 in the US, three in Canada, and two in Europe (see Table 2). Except for the site visits to Santa Cruz, Boulder, and Amsterdam, which only lasted one day, all site visits were at least three days in duration. All site visits involved either two or three project investigators or CDC personnel, except the brief visit to Boulder, which was conducted by a single investigator.

Identification of Sites and Interviewees

Programs were identified from a list of NEPs in a published article[22] and through the community and expert input process described above. They were selected in consultation with the CDC to reflect the range of existing NEPs with respect to size, legal status, geographical location, IDU HIV seroprevalence, and extent of prior evaluation research.

The Project Director initially called the NEP staff to explain the purpose of the project and to obtain permission to visit the NEP. In no case was permission denied. NEP staff members were also used as initial sources for identifying other key informants. We supplemented these sources by adding individuals known to the investigators through their reading or discussions with other key informants as important figures in the development of NEPs in that city. Key informants were selected in order to represent a diversity of views both in support of and opposition to NEPs.

Table 2

Project Site Visits

UNITED STATES	
Berkeley, CA	Portland, OR
Boston, MA	San Francisco, CA
Boulder, CO (partial assessment)	Santa Cruz, CA
New Haven, CT	Seattle, WA
New York City, NY	Tacoma, WA
CANADA	
Montreal, PQ	Vancouver, BC
Toronto, ON	
EUROPE	
Amsterdam, the Netherlands (partial assessment)	
London, England (partial assessment)	

Methodological Framework

In order to achieve internal and external validity for our study we utilized methodological triangulation:[23] multiple data collection methods with multiple iterations. This cross-checking helps to ensure a level of confidence in the results that would otherwise be lacking.[24-26] Interviews, focus groups, and NEP site observations used the Rapid Assessment Procedure (RAP) method as a general framework. RAP is a collection of qualitative research strategies used for quick evaluation of health interventions.[24]

Training

A training manual for conducting interviews, focus groups, and NEP site observations was produced and used as a guide by project members. In addition, a two hour training session was organized in which salient elements of the training manual were reviewed and interview role-playing conducted. Members of the CDC who participated in the site visits received a one hour training session by telephone. At least one project member who had attended the more comprehensive training session was present at all site visits.

Site Observations

Observations of NEP sites were conducted in all cities visited (see Table 3). These observations lasted from one to four hours and occurred in the presence of NEP staff. In the 13 US and Canadian cities visited, we visited 18 NEPs that provided services at 102 different sites. Six sites operated by five programs in London and Amsterdam were also observed.

Table 3

Observations, Interviews, and Focus Groups Conducted

Total site observations	33
Interviews with:	
NEP directors and staff	25
Public health officials	14
IDU researchers	22
Community leaders	49
Focus groups with:	
NEP clients (11 focus groups)	82
NEP non-clients (7 focus groups)	47
Total number of persons interviewed	239

In order to create as little intrusion into NEP services as possible, investigators followed the direction of the NEP staff in terms of dress, location from which to observe the NEP, and number of observers. In several cases, IDUs had been told that researchers would be visiting the site on that particular day. A list of items to be observed at each site guided the observation process.[24] These included physical characteristics of the site, the exchange process itself, and interactions with the local community. The observation guidelines were pre-tested at two sites and the results compared qualitatively for inter-rater reliability before adopting the final guidelines.

Key Informant Interviews

Interview protocols for four distinct types of interviews were developed: (1) NEP directors and staff; (2) public health officials; (3) IDU researchers; and (4) community leaders, including leaders from the following groups: law enforcement, ethnic minority groups, religious groups, local businesspeople, elected officials, and neighborhood groups. The protocols were designed as guides for the interviews; investigators were not expected to follow the questions in exact form or sequence. Rather, emphasis was placed on making the interviewee comfortable and allowing answers to emerge during the course of conversation.

For each interview, one project member was assigned responsibility for guiding the interview, although all project members had the opportunity to clarify respondent answers or add questions of their own; another investigator was responsible for recording respondent answers and writing up the interview. Except for the interviews of NEP directors and staff, which lasted up to three hours, most interviews were completed in one hour. A total of 231 interviews were conducted during the site visits (see Table 3). In eight cases, key informants were unavailable at the time of the site visit and were subsequently interviewed by telephone using the same procedures.

The purpose of the study was explained to key informants who were asked for permission for direct attribution of their comments. Except for one individual in the Boston area who had operated an illegal NEP, such permission was always granted, although some respondents provided additional "off the record" information which was not included in the Final Report. Permission to record the interviews on audio tape was sought; in only two cases was permission denied. The interviews also provided the opportunity to augment the data collection effort and to clarify local investigator's research findings.

IDU Focus Groups

IDU focus group guidelines were prepared and reviewed in a fashion similar to the interview protocols. These included inquiries into their use of the NEP, factors promoting or deterring use of the NEP, enforcement of exchange rules, and suggestions for program improvement. Separate interview protocols were designed for clients of the NEP and those not using the program.

In initial telephone contacts with NEP staff, the Project Director discussed conducting anonymous focus groups with IDUs who were clients of the NEP and with those not using the NEP. NEP staff provided guidance on how best to recruit client focus group members. In most circumstances, fliers or sign-up sheets were provided to the NEP staff, who then identified potential subjects from those volunteering, paying attention to achieving an appropriate mix of gender, ethnicity, and opinion of the NEP. Eighty-two clients from 11 NEPs were interviewed.

IDUs rarely or never using the NEP were recruited from the clientele of drug treatment programs and ongoing street-based research projects. Again, recruiters were asked to seek a representative group with respect to gender, ethnicity, and opinion of the NEP. Forty-seven non-clients from seven NEPs were interviewed.

One investigator took responsibility for leading the focus group session and explaining the purpose of the study. This was facilitated by providing focus group attendees with a participant information sheet. Individuals attending the focus groups were provided with refreshments and reimbursed between $10 and $15 for their time. The focus groups were attended by between two and 10 IDUs, lasted approximately one hour and were not recorded on tape, except in Montreal where the focus groups were conducted in

French and recorded for later translation. NEP staff were not present during the client focus groups.

Qualitative Analysis

Project members were provided with blank computer templates of the interview and focus group protocols and recorded the interviews by reporting interviewee responses in spaces on the template below the appropriate questions. Information provided by subjects that was not directly responsive to any protocol question was noted as an addendum to the interview write-up. These write-ups were completed using notes taken during the interviews and/or tape recordings of the interviews. Each interview and observation write-up was circulated to all investigators present at the interview to confirm the accuracy of recorded information and to identify additional information for inclusion. A binder with hard copies of all interview write-ups was provided to each investigator.

Interview write-ups were also entered into a computerized qualitative database software program called askSam.[27] This software is frequently used in ethnographic research and permits the categorization and indexing of data so that sections of separate interviews addressing the same research question can be easily assembled. The database was used in the synthesis of the site visit findings.

Mail Survey of NEPs Not Visited

In order to obtain as complete a description of US NEPs as possible, the site visits were supplemented by a mail survey of 20 NEPs not visited by project members. After the surveys were completed in May 1993, we identified four additional US NEPs. A five-page questionnaire seeking basic descriptive information was sent to the 20 NEPs. Phone follow-up was used to increase the response rate and to clarify any uncertainties regarding the responses received. The information obtained through the mail survey was integrated into the description of NEPs.

Cost-Effectiveness Modeling

Cost-effectiveness modeling involved a four-step process: (1) an assessment of NEP budgets; (2) the systematic evaluation of studies of NEP impact on HIV risk behaviors; (3) the assessment and further development of existing mathematical models of NEP impact on HIV transmission; and (4) the use of mathematical models to estimate the cost-effectiveness of NEPs, defined as cost per HIV infection averted. In this section, we describe only methods used to evaluate existing research.

We summarized the methods and findings of all available studies addressing the effects of NEPs on HIV risk behaviors and needle-borne disease rates using a similar format. Only information on behavior change was utilized in the mathematical modeling. The assessment of the overall usefulness of each study for answering the particular research question was ranked on a scale from 1 to 5: (1) completely inadequate or not relevant to research question; (2) unacceptable: contains flaws in design or reporting that make interpretation unreliable; (3) acceptable: provides credible evidence but has limited detail, precision, or generalizability; (4) well done: provides detailed, precise, and persuasive evidence; and (5) excellent: compelling and complete. The final ranking was determined by agreement of at least two project members.

CONCLUSIONS

How and Why Did NEPs Develop?

NEPs have continued to increase in number in the US and by September 1, 1993 at least 37 active programs existed. The evolution of NEPs in the US has been characterized by growing efforts to accommodate the concerns of local communities, increasing likelihood of being legal, growing institutionalization, and increasing federal funding of research, although a ban on federal funding for program services remains in effect.

How Do NEPs Operate?

About one-half of US NEPs are legal, but funding is often unstable and most programs rely on volunteer services to operate. All but six US NEPs require one-for-one exchanges and rules governing the exchange of syringes are generally well enforced. In addition to having distributed over 5.4 million syringes, US NEPs provide a variety of services ranging from condom and bleach distribution to drug treatment referrals.

Do NEPs Act as Bridges to Public Health Services?

Some NEPs have made significant numbers of referrals to drug abuse treatment and other public health services, but referrals are limited by the paucity of drug treatment slots. Integrating NEPs into the existing public health system is a likely future direction for these programs.

How Much Does it Cost to Operate NEPs?

The median annual budget of US and Canadian NEPs visited is relatively low at $169,000, with government-run programs tending to be more expensive. Some NEPs are more expensive because they also provide substantial non-exchange services such as drug treatment referrals. The annual cost of funding an average NEP would support about 60 methadone maintenance slots for one year.

Who Are the IDUs Who Use NEPs?

Although NEP clients vary from location to location, the programs generally reach a group of IDUs with long histories of drug injection who remain at significant risk for HIV infection. NEP clients in the US have had less exposure to drug abuse treatment than IDUs not using the programs.

What Proportion of All IDUs in a Community Uses the NEP?

Studies of adequately-funded NEPs suggest that the programs do have the potential to serve significant proportions of the local IDU population. While some NEPs appear to have reached large proportions of local drug injectors at least once, others are reaching only a small fraction of them. Consequently, other methods of increasing sterile needle availability must be explored.

What Are the Community Responses to NEPs?

Unlike in many foreign countries, including Canada, proposals to establish NEPs in the US have often encountered strong opposition from a variety of different communities. Consultation with affected communities can address many of the concerns raised.

Do NEPs Result in Changes in Community Levels of Drug Use?

Although quantitative data are difficult to obtain, those available provide no evidence that NEPs increase the amount of drug use by NEP clients or change overall community levels of non-injection and injection drug use. This conclusion is supported by interviews with NEP clients and by IDUs not using the programs, who did not believe that increased needle availability would increase drug use.

Do NEPs Affect the Number of Discarded Syringes?

NEPs in the US have not been shown to increase the total number of discarded syringes and can be expected to result in fewer discarded syringes.

Do NEPs Affect Rates of HIV Drug and/or Sex Risk Behaviors?

The majority of studies of NEP clients demonstrate decreased rates of HIV drug risk behavior, but not decreased rates of HIV sex risk behavior.

What is the Role of Studies of Syringes in Injection Drug Use Research?

The limitations of using the testing of syringes as a measure of IDUs' behavior or behavior change can be minimized by following syringe characteristics over time, or by comparing characteristics of syringes returned by NEP clients with those obtained from non-clients of the program.

Do NEPs Affect Rates of Diseases Related to Injection Drug Use Other than HIV?

Studies of the effect of NEPs on injection-related infectious diseases other than HIV provide limited evidence that NEPs are associated with reductions in subcutaneous abscesses and hepatitis B among IDUs.

Do NEPs Affect HIV Infection Rates?

Studies of the effect of NEPs on HIV infection rates do not and, in part due to the need for large sample sizes and the multiple impediments to randomization, probably cannot provide clear evidence that NEPs decrease HIV infection rates. However, NEPs do not appear to be associated with increased rates of HIV infection.

Are NEPs Cost-effective in Preventing HIV Infection?

Multiple mathematical models of NEP impact support the findings of the New Haven model. These models suggest that NEPs can prevent significant numbers of infections among clients of the programs, their drug and sex partners, and their offspring. In almost all cases, the cost per HIV infection averted is far below the $119,000 lifetime cost of treating an HIV-infected person.

RECOMMENDATIONS

These conclusions demonstrate that NEPs can provide a variety of public health services to significant numbers of IDUs who continue to inject drugs and who may otherwise not receive these services. Such services can be provided cost-effectively and are associated with diminutions in HIV drug (but not sex) risk behavior. Although the data available are limited, they provide no evidence that NEPs increase the amount of drug use by their clients or change overall community levels of injection and non-injection drug use. Any controversy in local communities can be minimized by involving all interested communities in the planning of needle exchange services, both prior to opening the NEP and after it is implemented, to address concerns such as program sites and hours of operation. NEPs should be conceptualized as an integral part of public health efforts to stem HIV infection among drug users and should be *part of a comprehensive approach to drug use*, that should also emphasize expanded access to drug treatment and school- and community-based interventions to prevent the initiation and continuation of drug use.

NEPs should be supplemented by the expanded sale of syringes by pharmacists, an approach that has the advantage of protecting client confidentiality while still guaranteeing the client that the syringe obtained is sterile. This is in marked contrast to the situation on the street, where syringes are often repackaged by unscrupulous dealers so as to appear new.[28] However, pharmacy schemes provide a weaker link to other public health services and pharmacists may be reluctant to participate because of concerns about syringe disposal and the effect of IDUs' presence on their businesses.

Although the research studies upon which this report's conclusions and recommendations are based cannot definitively prove that NEPs decrease HIV infection rates, four lines of evidence suggest that this is likely:

- Needle exchange is an intervention based on the sound theoretical principle of eliminating the vector (a contaminated syringe) that transmits infection from one person to another.[29] This is analogous to reducing the number of mosquitoes in an attempt to prevent malaria.

- There is clear evidence of decreases in HIV drug risk behavior among NEP clients, which should translate into decreased HIV infection rates.

- Hepatitis B infections appear to be reduced by NEPs.

- Mathematical modeling by this project and other researchers consistently estimate substantial decreases in HIV transmission rates.

We believe that the data reviewed in this report meet the two criteria established by the US Congress for lifting the ban on the use of federal funds for NEP services. Federal law currently requires that "the Surgeon General of the United States [determine] that such programs are effective in preventing the spread of HIV and do not encourage the use of illegal drugs."[30] With new HIV infections in IDUs and their offspring occurring daily, the time has arrived for federal, state, and local governments to remove the legal and administrative barriers to increased needle availability and to facilitate the expansion of NEPs in the US.

Recommendations for the Federal Government

- The federal government should repeal the ban on the use of federal funds for needle exchange services and substantial federal funds should be committed both to providing needle exchange services and to expanding research into these programs.

Recommendations for State Governments

- State governments in the ten states that have prescription laws should repeal these laws.***
- States should repeal the paraphernalia laws as they apply to syringes.****

Recommendations for Local Governments and Communities

- Local governments should enter into discussions with local community groups to develop a comprehensive approach to preventing HIV in IDUs, their sex partners, and their offspring. This approach should include NEPs and the expansion of drug treatment services.
- Local communities should seek to further increase sterile syringe availability by encouraging the sale, distribution, or exchange of syringes by pharmacists.

Recommendations for Researchers

- Descriptions of the "kinetics" and determinants of needle use patterns: IDUs' sources of needles, methods of disposal of needles, frequency of needle re-use, and needle-sharing patterns. How do these change when an NEP or other changes in needle availability are implemented?

*** Prescription laws preclude the purchase of a syringe without a prescription, limiting sterile syringe availability and creating a risk of arrest for needle exchange program staff and clients.

**** Paraphernalia laws exist in 46 states and require pharmacists to determine whether the purchaser intends to use the syringe for "legitimate medical purposes." Conviction under a paraphernalia law is a felony or a misdemeanor.

- Evaluations of "natural experiments" in which needle availability laws change or pharmacists expand the over-the-counter sales of syringes.
- Surveys of pharmacists to determine their willingness to participate in pharmacy-based syringe sale, distribution, or exchange and to identify the barriers to their participation.
- Assessments of the effects of design features of NEPs (e.g., administering bodies, site characteristics, opening hours, and program rules) upon process measures of NEP outcome (e.g., needles distributed, drug treatment referrals, discarding of needles).
- Ethnographic and other qualitative research to assess the factors involved in drug use initiation and in transitions between various routes of drug use.
- Case-control studies of the relationship between use of the NEP and acute hepatitis B, particularly in cities with active surveillance for the infection.
- Large, multicenter case-control studies within existing cohorts of IDUs to assess whether use of the NEP is associated with hepatitis B or HIV seroconversion.
- Mathematical modeling using program data and behavior change evaluations to determine which aspects of program design determine effectiveness and cost-effectiveness.

APPENDIX

Research Questions

1. NEP Descriptions
   a. How and why did NEPs develop?
   b. How do NEPs operate?
   c. Do NEPs act as bridges to public health services?
   d. How much does it cost to operate NEPs?
2. Populations Reached by NEPs
   a. Who are the IDUs who use NEPs?
   b. What proportion of all IDUs in a community uses the NEP?
3. Community Responses to NEPs
   a. What are the community responses to NEPs?
   b. Do NEPs result in changes in community levels of drug use?
   c. Do NEPs affect the number of discarded syringes?
4. NEP Effect on HIV Risk Behavior
   Do NEPs affect rates of HIV drug and/or sex risk behaviors?
5. Studies of Syringes
   What is the role of studies of syringes in IDU research?
6. NEP Effect on Disease Rates
   a. Do NEPs affect rates of diseases related to injection drug use other than HIV?
   b. Do NEPs affect HIV infection rates?
7. NEP Cost-effectiveness
   Are NEPs cost-effective in preventing HIV infection?

REFERENCES

1. Lurie, P, Reingold, AL, Bowser, B, et al. *The public health impact of needle exchange programs in the United States and abroad, Volume I.* University of California. September, 1993.

2. Lurie, P, Reingold, AL, Bowser, B, et al. *The public health impact of needle exchange programs in the United States and abroad, Summary.* University of California. October, 1993.

3. Lurie, P, Reingold, AL, Bowser, B, et al. *The public health impact of needle exchange programs in the United States and abroad, Volume II.* University of California. October, 1993.

4. Lurie, P, Chen, D, and Needle Exchange Program Evaluation Project. A review of programs in North America. In: Stryker, J, and Smith, MD. *Dimensions of HIV prevention: Needle exchange.* Menlo Park, CA: The Henry J. Kaiser Family Foundation, 1993:11-33.

5. Lane, SD, and Needle Exchange Program Evaluation Project. A brief history. In: Stryker, J, and Smith, MD. *Dimensions of HIV prevention: Needle exchange.* Menlo Park, CA: The Henry J Kaiser Family Foundation, 1993:1-9.

6. Anon. U.S. Department of Commerce, Bureau of the Census. *1990 census of population and housing: Summary population and housing characteristics.* 1990.

7. Wood, J. *Canada year book, 1992.* Ottawa, Ontario: Statistics Canada, 1991.

8. Anon. US Department of Health and Human Services. *Highlights from the 1991 National Drug and Alcoholism Treatment Unit Survey (NDATUS)* (and special computer runs for this project). September, 1992.

9. Anon. U.S. Department of Health and Human Services, Public Health Service, Alcohol, Drug Abuse, and Mental Health Administration, National Institute on Drug Abuse. *Data from the Drug Abuse Warning Network (DAWN): 1988 annual data* (and special computer runs for this project). 1989.

10. DeWitt, CB. National Institute of Justice. *Drug use forecasting: January to March 1990.* October, 1990.

11. DeWitt, CB. National Institute of Justice. *Drug use forecasting: April to June 1990.* April, 1990.

12. DeWitt, CB. National Institute of Justice. *Drug use forecasting: Drugs and crime 1990 annual report.* August, 1991.

13. DeWitt, CB. National Institute of Justice. *Drug use forecasting: First quarter 1991.* November, 1991.

14. DeWitt, CB. National Institute of Justice. *Drug use forecasting: Second quarter 1991.* February, 1992.

15. DeWitt, CB. National Institute of Justice. *Drug use forecasting: Third quarter 1992.* July, 1992.

16. Stewart, JK. National Institute of Justice. *Drug use forecasting: January to March, 1989.* September, 1989.

17. Stewart, JK. National Institute of Justice. *Drug use forecasting: Fourth quarter 1988.* June, 1989.

18. Stewart, JK. National Institute of Justice. *1989 drug use forecasting annual report*. June, 1990.
19. Stewart, JK. National Institute of Justice. *1988 drug use forecasting annual report*. March, 1990.
20. Anon. Federal Bureau of Investigation. *Uniform crime reports* (and special computer runs for this project). 1988.
21. Niles and Associates. *EndNote Plus*. Niles and Associates, 1990.
22. Drucker, E. Through the eye of the needle III: In a dark season, one million points of light. *The International Journal on Drug Policy.* 1990;2:6-8.
23. Crano, W. Triangulation and cross-cultural research. In: Brewer, M, and Collins, B. *Scientific inquiry and the social sciences. A volume in honor of Donald T. Campbell.* San Francisco: Jossey-Bass, 1981:317-344.
24. Scrimshaw, S, and Hurtado, E. UCLA Latin American Center. *Rapid assessment procedure for nutrition and primary health care.* 1987.
25. Pelto, P, and Pelto, G. *Anthropological research. The structure of inquiry (second ed.).* Cambridge: Cambridge University Press, 1978.
26. Naroll, R, and Cohen, R. *A handbook of method in cultural anthropology.* Garden City: Natural History Press, 1970.
27. SeaSide Software Inc. *DBA askSam Systems.* Perry, FL: 1985-1991.
28. Des Jarlais, DC, and Hopkins, W. "Free" needles for intravenous drug users at risk for AIDS: Current developments in New York City (letter). *New England Journal of Medicine.* 1985;313:1476.
29. Kaplan, EH, and O'Keefe, E. Let the needles do the talking! Evaluating the New Haven needle exchange. *Interfaces.* 1993;23:7-26.
30. Anon. *General Provisions of the Department of Labor, Health and Human Services, and Education and Related Agencies Appropriations Act (P.L. 102-321)*, 1993.

RISK FOR HUMAN IMMUNODEFICIENCY VIRUS AND HEPATITIS B VIRUS IN USERS OF THE TACOMA SYRINGE EXCHANGE PROGRAM

HOLLY HAGAN, Tacoma-Pierce County Health Department, Washington;
DON C. DES JARLAIS, Chemical Dependency Institute, New York;
SAMUEL R. FRIEDMAN, National Development and Research Institute, New York;
and DAVID PURCHASE, Point Defiance AIDS Projects, Tacoma, Washington

INTRODUCTION

In almost all developed countries, syringe availability programs have become a major component of public health programs to reduce transmission of HIV and other blood-borne infections via needle-sharing[1-3]. In the U.S., the controversy surrounding syringe exchange has limited opportunities for conducting research[4-6], and no large-scale controlled studies have been carried out to date. The approach taken by many researchers has been to collect different indicators of the effects of syringe exchange, including HIV risk behavior information, HIV and hepatitis B serology, and community incidence trends, and to determine whether the relationships between exchange programs and these indicators suggest reduction in blood-borne viral transmission[7-16]. The ongoing study of the Tacoma syringe exchange is an example of such a research strategy.

The current approach of the Tacoma study is to examine the association between exchange use and the incidence of hepatitis B. Because HIV and hepatitis B virus (HBV) have similar routes of transmission, and the incidence of HBV infection is higher than that of HIV[17-18], studies of hepatitis B will have greater statistical power to detect a difference in risk of infection attributable to exchange use[19]. Studies conducted in Europe and the U.S. have found that 65-95% of IDUs have serologic evidence of previous hepatitis B infection[20-25], and the Centers for Disease Control and Prevention (CDC) estimates that 10-20% of susceptible IDUs acquire hepatitis B every year[18]. In favor of studying hepatitis B as an outcome in Tacoma are that HIV seroprevalence in local IDUs is low, and a comprehensive hepatitis surveillance system has existed in the county since 1979.

In this paper, we summarize the methods and findings of the Tacoma study and examine the limitations. The preliminary results of the first analysis of the association between hepatitis B and the syringe exchange at the individual level are also described in this paper.

METHODS

The Intervention

The Tacoma syringe exchange began operating in August, 1988, and is the longest-running program in North America. It is estimated that the program serves 800-1000 clients per week -- approximately 30% of an estimated 3000 IDUs residing in the county. Between 50,000 and 60,000 syringes are exchanged each month in four locations: two stationary street-based sites, a pharmacy-based exchange, and a mobile delivery program. The staff of the program have sought to limit barriers to participation, and users are not required to show evidence of legal age or recent injection, or to register or participate in any research.

The syringe exchange has been the primary HIV prevention strategy for IDUs in Pierce County. Some HIV education is given to drug injectors when they enter drug treatment, but there is no other outreach education program for this segment of the population in the community.

Studies of Risk Behavior in Local IDUs

Interviews with injecting drug users in the county have been carried out since 1988. The details of the methods used in this study have been described elsewhere[26]. Exchange users were systematically sampled at exchange locations; IDUs who had never used the exchange (non-exchangers) were recruited from health and social service agencies and street locations where the exchange didn't operate. Risk behavior interviews and blood draws for HIV and HBV serology were conducted in the field. Variables included in the standardized instrument included demographic characteristics and injection risk behavior during the previous 30 days while participating (exchange users) or not participating (non-exchangers) in the program. Exchange users were also asked about behavior before first use of the program (pre-exchange), and this was compared to post-exchange behavior (while participating).

For variables with a continuous distribution (age, number of injections per month, number of unsafe injections per month), the median for the entire sample was used to create dichotomous categories. Prevalence odds ratios (P.O.R.) were used to estimate the relationship between syringe exchange use and injection behavior, and these P.O.R. were adjusted for duration of injection, a potential confounding variable, by use of the Mantel-Haenszel statistic[27].

Surveillance of Blood-Borne Viral Infections

Pierce County is one of four U.S. sentinel counties for hepatitis surveillance conducted by the Hepatitis Branch of the CDC. Stimulated reporting of hepatitis by the sentinel surveillance system has resulted in approximately 50% of all symptomatic cases of hepatitis B infections in Pierce County being reported, compared to 17% nationwide[28].

Since 1988, the Tacoma-Pierce County Health Department's drug-treatment program has enrolled newly admitted opiate users in the CDC Family of HIV Seroprevalence Surveys[29]. HIV risk behavior was recorded for each client, and HIV testing was done on sera remaining after routine blood tests were performed.

Case-Control Study of Incident HBV Infections

Cases of acute hepatitis B infection reported to the sentinel surveillance system from January 1991 to December 1992 who were IDUs were included in the case series. Demographic data and information relating to potential source of exposure were collected according to the sentinel county protocol[30]. Additional information obtained from cases included syringe exchange use and duration of drug injection (less than or five or more years). We excluded IDUs who also reported male-with-male sexual activity or sexual contact with a confirmed hepatitis B case, as HBV transmission may have occurred via a causal pathway other than the one of interest in this study. No other risk factors for hepatitis B were reported by the cases.

The control series was assembled from among IDUs enrolled in the HIV Family of Seroprevalence Surveys during the study period. Potential controls were screened for antibody to hepatitis B core antigen (anti-HBc), and hepatitis B surface antigen (HBsAg). Heterosexual IDUs who had neither of these serologic markers of immunity or infection were eligible to serve as controls.

IDUs with acute hepatitis B were compared with their controls for differences in demographic characteristics and injection behavior, and the independence of factors that were significant on univariate analysis was examined using multiple logistic regression with backward elimination.

RESULTS

In the interview study comparing 426 exchange users and 159 non-exchangers, there were no differences in the gender or racial/ethnic composition of the two IDU samples. Exchange users were significantly older than non-exchangers, and had been injecting longer (Table 1). One percent of exchange users and 4% of non-exchangers were new injectors, having begun injecting in the previous year ($p=0.12$).

Changes in injection practices among exchange users pre- and post-first use of the exchange are described in Table 2. There were no changes in the rate of injection by exchange users, but there were significant declines in unsafe injections. Fifty-eight percent of exchangers reported any unsafe injections pre-exchange, compared to 33% while participating (P.O.R.=0.36, 95% CI 0.26 to 0.49). Exchange users also reported fewer occasions when they passed a used syringe onto another injector.

Injection practices at baseline reported by exchange users and non-exchangers are compared in Table 3. Exchange users were more frequent injectors, with a median of 37 injections per month, compared to 17 for non-exchangers. However, fewer exchange users reported any injections with a syringe used by another injector. For both samples, heroin and speedball (an injection of heroin and cocaine together) were the primary injected drugs. The differences in injection frequency and unsafe injection persisted when the data were adjusted for duration of injection (Table 3). There were no differences in the frequency of passing on a used syringe to another injector.

The presence, at time of interview, of antibody to HIV, HBV and HCV is compared in Table 4. In both IDU groups, a high proportion of subjects had evidence of previous HBV or HCV infection. Fewer exchange users (2%) than non-exchangers (8%) were HIV-antibody positive. There have been no HIV seroconversions detected in either exchange users or non-exchangers in follow-up testing (66.9 person-years followup for non-exchangers, 223 person-years for exchange users).

Figure 1 shows HBV incidence trends in Pierce County from January, 1985 to December, 1992. An outbreak of drug-related hepatitis B infection began in 1985 that persisted until several months following the opening of the exchange program, and then rapidly declined. Hepatitis B in persons whose source of infection was not identified has followed a similar trend. Incidence in persons with other sources of infection, primarily heterosexual and homosexual transmission, have been relatively stable during this time period. HIV seroprevalence in opiate users entering methadone treatment in Pierce County has remained between two and five percent from 1988 to 1992[31].

In the case-control study, eligible cases included 34 heterosexual IDUs with acute hepatitis B, and 25 eligible controls with no hepatitis B markers. Control subjects were older than cases, but there were no differences with regard to gender or race. Cases of incident hepatitis B were eight times more likely to have injected for less than five years (95% CI 2.3 to 35.3), and five times more likely to never have used the syringe exchange (95% CI 1.4 to 20.0). In multiple logistic regression analysis, two factors, not using the syringe exchange (AOR 2.1, 95% CI 1.1, 4.2) and injecting for less than five years (AOR 2.5, 95% CI 1.1, 4.2) were independently related to acquisition of hepatitis B[32].

DISCUSSION

These studies have examined the relationship between the Tacoma syringe exchange and self-reported injection behavior, individual-level HIV-, HBV-, and HCV-seroprevalence, community-level HIV-seroprevalence trends and HBV-incidence trends, and acquisition of hepatitis B. All of these measures suggest that syringe exchange protects against blood-borne infection; each has limitations, which will be summarized.

Self-reported safer injection may have been influenced by subject-bias whereby exchange users would be motivated to report cessation of injection risk behavior. All interviews have been carried out by well-trained interviewers who are not affiliated with the exchange program, so subjects are unlikely to expect to gain by giving specific responses. We examined the influence of social desirability on report of safer injection in a previous analysis[33] by re-analyzing the data after excluding subjects who reported certain behaviors that could be viewed as socially desirable. The results were consistent with those reported for the entire sample, so it is unlikely that social desirability of respondents substantially biased the results.

Differences in injection practices between exchange users and non-exchangers may be due to volunteer bias, whereby IDUs motivated to inject safely would be attracted to the exchange. Klee et al.[34] have reported that IDUs may inject for several years before adopting safe injection practices. Because older IDUs may be safer injectors as a result of their longer experience, controlling for duration of injection may have eliminated some of this form of bias. Additionally, exchange users did report safer injection after beginning to participate in the program, so there was a change beyond that which may be attributable to baseline differences in the two groups.

Ecologic correlations between HIV prevalence and hepatitis B incidence trends and the opening of the syringe exchange program cannot be interpreted as an individual-level association. No "control" community with similar demographic and disease incidence features has been compared to the Pierce County trend. Other factors that may have contributed to the observed trends include community-wide HIV education campaigns, legal sale of injection equipment by pharmacists, use of disinfectant bleach, and saturation of susceptibles during the hepatitis B outbreak.

Separating the education and bleach distribution effect of the exchange from the single effect of syringe availability was not possible in these studies. Syringe exchange programs have always been "more than just needles", and work to achieve multiple public health objectives in the course of their interactions with IDUs. Condom and bleach distribution, screening for tuberculosis and other infectious disease, health and social service referrals, and facilitation of drug treatment admission have been elements in the majority of syringe exchange programs in the U.S.[2] It is also difficult to draw the line between the effects on individual users and community norms. It is conceivable that, by increasing awareness of injection-related HIV risk and establishing new norms of needle-hygiene, syringe exchange's influence extends far beyond the individual user. Within-community studies may be hampered by this "contamination" of potential controls.

With respect to the case-control study, the small sample size led to wide 95% confidence limits about the estimates. Additionally, there was limited data on covariates, and some residual confounding could be present in the final estimates. However, duration of injection was probably the most important potential confounder and was included in the analysis. There was little detail in quantification of use of the syringe exchange, but measuring exchange use as ever vs. never would tend to underestimate the protective effect. Similar studies should be carried out to address these methodologic concerns.

While these individual studies of the Tacoma syringe exchange each had their limitations, there was strong consistency among their findings, all indicating reduction of transmission of blood-borne viruses among participants in the exchange program.

REFERENCES

1. Des Jarlais DC, Friedman SR. AIDS and legal access to sterile drug injection equipment. *Ann Int Med* 1992; 521: 42-65.

2. Lurie P, Chen D. A review of programs in North America. In: Stryker J, Smith MD (eds.): *Dimensions of HIV Prevention: Needle Exchange* (pp. 11-34). Menlo Park, California: Henry J. Kaiser Family Foundation, 1993.

3. Stimson G. Syringe-exchange programmes for injecting drug users. *AIDS* 1989; 3:253-60.

4. Rogers DE, Osborn JE. AIDS policy: Two divisive issues. *JAMA* 1993; 270:494-95.

5. Anderson W. The New York needle trial: The politics of public health in the age of AIDS. *Am J Public Health* 1991; 81:1506-17.

6. Des Jarlais DC, Friedman SR. Missing the point: Science and politics in the American debate on syringe exchanges. *Pediatric AIDS and HIV Infection* 1993; 4:61-65.

7. Ljungberg B, Christensson B, Tunving K, et al. HIV prevention among injecting drug users: Three years of experience from a syringe exchange program in Sweden. *J Acq Immun Defic Syndr* 1991; 4:890-95.

8. Hagan H, Des Jarlais DC, Purchase D et al. Lower HIV seroprevalence, declining HBV incidence and safer injection in relation to the Tacoma Syringe Exchange. In: Volume 2, Abstracts of the 7th International Conference on AIDS, Florence, July 16-21, 1991: 368, abstr. W.C. 3291.

9. Hart GJ, Carvell ALM, Woodward N, Johnson AM, Williams P, Parry J. Evaluation of needle exchange in central London: behaviour change and anti-HIV status over one year. *AIDS* 1989; 3:261-65.

10. Van Haastrecht HJ, van den Hoek JA, Bardoux C, et al. The course of the HIV epidemic among intravenous drug users in Amsterdam, the Netherlands. *Am J Public Health* 1991; 81:59-62.

11. Des Jarlais DC, Goldberg D, Frischer M, Green S, Tunving K, Ljungberg B, Wodak A, Ross M, Hagan H, Purchase D, Friedmann P, Friedman SR. Characteristics of 'prevented' HIV epidemics. In: Volume 1, Abstracts of the 9th International Conference on AIDS, Berlin, June 6-11, 1993: 98, abstr. WS-C15-6.

12. Des Jarlais DC, Hagan H, Goldberg D, Frischer M, Green S, Tunving K, Ljungberg B, Wodak A, Ross M, Purchase D, Friedmann P, Friedman SR. Characteristics of 'prevented' HIV epidemics among injecting drug users. Manuscript submitted, September, 1993.

13. Hagan H, Des Jarlais DC, Purchase DC, Reid T, Friedman SR, Bell TA. The incidence of HBV infection and syringe exchange programs [letter]. *JAMA* 1991; 266:1646-47.

14. Buning EC. Effects of the Amsterdam needle and syringe exchange. *International Journal of the Addictions* 1991; 26:1303-11.

15. Wolk Hs, Wodak A, Morlet A, et al. HIV-related risk-taking behavior, knowledge, and serostatus of intravenous drug users in Sydney. *Medical Journal of Australia* 1990; 152:453-58.

16. Hart GJ, Woodward N, Johnson AM et al. Prevalence of HIV, hepatitis B, and associated risk behaviors in clients of a needle exchange in central London. *AIDS* 1991; 5:543-47.

17. Centers for Disease Control and Prevention. Public Health Service inter-agency guidelines for screening donors of blood, plasma, organs, tissues, and semen for evidence of Hepatitis B and Hepatitis C. *MMWR* 1991; 40, RR-4, 1-15.

18. Centers for Disease Control, Immunization Practices Advisory Committee. Update on adult immunization. *MMWR* 1991; 40 (RR-12):8-13.

19. Committee on Social and Behavioral Sciences. *Evaluating HIV Prevention Programs*. Washington D.C.: National Academy Press, 1992.

20. Margolis HS, Alter MJ, Hadler SC. Hepatitis B: Evolving epidemiology and implications for control. *Seminars in Liver Disease* 1991; 11:84-92.

21. DeCock KM, Jones B, Govindarajan S, Redeker AG. Prevalence of hepatitis delta virus infection: A seroepidemiologic study. Western Journal of Medicine 1988; 148:307-09.

22. Ponzetto A, Seeff LB, Buskell-Bales Z, Ishak KG, Hoofnagle JH, Zimmerman HY, Purcell RH, Gerin JL, & the Veterans Administration Hepatitis Cooperative Study Group. Hepatitis B markers in United States drug addicts with special emphasis on the delta Hepatitis virus. *Hepatology* 1984; 4:1111-15.

23. Rosenblum L, Darrow W, Witte J, Cohen J, French J, Gill, PS, Potterat J, Sikes K, Reich R, Hadler S. Sexual practices in the transmission of hepatitis B virus and prevalence of hepatitis delta virus infection in female prostitutes in the United States. *JAMA* 1992; 267:2477-81.

24. Piot P, Goilav C, Kegels E. Hepatitis B: Transmission by sexual contact and needle sharing. *Vaccine* 1990; 8:S37-39.

25. Bortolotti F, Bertaggia A, Cadrobbi P, Crivellaro C, Pornaro E, Realdi G. Epidemiological aspects of acute viral hepatitis in drug abusers. *Infection* 1982; 5:277-79.

26. Hagan H, Des Jarlais DC, Purchase D, Reid TR, Friedman SR. The Tacoma Syringe Exchange. In: Friedman SR, Lipton DS (eds.) *Cocaine, AIDS, and Intravenous Drug Use*. Binghamton, NY: Haworth Press, 1991.

27. Mantel N, Haenszel W. Statistical aspects of the analysis of data from retrospective studies of disease. *J NCI* 1959; 22: 719-48.

28. Alter MJ, Mares A, Hadler SC, Maynard JE. The effect of underreporting on the apparent incidence and epidemiology of acute viral hepatitis. *Am J Epidem* 1987; 125: 133-39.

29. Jones TS, Allen DM, Onorato IM, Petersen LR, Dondero TJ, Pappaooanou M. HIV seroprevalence surveys in drug treatment centers. *Public Health Rep* 1990; 105: 125-30.

30. Alter MJ, Hadler SC, Margolis HS, Alexander J, Hu PY, Judson FN, Mares A, Miller JK, Moyer LA. The changing epidemiology of hepatitis B in the United States. *JAMA* 1990; 263: 1218-22.

31. Hagan H, Hale CB. HIV-1 seroprevalence surveys in Pierce County. Report available from the Tacoma-Pierce County Health Department Office of Community Assessment, June, 1993.

32. Hagan H, Des Jarlais DC, Friedman SR, Purchase D, Alter M. The risk of hepatitis B in injecting drug users in relation to participation in a syringe exchange program. Manuscript submitted, September, 1993.

33. Hagan H, Des Jarlais DC, Purchase D, Friedman SR, Reid TR, Bell TA. An interview study of participants in the Tacoma syringe exchange. In press, *Addiction*, May, 1993.

34. Klee H, Faugier J, Hayes C, Boulton T, Morris J. Factors associated with risk behavior among injecting drug users. *AIDS Care*, 1990; 2: 133-45.

Table 1. Demographic characteristics of exchange users and non-exchangers, Tacoma syringe exchange study.

Characteristic	Exchange Users (n=426)	Non-Exchangers (n=159)	p*
Gender			
male	298 (70.1)	107 (67.7)	0.66
female	127 (29.9)	51 (32.3)	
Age			
younger than 37	198 (46.5)	108 (67.9)	<0.001
37 or older	228 (53.5)	51 (32.1)	
Race/ethnicity			
white	241 (56.6)	96 (60.4)	0.41
non-white	185 (43.4)	63 (39.6)	
Residence			
street/shelter	77 (19.3)	20 (13.3)	0.1
house/apt/other	321 (80.7)	130 (86.7)	
Duration of injection			
15 yrs or less	200 (47.0)	111 (69.8)	<0.001
more than 15 yrs	226 (53.0)	48 (30.2)	

*as determined by chi-square or Fisher's exact test

Table 2. Injection behavior pre- and post-first use of the exchange.

Behavior	Pre-exchange	Post-exchange	P.O.R.* (95% C.I.)
Injections/month			
fewer than 37	42.2%	46.9%	0.83
37 or more	57.8%	53.1%	(0.61, 1.12)
Injections w/used syringe/month			
none	42.4%	67.3%	0.36
at least one	57.6%	32.7%	(0.26, 0.49)
Passing on used syringe/month			
none	27.9%	53.7%	0.33
at least once	72.1%	46.3%	(0.24, 0.46)

*P.O.R. =prevalence odds ratio

Table 3. Injection behavior at baseline - exchange users and non-exchangers.

Behavior	Exchange Users (n=426)	Non-Exchangers (n=159)	P.O.R.* (95% C.I.)	A.O.R* (95% C.I.)
Injections/month				
fewer than 37	200 (47.0)	111 (69.8)	0.38	0.41
37 or more	226 (53.0)	48 (30.2)	(0.26, 0.56)	(0.28, 0.60)
Injections w/used syringe/month				
none	288 (67.3)	67 (43.2)	0.5	0.36
at least one	135 (32.7)	88 (56.8)	(0.25, 0.54)	0.25, 0.52)
Passing on used syringe/month				
none	223 (53.7)	70 (46.7)	0.73	0.72
at least once	192 (46.3)	80 (53.3)	(0.51, 1.07)	(0.49, 1.06)

*P.O.R. =prevalence odds ratio
*A.O.R.= adjusted for duration of injection, by Mantel-Haenszel statistic

Table 4. The presence of serologic markers for infection at baseline - exchange users and non-exchangers.

	Exchange Users (n=426)	Non-Exchangers (n=159)	p*
Percent anti-HBc positive	71%	62%	> .05
Percent anti-HCV positive	95%	84%	> .05
Percent anti-HIV positive	2%	8%	0.02

*as determined by chi-square or Fisher's exact test

Figure 1. Hepatitis B in Pierce County, 1/85 - 12/92.

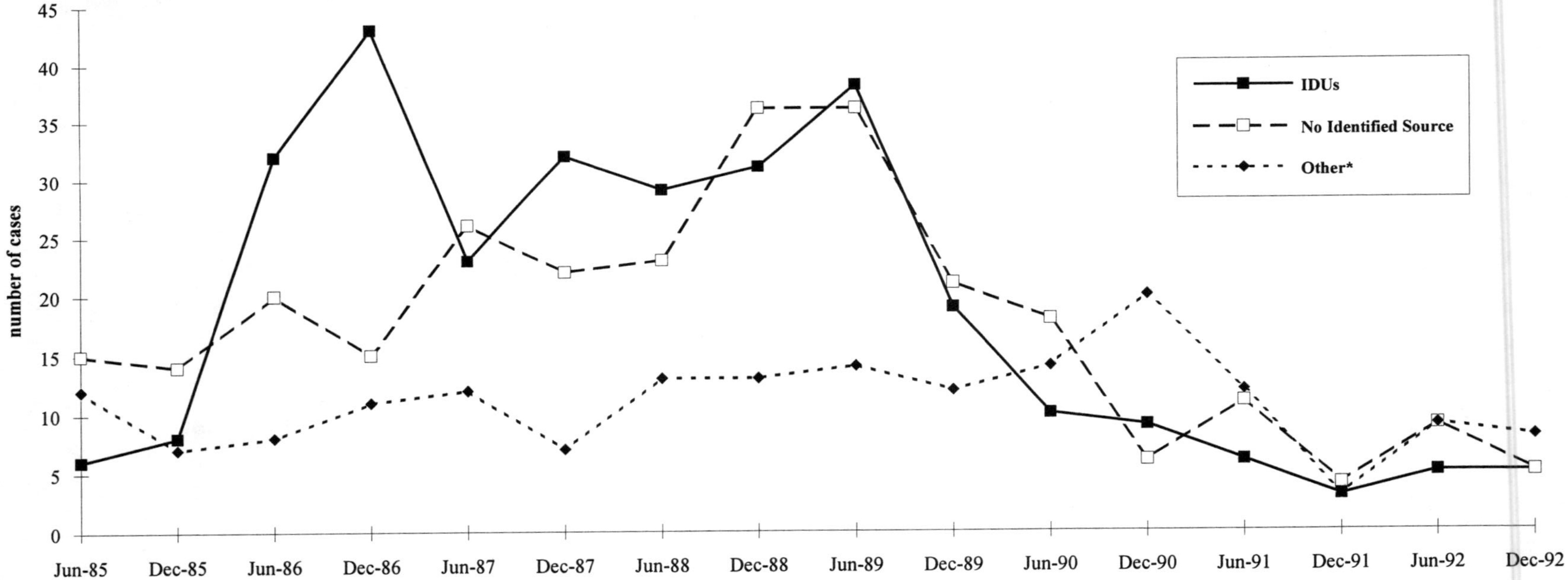

(Adapted from Hagan H et al., JAMA 1991; 266:1646-47.)

*primarily cases reporting male-male sex, and included IDUs reporting male-male sex

BEHAVIORAL AND COMMUNITY IMPACT OF THE PORTLAND SYRINGE EXCHANGE PROGRAM

KATHY OLIVER, Outside In; H. MAYNARD, Portland State University;
SAMUEL R. FRIEDMAN, National Development and Research Institutes, Inc.;
and DON C. DES JARLAIS, Beth Israel Medical Center

PROGRAM OVERVIEW

The Syringe Exchange in Portland, Oregon began November 1, 1989. The opening of the Exchange was delayed for two years because our insurance company refused to cover syringe exchange and threatened to withdraw coverage from our clinics and other programs if we started an exchange. Outside In operates medical and prenatal clinics and housing and emergency services programs for homeless youth.

At the time of the study, the Exchange operated out of a fixed site at Outside In. It now operates out of two fixed sites and one van.

At the time of the study, the Exchange operated 3-7 pm Monday-Friday. Clients were age 18 or over - it is illegal to give minors syringes in Oregon unless by order of a physician for an authorized use. Clients were asked to exhibit needle tracks at the first visit to ensure that only IV drug users were provided syringes. At the first visit clients were given three syringes - whether or not they brought any in. Thereafter, syringes were exchanged on a one-to-one basis. Outside In also gave out rinse water, cotton, alcohol swabs, condoms and information handouts.

METHODS

Of over 1,000 participants in the Exchange, 753 (67%) were enrolled in the research component. Subjects were interviewed at three month intervals using the AIA (for intake) and AFA (for follow-up) Questionnaires designed by NIDA for use in its national survey of drug injectors. Consenting subjects were also tested for HIV and Hepatitis B antibodies at three month intervals. To encourage use of the exchange, subjects were allowed to remain anonymous, which prevented active tracking for follow-up, and thus limited follow-up at the three and six month data collection points.

Behavior of Exchange clients was examined at intake and at six months to determine the extent to which clients changed their behavior. To determine differences between a syringe exchange program and an outreach program, Exchange clients were compared with clients of the Portland NIDA-funded NADR outreach project for IV drug users. Clients of both groups were those who were still shooting up at six-month follow-up. The same questionnaires were used with both groups. Change in risk behavior over time was compared between groups.

A substudy was conducted to determine the extent to which the existence of the Exchange would lead injectors to return syringes to the Exchange rather than discarding them in public places. Prior to the opening of the Exchange, staff began to count (and collect) syringes in the vicinity on a daily basis. The data on syringes found before opening were compared to data on syringes found after the exchange opened.[1]

RESULTS

In the first two years since the Syringe Exchange began, 1,145 clients made 6,368 visits. Nearly 49,000 syringes were given out, with over 45,000 returned. The syringe return rate for the two years was 93% (see Table 1).

A description of the first 700 injectors using the Exchange and participating in the study is provided in Table 2.

The HIV infection rate among clients at intake was 3.9%. There was only one HIV seroconversion in 162 person-years at risk, for an HIV seroconversion rate of 0.619 per 100 person-years at risk (95% confidence intervals 0.109, 3.506). The single seroconversion was noted at the six month follow-up, so it is possible that this person may have become infected prior to beginning to use the Exchange.

The infection rate for hepatitis B core antibody at intake was much higher - 54%. Thirteen subjects seroconverted in 63.3 person-years at risk, for an HBV seroconversion rate of 20.5 per 100 person-years at risk (95% confidence intervals 12.0, 35.1).

Syringe exchange clients showed a considerable reduction in risk behavior over a range of risk behaviors measured at intake and at six months. Significant and meaningful declines were reported in sharing of syringes, as well as renting works, borrowing works, and cleaning works. (See Table 3).

Of the 117 subjects for whom follow-up data were obtained at six months, 34 attended the Exchange three or fewer times, and 83 attended it four or more times. These two groups were distinguished to try to separate out clients who came in only to collect interview fees and not otherwise using the Exchange from those really using the Exchange. The frequent attenders report significantly greater risk reduction on borrowing and on throwing away used syringes. This latter result indicates that injectors are using the Exchange as intended, that is returning syringes for safe disposal rather than simply discarding them. (Table 4)

On the other hand, the analysis indicate that while all clients reduced drug injection frequency, frequent attenders reduced frequency of injection less than infrequent attenders. While this did not reach significance ($P < .099$), it is worthy of note. Further analysis is needed to determine whether this is a methodological artifact analogous to regression to the mean (since those who come to inject only rarely will have little reason to frequently attend the Exchange to get new syringes.); a result of personal characteristics of these subjects (such as the stage of their addiction); or is an unintended effect of the program.

The respondents had long histories of IV drug use; there is little evidence in our data to support the idea that syringe exchanges recruit new users. Less than 2% of our respondents had histories of injecting of less than a year. The average duration of IV drug use was 14 years, and over 75% of respondents had been injecting for 5 years or more. Those with the longest histories of injecting were likely to be the heaviest current IV drug users ($p<.004$).

Drug injectors using the Syringe Exchange were then compared to drug injectors not using the Exchange. Clients for the comparison group were drawn from the Portland NADR outreach project. This was not an ideal comparison group in that drug injectors in the project did receive interventions. All NADR clients received bleach and were provided with HIV education. A subset either participated in groups or received one-on-one counseling. They were also encouraged to buy and use sterile syringes (legally available over-the-counter in Oregon).

Seventy-seven Exchange clients who attended the Exchange four or more times were compared to 355 NADR clients. Demographic information for both groups is shown in Table 5.

The comparison between these projects in complicated by potentially different subject populations. While there were no differences between samples on most variables, there were some differences. For example, NADR subjects were considerably more likely to be African American and less likely to be Latino; more likely to live in their own place, and were engaged in less risky injection practices at intake (e.g., they were more likely to clean syringes after use). Perhaps because we were studying frequent attenders, exchange users at six months follow up injected more frequently than the NADR subjects. These differences between samples may limit the conclusions that can be drawn from the comparison.

Subjects in both projects report significantly lower levels of risk over a wide range of risk behaviors at follow-up than at intake. On most of these measures no statistically significant differences in the amount of risk reduction were found between projects. However, syringes exchange subjects were significantly better on two variable involving risky injection behavior (Table 6): reduction in the extent to which subjects re-used syringes without cleaning - a key goal of the project, and the extent to which they no longer threw away used syringes (but returned them to the Exchange).

Differences are of particular significance in that syringes are legally available in Oregon, and the bleach outreach program encourages drug injectors to buy and use sterile syringes. Differences between the Exchange and the outreach program are likely smaller than they would be between an Exchange and an outreach program in a state where purchase of syringes was illegal.

Of considerable importance is the fact that syringe exchange and bleach outreach projects seem to recruit different clienteles. There was little overlap between the samples, with the Portland NADR project finding that only 11% of its sample had ever used the syringe exchange. *Thus, it appears that syringe exchanges and outreach programs might best be seen as complementary strategies that recruit and produce risk reduction among different sub-populations of drug injectors, rather than as competing options that should be chosen among to find which is the best approach to HIV prevention.*

The substudy on discarded syringes assessed the impact of the Syringe Exchange on the community in terms of the number of potentially infectious syringes thrown away on the streets.[1] In order to provide baseline data, a daily syringe search was begun three-and-one-half months prior to the opening of the Exchange. Discarded syringes were collected, counted and disposed of safely. Using consistent search patterns, this syringe count was continued until June 30, 1991.

Table 7 presents data comparing the number of days on which syringes were and were not found prior to and subsequent to the opening of the Exchange. Syringes were significantly more likely to be found prior to its opening (chi-square = 4.048; $p < .05$).

In spite of the fact that syringe exchanges aim to increase the availability of (sterile) syringes for drug injectors, this exchange has not led to an increase in the number of discarded syringes with which children or others might stick themselves. Instead, it reduced the number of discarded -- and possibly contaminated -- syringes in the streets.

CONCLUSIONS

The data presented here support the growing body of evidence that exchanges produce behavioral risk reduction. They also provide evidence that the number of potentially infected syringes in public places can be reduced by opening syringe exchanges. Comparisons between Exchange subjects and NADR are preliminary, with further analyses needed to control for possible differences between samples. Syringe exchange and bleach outreach programs are best seen as strategies that complement each other. They recruit different populations of drug injectors, and both lead to risk reduction. Differences between programs are likely smaller than in a city where syringes were illegal and the bleach outreach programs could not encourage people to buy sterile syringes.

These data are of course not definitive evidence that syringe exchanges reduce the spread of HIV or other pathogens. Indeed, it is not likely that a truly definitive study can ever be conducted of syringe exchanges, any more than this is feasible with evaluations of drug abuse treatment, drug interdiction, or laws against drug use. The cumulative weight of the research, however, and the fact that no studies have found any indication that the exchanges are doing any damage, clearly puts the burden of proof on opponents of syringe exchanges. In the interim, given the dangers from HIV spread, syringe exchanges should become an important part of the public health response to AIDS.

ACKNOWLEDGMENTS

We would like to acknowledge the support by the American Foundation for AIDS Research and the Multnomah County Health Division.

We would also like to acknowledge the staff of Outside In and the volunteers from Portland State University and the Portland community who assisted in making the Portland, Oregon syringe exchange and this research possible.

REFERENCE

1. Oliver KJ, Friedman SR, Maynard H, Magnuson LJ, Des Jarlais DC. Impact of needle exchange program on potentially infectious syringes in public places. *J AIDS*. 1992;5:534-535.

TABLE 1

Portland Syringe Exchange
Opened November 1, 1989
after more than two years of effort

In its first two years:
1,145 clients made 6,378 visits
753 (67%) enrolled in this
research evaluation study

Syringe Distribution Summary:

Dispensed: 48,753
Returned: 45,208
Return Rate: 93%

Year 1: 87% (18,784/16,418)
Year 2: 96% (29,969/28,790)

TABLE 2

Demographics Among 700 Drug Injectors
Who Used the Exchange At Least Once

1. Age (Mean 34; Range 18 - 72)

18 - 20	6%
21 - 25	11%
26 - 30	18%
31 - 35	20%
36 - 40	22%
41 - 45	14%
46 - 50	6%
50+	3%

2. Sex

Male	86%
Female	14%

3. Ethnicity

African American	8%
Latino/a	3%
White	79%
Native American	9%
Asian/Pacific Islander	1%

4. Highest Grade Completed

1 - 8	6%
9 - 11	43%
High School Graduate	19%
Some College	29%
College Graduate	3%

5. Current Work Status

Full-time	9%
Part-time	10%
Occasional	21%
Unemployed	45%
Disabled	13%
Other	2%

TABLE 3

Risk Behaviors Among
77 Portland Syringe Exchange Clients

	(Intake) AIA Mean (%)	(6 Months) AFA Mean (%)
Not Sharing Works	56	65
Rented Works	9	3
Borrowed Works	20	7
Used Syringe and Threw Away	54	40
Cleaned Needles	51	65
Re-used works without cleaning	23	12

TABLE 4

Risk Behaviors Among Clients Who Used the Exchange Less than Four Times (N=32) and Clients Who Used It Four or More Times (N=83)

	Number Of Visits	AIA Mean	AFA Mean	Group P	Trial P	Group/ Trial P
Shooting Up Now	< four	28.7	8.9	.002	.039	.099
	four +	33.0	30.7			
Not Sharing Works	< four	.58	.60	.660	.164	.380
	four +	.56	.66			
Cleaned Needles	< four	.50	.52	.284	.177	.343
	four +	.53	.66			
Rented Works	< four	.14	.14	.004	.260	260
	four +	.08	.03			
Borrowed Work	< four	.19	.19	.109	.021	.021
	four +	.20	.07			
Used Syringe & Threw Away	< four	.50	.57	.214	.363	.026
	four +	.54	.38			
Re-used Works W/O Cleaning	< four	.19	.17	.978	.108	.228
	four +	.23	.12			

TABLE 5

	EXCHANGE	NADR	P<
Sex			
Female	20%	27%	.15
Male	80%	73%	
Sexual Orientation			
Heterosexual	86%	Unknown	
Gay	8%		
Lesbian	0%		
Bisexual Male	4%		
Bisexual Female	2%		
Ethnicity			
African American	6%	27%	.001
Latino/a	8%	1%	
White	83%	67%	
Native American	3%	4%	
Asian/Pacific Islander	0%	1%	
Highest Grade Completed			
1- 8	6%	5%	.86
9-11	50%	49%	
High School Graduate	16%	20%	
Some College	25%	24%	
College Graduate	3%	2%	
Major Source Of Income			
Job	47%	39%	.13
Unemployment	0%	1%	
Disability	13%	8%	
Welfare	6%	14%	
Spouse/Partner	4%	5%	
Family/Friends	6%	7%	
Illegal Means	16%	23%	
Other	8%	3%	
Where Respondent Lives			
Own Place	43%	30%	.01
Someone Else's Place	18%	38%	
Boarding House	12%	7%	
Shelter	6%	10%	
On the Street	13%	11%	
Other	8%	4%	

TABLE 6

Risk Behaviors Among
77 Portland Syringe Exchange Clients and 335 NADR Clients

	Program	AIA Mean	AFA Mean	Group P	Trial P	Group Trial P
Shooting Up Now	Exchange	33.6	27.5	.004	.001	.06
	NADR	29.2	12.2			
Not Sharing Works	Exchange	.56	.65	.324	.231	.08
	NADR	.59	.57			
Cleaned Needles	Exchange	.51	.65	.001	.008	.261
	NADR	.69	.75			
Rented Works	Exchange	.09	.03	.569	.001	.280
	NADR	.07	.04			
Borrowed Works	Exchange	.20	.07	.038	.001	.122
	NADR	.21	.14			
Used Syringe & Threw Away	Exchange	.54	.40	.810	.076	.002
	NADR	.44	.48			
Re-used Works W/O Cleaning	Exchange	.23	.12	.002	.001	.038
	NADR	.13	.09			

TABLE 7

Mean number of syringes found before and after Exchange opened.

Mean/Month

Prior to Exchange opening	5.19
After Exchange opened	1.9

Number of days on which syringes were and were not found prior to and subsequent to the opening of the Exchange.

	Before 7/14/89-11/1/89	After 11/2/89-3/2/90	Totals
No Syringe	52	62	114
Syringe	14	6	20
Total Search Days	66	68	134
% of search days on which a syringe was found	21.2%	8.8%	14.9%

NEW YORK CITY SYRINGE EXCHANGE: AN OVERVIEW

Denise Paone, Don C. Des Jarlais, Stephanie Caloir, Patricia Friedmann, and Immanuel Ness, Beth Israel Medical Center, New York;
Samuel R. Friedman, National Development and Research Institutes, New York

INTRODUCTION

New York City has experienced the largest HIV epidemic among injecting drug users (IDUs) of any city in the world. Approximately one-half of the estimated 200,000 IDUs in New York are already infected with HIV. 19,792 cases of AIDS among IDUs in New York City (including IDUs who also report male-sex-with-males) had been reported through December 1992 (NYC AIDS Surveillance Report). If one adds the 1,809 New York City cases of AIDS that resulted from heterosexual transmission from IDUs to persons who did not inject and the 815 cases of perinatal transmission of AIDS attributed to the mother's drug use or that of her sexual partner, then injecting drug use in NYC is associated with almost ten percent of the 250,000 total cases of AIDS reported in the U.S. through December 1992 (Centers for Disease Control, 1993).

Syringe exchange programs have become a primary method of preventing HIV infection among injecting drug users in almost all developed countries (Des Jarlais & Friedman, 1992), although they have remained quite controversial in the United States. Most syringe exchange evaluation studies have been conducted in areas with low HIV seroprevalence among the local population of IDUs. All syringe exchange evaluations conducted to date have shown reductions--but not elimination--of injection risk behavior and stability of the low HIV seroprevalence. In a high seroprevalence area, these residual levels of risk behavior may still leave an unacceptably high rate of HIV seroconversions. Only two studies of syringe exchanges have been conducted in moderate to high seroprevalence areas. The New Haven evaluation has estimated a one-third reduction in new HIV infections among IDUs attending the syringe exchange in that city, but it was not possible to directly measure the HIV seroconversion rate (Kaplan & O'Keefe, 1992). In Amsterdam, the HIV seroconversion rate was directly measured among participants in the exchanges, but the rate did not differ from that observed in IDUs not utilizing the exchanges (although many of the comparison subjects were probably obtaining sterile injection equipment from pharmacies or from exchangers).

Most syringe exchange programs that have been studied in the U.S. have also been relatively small exchanges, with a few exchange sites and open for a limited number of hours per week. If syringe exchanges are to become an important method of HIV prevention in the U.S., it will be necessary to operate them on a much larger scale. Given the importance of syringe exchanges being sensitive to the needs of the local population of IDUs, it is very unlikely that a single "standard" model of syringe exchange will be applicable to all locations. Instead, some form of "integrated system" of syringe exchanges that would be sufficiently flexible to meet the needs of the local mix of IDUs, but sufficiently uniform to meet the demands for accountability that will inevitably come with federal or state government funding. The present system of syringe exchanges in NYC, with five different exchanges currently operating, may serve as a model for how such a multi-exchange system might operate.

OVERVIEW OF EVALUATION

The New York City syringe exchange programs are required by the State Department of Health to participate in our evaluation study. This requirement is similar to the situation in Honolulu, HI, New Haven, CT, and Washington, DC. In all these cities, establishment of syringe exchange was controversial, and the requirement for an evaluation study was both part of the political process for obtaining legal authorization and part of a larger concern of public-health officials with assessing the extent to which the multiple goals of syringe exchanges were being achieved. We are currently conducting an evaluation study of the recently legalized syringe exchange programs in New York City. This evaluation study will address two fundamental questions: the potential effectiveness of syringe exchange in a high HIV seroprevalence environment, and the New York exchanges as a prototype for an integrated system of syringe exchanges.

METHODS

The design of the NYC needle exchange evaluation consists of two major components: (1) Ethnographic Study and (2) Behavioral Change and Seroconversion Study.

Ethnographic Study

The ethnographic component has been designed to provide a description of the operations of the syringe exchanges and to study the organizational issues. The ethnographic methods in this evaluation study include direct observation of the syringe exchanges in operation, and semi-structured interviews to document the past and ongoing decision-making of the syringe exchange staff.

These ethnographic methods have produced the types of descriptions of the everyday operation of the programs that can be readily understood by decision-makers who would otherwise have little familiarity with the "front line" work of preventing HIV infection among IDUs.

A key area for ethnographic inquiry has been an examination of how semi-legal syringe exchange programs make the transition from underground to legal status and how community based organizations integrate syringe exchange into their pre-existing services.

Ethnographic research methods, with their great flexibility and ability to probe beneath "surface" events for underlying contradictions and hidden inconsistencies, are ideally suited for addressing the types of organizational questions faced by the syringe exchange programs in New York City. Ethnographic research methods are also highly likely to produce the types of scientific reports that will be useful for replication of effective syringe exchange programs in other areas, particularly other high-seroprevalence areas.

Behavioral Change and Seroconversion

The fundamental goal of syringe exchange programs is to reduce AIDS risk behavior and actual transmission of HIV. Changes in AIDS risk behaviors and HIV transmission among participants are examined through a series of cross-sectional studies with recapture of subjects who participated in previous cross-sectional studies.

Each cross-sectional study includes an interview concerning AIDS risk behavior and a saliva sample for HIV testing. Subjects for interviewing are randomly selected from those attending the exchanges within a given week. To be eligible for inclusion in the study, subjects must: (1) have been an active injecting drug user; (2) have used syringe exchange on at least one occasion; (3) have just made an exchange. Verbal informed consent is obtained in order to protect subjects' confidentiality. Two separate interview questionnaires are administered, one for the initial interview with a subject and one for subsequent interviews with the same subject. Subjects are paid a modest honorarium ($10) each time they participate in the study. A "unique identifier" anonymous coding system is utilized for tracking multiple interviews with the same subjects across the different cross-sectional studies.

In the initial interview, subjects are asked about their drug use and AIDS risk behavior during the month before they started to use the exchange, as well as for the past 30 days while using the exchange. Comparison of the "pre-exchange" and "during exchange" levels of illicit drug use and AIDS risk behavior has permitted inferences (Paone et al., 1993) about behavior change associated with use of the exchange.

Subsequent interviews of previously interviewed subjects include risk behavior since the last time interviewed. The questionnaire is also used to monitor any changes in the frequency of drug use and risk behavior over time among "regular" users of the exchanges. These questionnaires also permit comparison of AIDS risk behavior among participants in syringe exchange in the New York City exchanges with AIDS risk behavior among participants in syringe exchanges in cities of lower background seroprevalence.

Seroprevalence and Seroincidence

In order to determine the effectiveness of syringe exchanges to reduce HIV transmission, this study directly measures HIV seroprevalence and HIV seroconversions among regular participants of the exchanges.

Saliva samples are collected at the time of each research interview. The saliva samples are tested for HIV using GACELISA and Western blot assays. Although the saliva tests are not currently licensed in the United States, they have shown considerable accuracy. Compared with serum tests for HIV antibody, saliva tests are at least 95% sensitive and 100% specific. Saliva testing has been successfully utilized in the United Kingdom HIV seroprevalence studies (Johnson et al., 1988) and in United Kingdom syringe-exchange evaluations (Hart et al., 1989).

We have estimated that approximately 1000 (20%) of the first 5000 interviews and saliva samples will be "subsequent" interviews of persons who have already been interviewed and who have given a previous saliva sample. Using an estimate of 50% seroprevalence among persons using the syringe exchange, there will be an estimated 500 subjects with multiple saliva samples who are at risk for seroconversion. Assuming an average period of between 6 and 9 months between the first and last saliva sample among the matched saliva samples, there will be an estimated 250 to 375 person years at risk for determining the rate of HIV seroconversion among regular participants in the syringe exchanges.

RESULTS

Organizational-System Issues

Space limitations do not permit a full analysis of the complex issues involved in establishing a network of syringe exchanges within the politically complicated environment of New York City. It will be helpful, however, to start with brief descriptions of the different organizational players. There are four different types of organizations actively involved in syringe exchange work in New York City.

Health Departments

Both the New York State and the New York City Health Departments are involved in the syringe exchange system. The City Health Department provides moral and political support to the legal exchanges, but does not contribute financial resources to the programs. The State Department of Health, in contrast, occupies a dominant role within the syringe exchange system. New York State law permits the State Health Commissioner to waive the requirement for written prescriptions for dispensing of needles and syringes. This waiver was originally included in the law in order to reduce the need for prescriptions in State operated hospitals, and was not intended to include syringe exchange programs. Operating under a public health emergency provision, this waiver has been extended to syringe exchange programs that file the appropriate applications with the State Health Department and agree to abide by the 27 page set of Department regulations for legal syringe exchanges.

The State Health Department also provides funding for syringe exchange work in New York. The funding is provided under an explicit comprehensive "harm reduction" (NYS Dept. of Health, 1993) philosophy which emphasizes using syringe exchanges not only to reduce HIV risk behavior but also as a linkage mechanism for providing additional health and social services to the drug injecting population.

Both Health Departments can be considered traditional bureaucracies, with clearly defined roles within the organization and well-articulated authority structures. Both need to be responsive to community concerns and the concerns of New York State Legislature, which must approve funding for the State Health Department and whose laws govern the operations of both departments. Both Health Departments are concerned that their activities be consistent with the relevant state laws and frequently rely upon the advice of their counsels.

Both Health Departments also have a tradition of regulating and/or inspecting health care facilities. The State Health Department, for example, has the authority not only to license health care facilities but to set reimbursement rates for hospitals. The HIV/AIDS epidemic has extended the regulatory/inspection responsibilities to areas beyond traditional health care facilities. The State Health Department is currently regulating the syringe exchanges and the City Health Department is inspecting bath houses and sex clubs for unsafe sexual activities. The State Health Department has provided technical assistance to programs. The State Health Department's, AIDS Institute Staff, has worked closely with law enforcement community, providing education in order to gain acceptance for the programs.

The American Foundation for AIDS Research (AmFAR)

AmFAR is a not-for-profit foundation that funds AIDS related research and that advocates for AIDS policies. AmFAR has been the most important source of funding for syringe exchange research in the United States. Until 1992, the federal government had not funded any research on syringe exchange programs. AmFAR is funding the current syringe exchanges in New York, with privately obtained money and money from the State Department of Health. AmFAR provides technical assistance to the syringe exchange programs and centralized purchasing of supplies for the programs. AmFAR is also funding the evaluation of the syringe exchange programs.

Two of the syringe exchange programs that received legal operation authority in the summer of 1992 had been operating previously as "underground" exchanges. A third program with a variation on the model noted below received authorization in (February) 1993. Prior to receiving this authority, these exchanges had no paid staff; necessary supplies were provided by private donations, mostly from the AIDS Coalition to Unleash Power (ACT UP or the volunteers themselves). Decision making was made primarily through developing a consensus among the volunteers who were present at the meeting when an issue was raised. This method of decision-making provides for maximum egalitarian participation among the totally volunteer staff. It also meant that no single person "representing" these two exchanges had authority to make commitments for the exchange.

With legal authorization to operate syringe exchanges and funding from AmFAR and the State, these exchanges were required to affiliate legally with a 501 (C) 3 not-for-profit corporation in the neighborhoods where they were to continue operations. Funding would go through the sponsoring organization, which would have legal control and legal responsibility for expenditures. These three exchanges had considerable difficulties in finding suitable sponsoring organizations and have moved towards incorporating as 501 (C) 3 organizations themselves, with their own boards of directors and formal organizational hierarchies.

These underground exchanges were able to expand greatly when they received legal authorization and funding support. They expanded from providing exchange services to 1,000 IDUs one year prior to legalization in June 1992, to 8,379 IDUs by June 1993. This expansion brought with it many of the problems that occur with rapid growth in any organization. (Space limitations do not permit examination of these problems and their solutions here.)

The three other syringe exchanges that were initially approved for funding in the summer of 1992 were to be operated by existing community based organizations that already held 501 (C) 3 status. These organizations were already providing AIDS related services to injecting drug users, but were not providing syringe exchange. Thus, they had to integrate syringe exchange into their existing services. (Space limitations do not permit presentation of the complicated issues raised during this integration process.) We should mention, however, that some staff in these organizations were philosophically committed to assisting IDUs to stop using drugs, and did not accept the harm reduction rationale for syringe exchange. Although these organizations already had 501 (C) 3 status, they also had undergone (or were still undergoing) problems associated with rapid growth, overdependence upon key personnel, and the staff burnout common in many CBOs in the AIDS field.

Not unexpectedly, these existing non-exchange service organizations encountered many difficulties in starting exchange services. One of them never officially obtained authorization to operate a legal syringe exchange, and subsequently AmFAR funding was withdrawn from that organization.

Evaluation

The evaluators must also be considered one of the organizational players within the syringe exchange system. As noted above, participation in the evaluation study was required for both AmFAR funding and for obtaining State Health Department authorization for operating a legal exchange. The evaluators have considerable experience in research on syringe exchanges, having consulted on several studies of European and American syringe exchanges and on the evaluation of the first legal exchange in New York City, and served as co-investigators on studies of the Portland, Tacoma and Boulder syringe exchanges in the U.S. This experience, as well as the research literature on syringe exchange, has led them to believe that syringe exchanges can be important components of AIDS prevention effort for IDUs, but that as a human service operation, syringe exchanges will not always be properly implemented, and even if properly implemented, may not necessarily be effective in all environments.

The purposes of the evaluation (as seen by the evaluators) were to advance scientific knowledge about the operations and potential effectiveness of syringe exchange, particularly in a high HIV seroprevalence environment; to utilize biological marker data as one outcome measure in this evaluation because of the greater perceived "objectivity" of such data; and to provide the exchanges with information that could be utilized to improve operations.

PROBLEM SOLVING

Another important aspect of the first year was the development of positive working relationships among the different organizations. Given the differences in organizational cultures, this in itself can be considered a major accomplishment (Broadhead & Margolis, 1993). Much of the development of positive working relationships occurred during monthly meetings hosted by AmFAR and attended by representatives of the syringe exchanges, the State Health Department and the evaluators. These meetings consisted primarily of problem identification followed by protracted, but usually successful, group problem solving.

The "tagging" of the syringes to be distributed by the exchanges is a good example of an identified problem with an eventual resolution. When the two underground exchanges were operating as underground exchanges, they usually "tagged" the syringes they distributed by painting a small mark on them. This tagging had several advantages. It permitted the exchanges to determine how many of their own syringes were being returned versus how many syringes from other sources were being brought in to the exchanges. The visible tag also served an educational/reminder function for the IDUs, indicating that it was possible to obtain HIV-free syringes from the exchanges.

When the exchanges were given legal authorization in the summer of 1992, it was expected that the tagging would continue. Tagging would have additional advantages for the legally authorized exchanges. Since it was now legal for an IDU to possess syringes obtained from an authorized exchange, tagging could assist law enforcement officials in distinguishing between legal and illicit syringes. (Though this would obviously not be foolproof, since illicit syringes could also be marked by anyone who chose to do so.) When the regulations for legal exchanges were first drafted, tagging of syringes to be distributed was included, and State Health Department officials made several public statements that tagging would be included in the final regulations.

The rapid expansion of the legalized exchanges brought forth the difficulties in attempting to tag syringes. Discussions with syringe manufacturers led to a quick conclusion that it would not be economically feasible for manufacturers to modify their production processes to produce relatively small lots of "pre-tagged" syringes. The manufacturers also noted that post-production tagging compromised the sterility of the syringes. The two large-scale legal exchanges (formerly underground exchanges) found that the tagging operation rapidly became the rate limiting factor in their ability to deliver syringe exchange services. The funding level of the syringe exchanges required the exchanges to use volunteers for the task of tagging syringes. Large scale tagging was creating a severe morale problem among the volunteers. The leaders of the two large exchanges reached a point where they believed it would be impossible to continue large-scale operations if the tagging was required.

As the exchanges proceeded during the first year, there were persistent reports of police harassment of IDUs participating in the exchanges, including confiscation of legally obtained tagged syringes and taking of the cards that identified the IDUs (by a code number) as participants in the legal exchanges. These reports undermined the rationale for having syringes that could be easily identified as legal. Concerns about liability issues if a tagged syringe should be involved in a needlestick injury of a person who did not inject illicit drugs were also raised, although there were no reports of needlestick injuries.

The need to know the percentage of distributed syringes that were returned to the exchanges was still considered important by the State Health Department and several of the exchanges themselves. The eventual resolution to the problem of continued tagging of syringes was to omit tagging from the regulations and to have the evaluators conduct a "Tagging Alternative Study" (TAS). In this study, a sample of syringes will be tagged, with systematic measurement of the returned syringes over the next month. This study will provide an estimate of the percentage of syringes returned for each of the different exchanges over the one month measurement period. The study could be repeated for either all exchanges or for selected exchanges if a need should arise in the future.

The "tagging question" is an example of an issue where the perceived needs of the different organizations within the system were in sharp conflict. This issue reflects a more general conflict between having tightly regulated exchanges and the HIV prevention goal of providing sterile injection equipment to as many injecting drug users as possible. This more general conflict has been a dominant theme during the first year of operation, and we expect it to continue as a dominant theme for the indefinite future.

Subject Characteristics

To date 2849 interviews have been conducted; this analysis is based on 1752 baseline interviews conducted between the months of October 1992 and June 1993. Less than one percent of the interviews have been excluded from this analysis due to unreliability of the responses (as determined by the interviewer who recorded reliability on a Likert scale based on consistency of respondents' answers and on face-to-face judgment of the validity of the data.

Of the 1752 subjects included in this analysis 70% were male and 30% were female. IDUs participating in this study were racially/ethnically diverse (38% Latino, 35% African American, 28% White). The mean age of participants was 36 (SD=8) and ranged from 18 to 67 years old (Table 1).

Seventy-two percent (1256) of participants reported having been tested for HIV. Of these, 1112 reported knowing the results, 70% reported testing negative, 27% reported testing positive, 1.5% of the test results were inclusive and 1% of the participants refused to reveal their status.

The mean age of first injection was 19 (SD=5.5). Respondents had long histories of injecting drug use; the average length of injection was 16 years (SD = 9.0) (Table 2). Only 59 respondents (3%) had been injecting for 1 year or less. Participants had been using syringe exchange for an average of 5.8 (SD=9.0) months, and reported an average use of 15.2 (SD=13.1) syringes per week. Respondents reported obtaining 14 (93%) of their syringes from the exchange per week (Table 2).

Self-Reported Change in Risk-Taking Behavior

Participants reported that in the 30 days prior to using the syringe exchange, they injected with previously used works an average of 11.6% of the time compared to 3.9% of the time in the last 30 days while using the needle exchange ($p<.001$). Prior to using the exchange, respondents reported injecting an average of 95.2 times per month compared with 85.6 times per month during the last 30 days ($p<.0001$). There was a significant decrease in the number of participants who reported injecting with syringes used by others in the last 30 days compared with 30 days prior to using the exchange: with rented or bought used syringes, 21.7% prior, 5.8% current; with borrowed works, 29.3% prior, 12.1% current. The number of IDUs who reported using alcohol pads to clean their skin when injecting increased significantly, from 33.0% prior to 80.0% current (Table 3).

A total of 1337 participants responded to questions about renting or buying used syringes both 30 days prior to using the exchange and during the past 30 days. Of these, 1047 (78%) did not rent or buy used works prior to using the exchange and 290 (22%) did. In the last 30 days since using the exchange, 1259 (94%) did not inject with works used by others and 78 (6%) did. Among the 1047 who did not practice this behavior previously, only 11 (1%) began to do so. In comparison, among the 290 who did rent or buy used works prior to using the exchange, 223 (77%) no longer did (McNemar Chi square, $p<.001$).

A total of 1328 participants responded to questions about borrowing or using used works. Of these, 939 (71%) did not practice these behaviors in the 30 days prior to using the exchange and 389 (29%) did. Among those who did not, only 23 (2%) initiated this behavior. In the last 30 days while using the exchange, 1167 (88%) reported not borrowing or using used works and 161 (12%) did. In comparison, among those who previously borrowed or used works, 251 (65%) have not in the last 30 days (McNemar Chi square, $p<.001$).

A total of 1269 participants responded to queries about using alcohol pads while injecting. Of these, 851 (67%) did not use alcohol pads prior to using the exchange and 418 (33%) did. Among those who did not, only 9 (2%) still do not. During the last 30 days while using the exchange, 1015 (80%) reported using alcohol pads, and 254 (20%) reported not using them. Among those who did not previously use alcohol pads, 606 (71%) have begun since using the exchange (McNemar Chi square, $p<.001$).

Of the 1752 participants interviewed, 60% reported that they had anal, oral, or vaginal sex in the last 30 days. Table 4 presents the sex risk behaviors of these 1055 sexually active participants.

DISCUSSION

In contrast to questions about the use of bleach by IDUs to disinfect syringes (Center for Disease Control, 1982; Contoreggi et al., 1992; Vlahov et al., 1991), there is no need to conduct research on the efficacy of commercially manufactured needles and syringes in preventing HIV transmission. If only one person uses the needle and syringe, the chances of HIV transmission are as close to zero as anything in epidemiology. The effectiveness of syringe exchanges in reducing HIV transmission among injecting drug users is thus solely a question of the ability of the service providers to provide exchange services and the subsequent behavior of the persons utilizing the services.

The ability to provide services is largely determined by the specific operational procedures of the syringe exchange program, which in turn are substantially determined by the other organizations within the syringe exchange system and the availability of volunteers, and indirectly determined by a wide variety of supporters and opponents of syringe exchange. The New York syringe exchange system is the first attempt to establish a multi-exchange system within the United States. If syringe exchanges are to be an important factor in preventing HIV infection in the United States, it is very likely that they will operate within state-wide systems (or possibly a federal system). The systems issues that have arisen in New York are thus likely to be replayed in other states and possibly at a federal level.

The different organizations involved in the New York syringe exchange system have many differences in their organizational cultures. The potential for miscommunications and organizational cultural conflict, or serious conflicts of interest cannot be underestimated. That most of the problems have been successfully resolved so far is something we attribute to the skills and good will of the individuals who have been devoting many long hours to the system issues.

There also have been recurrent problem themes, such as the conflict between having tightly regulated, legally compliant exchanges and reaching the largest number of IDUs per dollar of funding. This conflict also occurs for single, isolated exchanges, but is much more complicated within a system of exchanges. (The smallest exchange in the New York system currently has 85 enrolled participants, while the largest has 5,888 enrolled participants.)

The effectiveness of the exchange will also depend upon the behavior of the participants. Similar to other studies (Buning, 1989; Hagan et al., 1991; Hart et al., 1989), participants in the NYC syringe exchange have demonstrated a reduction, but not elimination, of some high risk behaviors. This is particularly evident for syringe sharing behaviors. Overall the data indicate that there has been a significant reduction in renting and buying used syringes and a marked decrease in borrowing used works. These findings are consistent with international studies which have shown that exposure to harm reduction strategies and access to clean equipment reduces some high risk behaviors associated with HIV infection. However, despite the evidence of drug related risk reduction among participants of syringe exchanges in NYC, sexual risk reduction still lags behind (Abdul-Quader et al., 1990; Deren et al., 1993; Des Jarlais, 1992). Our data indicate that participants are having unprotected sex more than half of the time, whether with primary or casual partners. This suggests that syringe exchange programs may need to expand their efforts at sexual risk reduction education, but will more than likely require increased funding in order to accomplish this expansion. Research is still needed which will explore the determinants of consistent use of condoms among this population.

These data from the first year of the NYC syringe exchange evaluation, are consistent with data from other studies which have shown that syringe exchanges are not attracting new injectors (Des Jarlais et al., 1988). Our data indicate that the majority of IDUs attending syringe exchange are long time injectors (average length of injection 16 years) and that only 59 (3%) have been injecting for less than one year.

The most important single datum for assessing the New York syringe exchanges will obviously be the HIV seroconversion rate among the participants. Previous studies have shown seroconversion rates from 6 to 11 per 100 person-years at risk among persons continuing to inject illicit drugs in high seroprevalence areas. We will eventually be able to compare the rate observed among New York syringe exchangers to these other studies, with appropriate multivariate controls. The important question, however, will not be a statistically significant difference, but an epidemiologically substantial difference. It is quite possible that in an area like New York, both more extensive and more intensive prevention services will be needed in addition to syringe exchanges.

ACKNOWLEDGMENTS

This study was funded by the American Foundation for AIDS Research (AMFAR). We would like to acknowledge all syringe exchange staff who have cooperated with this evaluation and who have provided access to the participants, our interviewing staff, Judith Milliken for her work on this manuscript, and Lee Kochems for his comments.

REFERENCES

Abdul-Quader, A.S., Tross, S., Friedman, S.R., Kouzi, A.C., & Des Jarlais, D.C. (1990). Street-Recruited Intravenous Drug Users and Sexual Risk Reduction in New York City. *AIDS*, 4:1075-1079.

Broadhead, R.S., & Margolis, E. (1993). Drug Policy in the Time of AIDS: The Development of Outreach in San Francisco. *The Sociological Quarterly*, 34(3):497-522.

Buning, E.C. (Oct, 1989). The Role of the Needle Exchange Project in Prevention HIV Infection among Drug Users in Amsterdam. (*Paper delivered at the "What Works Conference: An International Perspective on Drug Abuse Treatment and Prevention Research, New York*).

Centers for Disease Control and Prevention. (1982). Acquired Immune Deficiency Syndrome (AIDS) Precautions for Clinical and Laboratory Staffs. *Morbidity and Mortality Weekly Report*, 31:557-580.

Centers for Disease Control, Atlanta, GA. (January 1993). *HIV/AIDS Surveillance, Year-End Edition. U.S. AIDS Cases Reported through December 1992.*

Contoreggi, C., Jones, S., Simpson, P., Lange, W., & Meyer, W. (1992). A Model of Syringe Disinfection as Measured by Polymerase Chain Reaction for Human Leukocyte antigen and HIV Genome. *VIII International Conference on AIDS, Amsterdam, The Netherlands. Abstract P.C. 4280;2:291.*

Deren, S., Paone, D., Friedman, S., Neaigus, A., Des Jarlais, D.C., & Ward, T. (Autumn, 1993). Berlin Conference Summary on IDUs and HIV/AIDS: Interventions, Behavior Change and Policy. *AIDS Care*, 5(4).

Des Jarlais, D.C. (1992). The First and Second Decades of AIDS among Injecting Drug Users. *British Journal of Addiction*, 87:347-353.

Des Jarlais, D.C., & Friedman, S.R. (1992). AIDS and Legal Access to Sterile Drug Injection Equipment. *The Annals of the American Academy of Political and Social Science*, 521:42-65.

Des Jarlais, D.C., Friedman, S.R., Sotheran, J.L., & Stoneburner, R. (1988). The Sharing of Drug Injection Equipment and the AIDS Epidemic in New York City: The First Decade. In: *Needle Sharing among Intravenous Drug Abusers: National and International Perspectives*. R. Battjes, & R. Pickens, R. (eds.). Pp. 1160-1175.

Hagan, H., Des Jarlais, D.C., Purchase, D., Reid, T., Friedman, S.R. (1991). The Tacoma Syringe Exchange. *Journal of Addictive Diseases*, 10(4):81-88.

Hart, G.J., Andrea, Carvell, A.L.M., Woodward, N., Johnson, A.M., Williams, P., & Parry J.V. (1989). Evaluation of Needle Exchange in Central London: Behavior Change and Anti-HIV Status Over One Year. *Current Science Ltd.*, 0269-9370: 261-265.

Johnson, A.M., Parry, J.V., Best, S.J., Smith, A.M., de Silva, M., & Mortimer, P.P. (1988). HIV Surveillance by Testing Saliva. *AIDS*, 3:369-371.

Kaplan, E.H., O'Keefe, E. (1993). Let the Needles do the Talking! Evaluating the New Haven Needle Exchange. *Interfaces*, 23:7-26.

New York City Department of Health, Office of AIDS Surveillance. (January 30, 1993). *New York City AIDS Surveillance Report*.

New York State Department of Health AIDS Institute (1993). *Authorization to Conduct Hypodermic Syringe and Needle Exchange Programs* (10 NYCRR Section 80.135, p. 5).

Paone, D., Des Jarlais, D.C., Caloir, S., & Friedmann, P. (1993). *AIDS Risk Reduction Behaviors among Participants of Syringe Exchange Programs in New York City, USA*. (Abstract) IXth International Conference on AIDS, Berlin, June 7-11.

Vlahov, D., Munoz, A., Celantano, D. et al. (1991). HIV Seroconversion and Disinfection of Injection Equipment among Intravenous Drug Users, Baltimore, Maryland. *Epidemiology*, 2(6):444-446.

TABLE 1 - Demographic Descriptors of Needle Exchange Participants
n=1752

Mean Age	35.7 (SD=8.0)
Gender	
Male	1192 (70%)
Female	557 (30%)
Ethnicity	
Latino	668 (38%)
Black	604 (35%)
White	443 (25%)
Other	33 (2%)
Marital Status	
Married/Common Law	415 (24%)
Never Married	805 (46%)
Divorced/Separated	447 (26%)
Widowed	70 (4%)
Have Children	
Yes	1297 (74%)
No	449 (26%)
Ever in Prison/Jail Overnight	
Yes	1238 (71%)
No	503 (29%)
Living Arrangements - Past 6 months[1]	
Own House/Apartment	738 (43%)
Someone else's House/Apt	647 (38%)
Hotel/Rooming House	130 (8%)
Shelter/Welfare Hotel	90 (5%)
Streets	259 (15%)
Jail	49 (3%)
Shanty	36 (2%)
Other	36 (2%)
Source of Income - Past 6 months[1]	
Regular Job	165 (10%)
Temporary Work	183 (11%)
Self-Employed/Panhandling	339 (20%)
Welfare	834 (49%)
Other Benefits	349 (21%)
Income from Spouse/Friends	129 (8%)
Sex for pay/Sex for drugs	101 (6%)
Illegal/Possibly illegal Sources	525 (31%)
Other	43 (3%)
Education (N=1735)	
Did not complete High School	732 (42%)
Completed High School	1006 (58%)

(1) Percents may add up to more than 100 since more than one response may apply.

TABLE 2 Drug Use Characteristics of Needle Exchange Participants
N=1752

Mean Age of First Drug Injection		19.4 (sd= 5.5)
Mean Number of Years Injecting		16.4 (sd= 9.0)
Mean Number of Months Using Exchange		5.8 (sd= 6.5)
Mean # of Syringes Used Per Week		15
Mean # of Syringes From Exchange (%)		14 (93%)
Type of Drug Injected		
	Heroin only	362 (24%)
	Cocaine only	121 (8%)
	Speedball only	261 (18%)
	Multiple drugs	712 (49%)
History of Drug Treatment		
	Yes	1322 (76%)
	No	414 (24%)
Currently in Drug Treatment		
	Yes	644 (46%)
	No	751 (54%)

TABLE 3- **Sharing Behaviors of Participants 30 Days Prior to Using the Needle Exchange and in the Last 30 Days (N=1269)**

Sharing behavior	30 days prior to using the exchange	In the last 30 days	p value
rent/buy used works			
yes	290 (22)	78 (6)	
no	1047 (78)	1259 (94)	p<.001
borrow/use used works			
yes	389 (29)	161 (12)	
no	939 (71)	1167 (88)	p<.001
use alcohol pads			
yes	418 (33)	1015 (80)	
no	851 (67)	254 (20)	p<.001

TABLE 4 - **Risk Behaviors Practiced by Sexually Active Needle Exchange Participants in the Last 30 Days n=1055**

Sexual Behaviors		# (%)
Same Sex Primary Partner		44 (4)
Primary Partner of the Opposite Sex		
	Yes	753 (71)
	No	303 (29)
Condom Use With Primary Partner		
	always	231 (31)
	sometimes	123 (17)
	never	379 (52)*
Casual Partner of the Opposite Sex		
	Yes	292 (28)
	No	764 (72)
Condom Use With Casual Partner		
	always	143 (50)
	sometimes	68 (24)
	never	77 (27)*

* May not equal 100% due to rounding

DISCUSSION: U.S. NEEDLE EXCHANGE DATA

ANDREW MOSS

Andrew Moss observed that almost a decade has passed since the first open operation of needle exchanges, yet the issue is still being hotly debated and the same arguments for and against needle exchanges are still being made. Now, however, much more is known about the operation and impact of individual needle exchange programs, and systematic studies of needle exchanges are beginning to emerge. He noted that, first, needle exchanges attract a large clientele. Second, they tend to attract older users, many of whom have long histories of injection drug use. Third, they do not seem to increase injection drug use in any way that can be observed or measured. Fourth, they may reduce needle sharing among injectors. Fifth, data are lacking--and may never be available--with which to isolate the impact of needle exchanges on HIV incidence from other factors. He remarked with interest on the finding that the Tacoma needle exchange had an individual-level protective effect against needle-borne transmission of hepatitis-B. Sixth, the data presented do not all point uniformly in the same direction: in particular, although needle exchanges attract older injectors, the data from the San Francisco presentation indicate a decline in sharing associated with needle exchange use by younger, not older, people. In addition, although many of the needle exchanges attracted a largely white clientele, African-Americans are known to be a high-risk group among injectors.

Given the data, Moss asked, should a push be made for large-scale federal and state funding of needle exchanges? His own response to the question was a qualified yes, for two reasons: first, the United States does not have a unified strategy for reducing HIV infection among injecting drug users, despite the fact that injection drug use is a major HIV risk factor in this country. Second, other serious diseases prevalent among the injector population, especially tuberculosis, are associated with HIV transmission, and reducing the incidence of HIV will have a positive impact on the incidence of those diseases as well. If the United States does move to the big model of federal and state funding of needle exchanges, Moss pointed out, the question then becomes how to do it in a way that does not destroy what has largely powered needle exchanges to date--social activism by people who have knowledge of and sympathy for people who inject illegal drugs.

INTERNATIONAL EVALUATIONS
OF NEEDLE EXCHANGE PROGRAMS

EVALUATION OF THE NEEDLE/SYRINGE EXCHANGE IN AMSTERDAM, THE NETHERLANDS

ANNEKE VAN DEN HOEK and ROEL COUTINHO, Municipal Health Service, Department of Public Health and Environment, The Netherlands

AIDS AND HIV IN THE NETHERLANDS AND AMSTERDAM

Through June 1993 a cumulative total of 2678 cases of AIDS have been reported in the Netherlands (circa 15 million inhabitants). Homosexual men are the most important risk group (78%), followed by injecting drug users (9%); 93% of the cumulative AIDS cases are men. In 1992 481 new cases were diagnosed and in 1991 437. Most of the AIDS cases in the Netherlands were reported from Amsterdam (700,000 inhabitants).

The total number of HIV infected persons in the Netherlands is estimated at 6,000-10,000. In Amsterdam the total number of homosexual men between 18 and 55 is estimated at 20,000 of whom 2,000-4,000 are infected with HIV. The number of drug users in the city is estimated at 7,000 of whom approximately 800 are HIV infected.

BACKGROUND INFORMATION ON AMSTERDAM DRUG POLICY

The estimate of the number of hard drug users in Amsterdam is based on a capture - recapture method and is a year prevalence. The estimated number of drug users staying on a regular day in Amsterdam is lower, approximately 5,500. This smaller number is due to the large number of foreign drug users who only stay briefly in Amsterdam.

Based on data of participants of the low threshold methadone programs, it is estimated that about 40% of the drug users in Amsterdam inject their drugs. The prevalence of the current injection of drugs among drug users differs according to country of origin: circa 40% of the Dutch drug users inject their drugs, compared to circa 70% of drug users of foreign origin (mainly German and South-European) and circa 5% of the ethnic drug users (from Surinam, the Netherlands Antilles, Morocco, and Turkey).

The assistance system for drug users in Amsterdam can be described in three phases: getting in contact, harm reduction and treatment.

Contact with drug users is made by 1) streetcorner workers, 2) physicians visiting drug users arrested in police-cells and 3) social nurses visiting all hospitalized drugs patients.

Through regular contact appropriate medical and social care can be given, which is considered "to be beneficial for drug users themselves and the society at large". This policy is called the harm reduction approach.

The main instrument for harm reduction (as long as the drug user is not able or willing to stop his/her drug use) is the large methadone program with a low level of threshold.

Another activity of the harm reduction approach is the needle and syringe exchange program, aimed at the reduction of the harm by injecting. This program was initially started in 1984 - through an initiative of the drug users organization, the "Junkiebond"- to prevent hepatitis B, but was soon overshadowed by the more important goal of AIDS prevention. In 1985, 100,000 needles and syringes were handed out and this number has gradually risen to circa 700,000 in 1988 and to approximately one million in 1991 and 1992. In 1992, 92% of the distributed needles/syringes had been exchanged for a used needle/syringe. Presently Amsterdam has 14 needle exchange locations. It is possible to exchange needles and syringes from 10 a.m. till 4 a.m. the next day. During the night, two slot machines are in operation for purchasing syringes. Participation in the exchange program does not require identification or registration. For this reason, no information is available on the number of participants or on their demographic characteristics.

As the needle/syringe exchange program is a low threshold project, there is no registration or monitoring of clients. Evaluation of the impact of the exchange program on injecting behavior and the spread of HIV, has therefore mainly taken place in our cohort study on HIV infection and AIDS.

THE AMSTERDAM COHORT STUDY ON HIV INFECTION AND AIDS AMONG DRUG USERS

The open cohort study started at the end of 1985. At that time only one drug user with AIDS had been reported in the Netherlands.

The aims of the study are

(a) to study the prevalence and incidence of HIV infection and AIDS in relation to (changes in) drug use and sexual behavior;

(b) to evaluate the impact of various HIV-prevention programs for drug users;

(c) to study determinants of risky injecting and sexual behavior; and

(d) to study the natural history of HIV infection.

Participants are recruited at methadone outposts, the special STD-clinic for drug using prostitutes and by word of mouth. Eligible for the study are men and women who use or have used drugs, either by injection or otherwise. Blood samples for serology, virology and immunology are taken and participants are interviewed using a standard questionnaire which includes questions concerning clinical symptoms, medical history, lifestyle, use of oral and intravenous drugs (methadone included), and prostitution. Participants are asked to return for a follow-up visit every four months. Twenty five Dutch guilders are paid per follow-up visit to encourage continued participation.

PREVALENCE AND INCIDENCE OF HIV INFECTION

Through July 1993 a total of 1,012 drug users had entered the study, 258 HIV positives and 754 HIV negatives. The HIV prevalence among drug users with a history of injecting drug use was approximately 30% (1) and remained more or less stable among new intakes in this group in following years (2). The annual HIV incidence per 100 person-years was 9.2 in 1986, varied between 2 and 5% in the years 1987-1991 (3) and was 2.5 in 1992. To date a total number of 52 seroconversions have occurred.

RISK REDUCTION AND THE EXCHANGE PROGRAM

The first study on risk reduction among the participants (December 1985-April 1988) showed that during follow-up, a strong reduction in borrowing and lending occurred, and that this behavioral was not dependent on being informed of HIV serostatus (4). Over time, the use of the needle and syringe exchange program increased. However, reduction in needle sharing was not seen among new entrants to the study. Therefore, we concluded that the risk reduction observed during follow-up was mainly an effect of the study (with counselling), with the exchange program only having a limited effect.

The next study (5) looked into factors related to regular participation in the exchange program and the borrowing of syringes in 131 HIV seronegative current injecting drug users (1989-1990). A total of 29% of the users reported borrowing syringes in the past 4-6 months. Users at increased risk of borrowing are previous borrowers, long term moderate-to-heavy alcohol users, current cocaine injectors, and drug users without permanent housing. Regular clients of the syringe exchange, when compared with other injecting drug users, were found more often to be frequent, long term injectors. They borrowed slightly less often than other users, but this was not statistically significant, even after controlling for frequency of injecting or other potential confounders. These results suggest that 5 years after the start of the exchange program, drug use characteristics govern an individual injecting drug user's choice of exchanging or not exchanging. We concluded that it seems more important to direct additional preventive measures at injecting drug users with an increased risk of borrowing rather than at users who do not participate in the syringe exchange or who do so irregularly.

Another study (3) assessed risk factors for seroconversion to HIV, between December 1985 and November 1991. The behaviors of 31 seroconverters were compared with those of 202 seronegative injecting drug users (controls). Three independent risk factors for seroconversion were found in logistic regression: 1) living >10 years in Amsterdam (OR=2.45, 95%CI 1.09-5.53); 2) first injection < 2 years ago (OR=3.43, 95%CI 1.20-9.81); and 3) injecting mainly at home (OR=0.39, 95%CI 0.18-0.88). No evidence was found that obtaining new needles/syringes via the exchange program was protective. However, the data suggest that exchanging needles/syringes may have been protective at the start of this program. In the discussion of this finding we mentioned that this may be explained by an overall increased availability of needles/syringes, which enabled non exchangers to more easily obtain new needles/syringes. Another explanation we mentioned was that, at the beginning of the program, a desire for risk reduction was the motive for exchanging, while later on exchanging became just a way to obtain injection equipment.

The methodological problems encountered in evaluating prevention programs are many. In general, little is known about the representativeness of the study sample of drug users. Furthermore, participants are self selected, and self selection occurs again with respect to participation in the follow-up study. Self-reports on injecting and sexual behavior may be unreliable and are difficult to validate.

To evaluate the impact of prevention-programs, random allocation of drug users to the various programs would be the best study design. However, this allocation would be in conflict with the harm reduction policy which includes large accessibility of the programs for all drug users. Another problem in evaluating the impact of the programs on risk-reduction is that drug users may attend programs for other reasons than risk reduction and the longer low threshold programs exist, the more this may be the case. On the other hand, health education messages have also reached drug users who do not want to use the needle and syringe exchange program to obtain clean needles and syringes and prefer to buy their needles and syringes at pharmacies and certain shops. These considerations may imply that the impact of a prevention-program cannot be assessed by studying differences in risk behavior between attenders and non-attenders.

Indeed, a last study (6) that studied serial, cross-sectional trends in injecting behavior from 1986 to 1992 showed that the proportion of drug users who reported borrowing and lending used injection equipment and re-using needles/syringes (in the 6 months preceding intake) continuously declined from 51% to 20%, from 46% to 10% and from 63 to 39%, respectively and that non-attenders of exchange programs reduced their risk behavior to the same extent as attenders. This finding explains why, in comparing attenders with non-attenders we were not able to demonstrate any impact of the exchange (and other prevention) programs on risk reduction*.

---

* For a part of the Amsterdam drug users the exchange program may have started too late, shown by the fact that in 1986 already 30% of the drug users in Amsterdam appeared to be infected with HIV. But for the rest of the Netherlands the exchange programs may have been in time. Recent HIV prevalence studies among drug users in four other cities (only 1 to 2 hours' drive from Amsterdan), showed that the prevalence of HIV among drug users outside Amsterdam is still low (less than 4%).

CONCLUSIONS

We conclude, therefore, that the evaluation of specific measures is difficult. Although we have not been able to demonstrate any impact of specific prevention measures, we think that all prevention activities taken together in Amsterdam (exchange programs, over-the-counter sales of needles/syringes by pharmacies, low threshold methadone programs, counselling projects, and information campaigns) have been responsible for the decline in high-risk injecting behavior.

However, it must be realised that a considerable number of drug users from time to time borrow an used needle/syringe and that transmission of HIV among drug users still occurs.

LITERATURE

1. van den Hoek JAR, Coutinho RA, van Haastrecht, van Zadelhoff AW, Goudsmit J. Prevalence and riskfactors of HIV infections among drug users and drug using prostitutes in Amsterdam. *AIDS* 1988;2(1):55-60

2. Van Haastrecht HJA, van den Hoek JAR, Bardoux C, Leentvaar-Kuijpers, Coutinho RA. The course of the HIV epidemic among intravenous drug users in Amsterdam, The Netherlands. *Am J Public Health* 1991;81:59-62

3. Van Ameijden EJC, van den Hoek JAR, van Haastrecht HJA, Coutinho RA. The harm reduction approach and riskfactors for HIV seroconversion in injecting drug users, Amsterdam. *Am J Epidemiol* 1992;136:236-43

4. Van den Hoek JAR, Van Haastrecht HJA, Coutinho RA. Riskreduction among intravenous drug users in Amsterdam under the influence of AIDS. *Am J Public Health* 1989;79:1355-1357

5. Hartgers C, van Ameijden EJC, van den Hoek JAR, Coutinho RA. *Public Health Reports* 1992;107:675-682

6. van Ameijden EJC, van den Hoek JAR, Coutinho RA. A substantial decline in injecting risk behavior among drug users in Amsterdam from 1986 to 1992, and its relationship to AIDS-prevention programs. *Am J Public Health* 1994;84:275-281.

EVALUATION OF HUMAN IMMUNODEFICIENCY VIRUS PREVENTION PROGRAMS FOR INJECTION DRUG USERS IN CANADA

MARGARET MILLSON, Department of Preventive Medicine and Biostatistics, University of Toronto, Canada, and City of Toronto Department of Public Health; and CATHERINE HANKINS, Centre for AIDS Studies, Montréal-Centre Regional Public Health Team, Canada

THE PILOT PROGRAMS

The first official HIV prevention program for injection drug users in Canada which included needle exchange opened in Vancouver in January 1989. It was quickly followed by programs in Montreal, Toronto, and several other major cities, so that by the end of 1990 there were 8 such publicly-funded programs involving needle exchange in operation. These programmes had not seen the light of day spontaneously but rather, with the exception of the Vancouver needle exchange, were part of a federal government strategy to stimulate the development of pilot intervention programmes for injection drug users.

The overall objectives for this initiative on the part of Health Canada were two-fold. First, the federal government aimed to collaborate with provincial governments in the support of pilot prevention programmes designed to reduce the transmission of HIV among injection drug users and their sexual partners. The second objective was to acquire national data concerning the risk of HIV infection among injection drug users and the efficacy of prevention strategies.

The funding criteria for the pilot prevention programmes were clearly spelled out. In order to be eligible, pilot studies had to take place within the context of a collaborative multidisciplinary network involving local public health officials, addiction treatment agencies, law enforcement, community groups and, where possible, academic or research institutions. A variety of collaboration mechanisms were considered to be acceptable, ranging from inter-agency committees to direct multi-agency programme delivery.

In addition to this multidisciplinary context, pilot studies had to embody a multi-faceted approach to prevention[1]. Proposed programs had to include risk reduction education and counselling, as well as linkage to addiction treatment services and to other existing health and social services. Prevention programs could opt to include a carefully monitored needle-syringe exchange component.

With respect to evaluation, in order to be eligible for funding, pilot studies were required to include a comprehensive and methodologically sound as well as ethically approved evaluation component. The evaluation research protocols had to receive the approval of a constituted ethics review committee and follow the Medical Research Council of Canada's guidelines on research involving human subjects, 1987[2].

With respect to the funding strategy, the federal government of Canada offered to cost-share the service delivery component on a 50-50 basis with the provinces during the pilot study period, up to a maximum of two years. The federal share of the programme funding was completely administered through those provinces agreeing to participate. The federal government bore the full cost of the programme evaluation component during the same pilot period.

What was the outcome of Health Canada's initiative to support pilot intervention programs for injection drug users? Five provinces participated with federal funding for the last of the pilot projects ending in March of 1993. Recognizing the importance of a long term integrated HIV prevention strategy in the injection drug using population, many provincial and local governments not only assumed the responsibility for ongoing funding but proceeded to increase the number of outreach programmes. More than 30 intervention projects are now operating and an additional 10 projects are slated to come on stream by the spring of 1994.

Publically funded programmes involving needle exchange in Montréal, Toronto, Vancouver and several major cities were opened in 1989 and 1990, eight of which form the basis for this national evaluation. Although a series of meetings was held to discuss evaluation of the projects and promote the use of common methodology and instruments in order to seek comparability, there were significant differences in the evaluation approaches utilized, and to some extent these have limited the ability to compare and attempt to generalize findings. This paper will provide a brief overview of key program features, evaluation methodologies employed, their strengths and limitations, and the major findings so far. This overview will be followed by a more detailed description of the evaluations carried out in Montreal and Toronto.

The programs which were established in different cities varied substantially in their organizational features. Although all were required to be multiagency collaborations, some programs were established within agencies already serving the target population, with pre-established credibility with their clients, while others were established as new services which needed to become known and accepted by potential clients. The cities involved also varied in the degree of acceptance by the police, politicians, and the public of the services, particularly of needle exchange. There were also important differences in the size and characteristics of the client population and in the drugs being used. For example, at the outset of these programs, injection of a combination of talwin and ritalin ("T and Rs") was very common in Western Canada, but was almost unheard of in Toronto and Montreal, where heroin and especially cocaine were the drugs of choice. There were police reports of shooting galleries in Montreal, but these were said to be quite uncommon in Toronto. Therefore each city represented a unique set of circumstances which influenced both the program and the evaluation undertaken.

An important difference among different services was the mix of outreach services undertaken. Some services relied heavily on a mobile van to reach potential clients, others conducted considerable street outreach on foot, while others relied primarily on a fixed site in a location judged to be appropriate for attracting potential service users. In some cities these fixed site(s) were in pre-existing agencies, in others they were newly established locations.

A common feature of all services was the effort to provide a range of services, including counselling and referral to drug treatment. In some sites where the volume of clients seen was high, the ability to carry out indepth counselling may sometimes have been compromised.

EVALUATION APPROACHES

All the evaluations undertaken as part of these projects attempted to collect process measures documenting numbers of clients served, numbers of needles given out and exchange rates, client characteristics including age, sex, drugs used and frequency, length of time injecting, needle-sharing frequency, reasons for needle-sharing, disinfection techniques used when taking used needles and their frequency of use, as well as frequency and gender of sexual partners, condom use, how the client heard of the service, and distance travelled to the service. Evaluators agreed to ask questions in a standardized way as much as possible, based on questionnaires developed for the World Health Organization/European Economic Community collaborative studies, which have been used in several cities, including New York, for research on the epidemiology of HIV and injection drug use.

Several of the evaluations undertaken attempted to measure impact through tracking individuals in some fashion to allow for one or more follow-up comparisons over time looking for reported behaviour change as well as repeated measures of HIV status using saliva +/- fingerprick blood samples. Generally speaking these approaches included a comparison group of injection drug users who were not in treatment and not attending needle exchange. Most of the evaluations using this approach experienced difficulty following up individuals, due in part to the policy of allowing participants to remain anonymous, which made repeated participation dependent on the individual to return, or workers/interviewers to recognize previous participants and encourage them to participate again. From the beginning, there was agreement that studies requesting lengthy interviews would need to pay participants; most studies such as the one in Toronto have paid $20 for a personal interview requiring 45 minutes or more; the payment is given to those completing the interview regardless of whether they agree to provide samples for testing. Despite this incentive, this study and some others had difficulty obtaining follow-up data on the same individuals; in the first year of the study, 3 month follow-up rates were only 20%, so that it was necessary to modify the design to focus on repeated cross-sectional measures of the population as a whole rather than individual follow-up. The implications of this will be discussed further below.

In general, researchers who were external to the program and trying to collect impact measures in some cases experienced difficulties in collaborating effectively with project staff who were asked to collect process measures. In some instances, staff considered collecting even minimal information such as age or drug of choice to be too intrusive to clients, and feared that clients would be driven away be being asked any questions. In many instances this problem was more acute at the beginning when programs were being launched, and became less problematic once client comfort with the service was established.

SELECTED FINDINGS OF PROCESS EVALUATIONS

Table 1 summarizes the findings of a key impact measure, numbers of needles distributed annually by some of the larger programs. It should be noted that each of these cities was estimated to have several thousand injectors at the time these programs were undertaken.

TABLE 1

Needles Given Out by Year by 5 Urban Canadian Needle Exchange Programs

YEAR			CITY			
	Toronto	Montreal	Vancouver	Winnepeg	Edmonton	Total
1989	4,387	24,267	127,806			156,460
1990	58,281	146,211	343,995	616	15,000	564,103
1991	130,442	169,423	527,248	36,624	183,000	1,046, 737
1992	120,637	193,740	607,385	24,831 (to Aug)	392,080	1,338, 673

In addition to needles, most programs provided alcohol swabs, sterile water for injection, and condoms; many also provided bleach kits and instructions on needle disinfection for use in situations where sterile needles were not immediately available. Some programs found a very high demand for condoms, in some cases by clients who did not request needles, reflecting the mix of sex trade workers attending services. Another key measure was demand for referral to other services, in particular to drug treatment. Some programs, for example Vancouver, reported that requests for treatment outstripped availability, and pressed for more treatment to be made available. In Toronto, experiences of the needle exchange and other community services in seeking treatment for their clients lead to concern about difficulty in finding treatment slots. The Ministry of Health responded with development of a registry of available treatment slots to allow counsellers to more readily refer their clients.

Over time, most services reported attempts to improve client access and to reach more clients through approaches such as alteration of hours, street outreach, and use of vans to provide a mobile service. Several cities identified an over-representation of males, especially older, long-term injectors, among their IDU clients, and in some cases also absence of certain ethnic groups known to have injectors. The response was generally to develop special outreach strategies, in some cases involving health, social service, or AIDS prevention organizations dealing with these populations in promoting or delivering services.

CLIENT SATISFACTION MEASURES

Most evaluators found high reported client satisfaction with the services, except in some cases for a desire for different or longer hours of service, a more convenient location, or, in a few cases, a more liberal exchange policy. Programs differed in exchange policy, with some adhering more strictly to 1:1 exchange or to limitations of the total number of needles provided at one visit; clients tended to prefer less strict policy in these matters.

KEY FINDINGS ABOUT IMPACT

Behaviour Change

Most programs demonstrated declines in needle sharing and increases in use of bleach to clean needles. Generally the improvements in safe needle use were greater among users of needle exchange than non-users; however in some studies, including the one in Toronto, there is some difficulty with interpreting trends in non-attenders of needle exchange, because trends in the population as a whole may be influenced by the work of the needle exchange, as well as by other services doing HIV education and counselling in the same population, so that the non-attenders are not truly without services, and the impact of the needle exchange in isolation is very difficult to determine. Indeed our own outlook has been that needle exchange should not be considered in isolation, but as part of a multi-service strategy; the reductions seen in risky needle use behaviour in the overall population suggest that the program as a whole is having beneficial impact.

The evidence for reduction in sexual risk behaviour is less clear-cut; although there is some suggestion of increased condom use with casual partners, most programs have not demonstrated statistically significant changes. This is a finding which has been identified elsewhere in the world, and requires further examination and program focus.

Infection Rates

With the possible exception of Montreal, which will be discussed further below, most cities in Canada have demonstrated HIV infection rates under 10%; some cities have been able to demonstrate maintenance of steady seroprevalence rates over two or more years.

Future Evaluation

The programs which began as pilots have now been continued, usually with provincial funding from AIDS prevention budgets, and the provinces of British Columbia and Ontario in particular have funded several more programs in smaller cities; the province of Quebec has made a particular effort to enhance needle availability in pharmacies as a strategy to complement ongoing needle exchange activities. It is highly desirable that ongoing core measures of process and impact be collected in order to assess the longer term results of these programs, and modify them as needed in response to changing circumstances.

ACKNOWLEDGMENT

The support and assistance of the National Health Research and Development Program and Ms. Betsy MacKenzie, AIDS Education and Prevention Unit, Health Canada, as well as the principal investigators of the evaluations mentioned are gratefully acknowledged.

REFERENCES

1. Health and Welfare Canada. Health and Welfare Initiative to Support Pilot Intervention Programs for Injection Drug Users, Ottawa, July 1989.

2. Medical Research Council of Canada. Guidelines of research involving human subjects. Minister of Supply and Services Canada, Ottawa, 1987.

TORONTO'S HIV PREVENTION PROGRAM FOR INJECTION DRUG USERS: TRENDS IN RISK BEHAVIOUR AND HIV SEROPREVALENCE OVER TWO AND A HALF YEARS

Margaret Millson, Department of Preventive Medicine and Biostatistics, University of Toronto, and City of Toronto Department of Public Health, Canada;
Ted Myers, City of Toronto Department of Public Health and Department of Health Administration, University of Toronto, Canada;
James Rankin, Department of Preventive Medicine and Biostatistics, University of Toronto, and Addiction Research Foundation, Toronto, Canada;
William Mindell, City of Toronto Department of Public Health, Toronto, Canada;
Bernadette McLaughlin, Carol Major, and Margaret Fearon, Ontario Ministry of Health, Toronto, Canada;
Janet Rigby and Steffanie Strathdee, Department of Preventive Medicine and Biostatistics, University of Toronto, Canada;
and Randall Coates, Department of Preventive Medicine and Biostatistics, University of Toronto, Canada (deceased)

INTRODUCTION

From October of 1989 to October 1990, we conducted anonymous interviews with out-of-treatment injection drug users in Toronto as part of an evaluation of the City of Toronto Department of Public Health's HIV prevention program for injection drug users. A key element of this program was the needle exchange called "The Works." In May 1991, we began another year of interviews with out of treatment IDUs recruited in the same sites as in the first year of study; this research represented the first year of a three year study in collaboration with the WHO multicentre study of HIV and injecting drug use. This drug user research has been funded by the National Health Research and Development Program of Health Canada.

This report, therefore, represents a comparison of the results of these repeated cross-sectional surveys conducted over two and a half years among injection drug users who had injected within 2 months of the time of interview, and who had not received treatment for drug problems within the preceeding 3 months. Subjects were recruited from agencies serving IDUS in the downtown area of Toronto in both years; in the second year, recruitment was expanded in one particular area which is well known for prostitution and drug use. Recruitment was through posters and word of mouth, and subjects were paid $20 for the interview. HIV testing was conducted in an anonymous fashion using saliva and finger prick blood samples; results were not provided to interviewees, who were instead encouraged to seek testing with counselling at appropriate clinics.

RESULTS

Fewer young subjects were interviewed in the second year; this was attributed to a combination of another study going on among street youth during part of our study period in the second phase, as well as a reported drop in injecting as a mode of drug taking among some young drug users. As a result of this age variation, we controlled for age in the analyses reported.

In both study periods the majority of interviewees were male, but there was a small (non-significant) increase in the proportion of females in the second year.

The drug of choice most commonly reported in both years was cocaine, but there was an increase in the proportion reporting heroin as their drug of choice in year 2.

Of particular note in our study population is the high rate of reported incarceration. In both years, about 80% reported having been in jail at least once since they began to use drugs. We also documented reported needle sharing while in custody.

Key Findings

Needle Use

1. There was a statistically significant ($p<.05$) move away from sharing needles, for both giving and receiving used needles, in this population between 1989 and 1991, such that in the second year of the study, 65% of IDUs reported never using someone else's needles in the preceding 6 months; 68% reported never giving someone else their used needles. A small but fairly stable percentage of 10-14% reported sharing at least weekly in the preceding 6 months in both years, with the remainder reporting infrequent sharing (i.e. monthly or less).

2. There was also an increase in cleaning of used needles with bleach reported by year two, with 75% of all those who took used needles reporting some use of this cleaning method, up considerably from the 51% reported for the 1989 sample.

3. Sources of new, sterile needles also shifted between the two study periods, with needle exchange being reported as the most important source by 46% in year two as compared with 18% in year one, with a drop occurring between the years in the proportion reporting pharmacies or friends as their most *important* source. This was the case even though approximately equal proportions of those interviewed mentioned pharmacies and needle exchange as one source they used (69% and 63% respectively). This may reflect the degree of access perceived to the two sources by IDUs. It should be pointed out that by the second year of study, the City of Toronto Dept. of Public Health had begun funding needle exchange in some of the community agencies in which we were doing recruitment, in addition to its own service, so these figures may reflect to some extent an increase in access within these agencies.

Sexual Behavior Over the Study Period

1. For males, consistent use of condoms with casual partners did rise from 30 to 40%, mainly associated with a drop in those reporting never using condoms with casual partners. However, for those with a regular partner, the proportion always using condoms dropped slightly over the two years, with a corresponding increase in those who never used condoms. This finding requires further detailed analysis to attempt to determine the factors involved in this behaviour.

2. For females, although the numbers are smaller, the trend with regular partners is similar to that for males; reporting of consistent use of condoms with casual partners did increase, but the numbers were small and this was not statistically significant.

HIV Testing

Self-report By the second year, nearly three-quarters of our interviewees reported at least one previous HIV test; 5.2% of those tested reported that they were positive.

Anonymous, Unlinked Testing We have found very good compliance with being tested in our studies, such that in year two, only 1.5% of those interviewed failed to provide any specimen for testing. There has also been a drop in the proportion providing only saliva or only blood, although 5% continue to refuse to provide a dried blood spot. We have found saliva to be safe, accurate, and convenient as a tool for these seroprevalence studies in the field, provided it is tested by a lab able to carry out the techniques required.

The results of testing showed a small increase in seropositivity in the year two sample when compared to year one, from 4.3% in year one to 5.7% in year two, however the confidence limits for the second year are 2-10%, so there is clear overlap between the two years, and no statistically significant increase. We have completed testing on specimens collected during our third year of study, ending in May 1993, and although we have not completed detailed analysis, the crude seroprevalence rate appears to be approximately the same as in years one and two.

CONCLUSIONS

We conclude that there has been significant decline in needle use related risk behaviour in this population, at the same time that ongoing HIV prevention efforts have been introduced and expanded. There is also some modest improvement in condom use with casual partners, although not with regular partners. These patterns and their significance require further exploration.

Seroprevalence in this population is high enough to be worrisome, and mandates ongoing intensive prevention efforts. We are encouraged by the finding that there is no increase apparent in seroprevalence in our ongoing studies; we intend to continue to monitor the situation as our city's prevention program continues to be active.

The accompanying copy of the poster presented at the IXth International AIDS Conference in Berlin illustrates the findings presented here.

TRENDS IN HIV SEROPREVALENCE AND RISK BEHAVIOUR IN IDUS IN TORONTO, CANADA

Millson, P.[12], Myers, T.[23], Rankin, J.[14], Major, C.[5]; Fearon, M.[5], Rigby, J[1]; Strathdee, S[1]
[1]Dept. of Preventive Medicine and Biostatistics, University of Toronto; [2] City of Toronto Dept. of Public Health;
[3] Dept. of Health Administration, University of Toronto; [4]Addiction Research Foundation, Toronto; [5]Ontario Ministry of Health, Toronto

OBJECTIVES

To examine trends in HIV prevalence and associated risk behaviours among injecting drug users (IDUs) in Toronto, Canada who were not in treatment.

METHODS

From Nov. 1989 to May 1992, we conducted interviews about HIV risk behaviour with IDUs, not in treatment, using the questionnaire developed for the WHO Multicentre Study on Injecting Drug Use and Risk of HIV Infection. Interviewees provided saliva and finger-prick blood samples for unlinked HIV testing.

RESULTS

We compared results from the one year period Nov. 1989 to Nov. 1990 (N=582) to those from the one year period May 1991 to May 1992 (N=342).

- There were fewer IDUs under 20 in year 2 than in year 1.

Figure 1:

Age

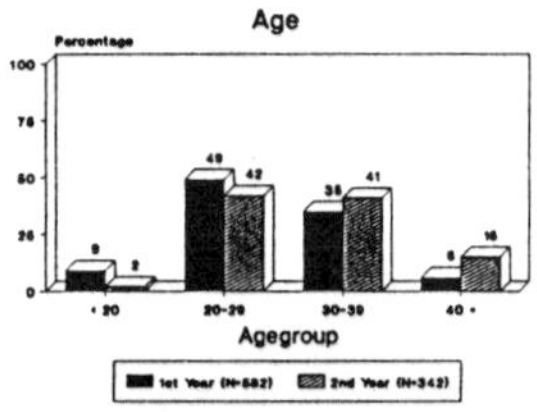

- As in year 1, there were fewer women than men in the sample in year 2.

Figure 2:

Gender

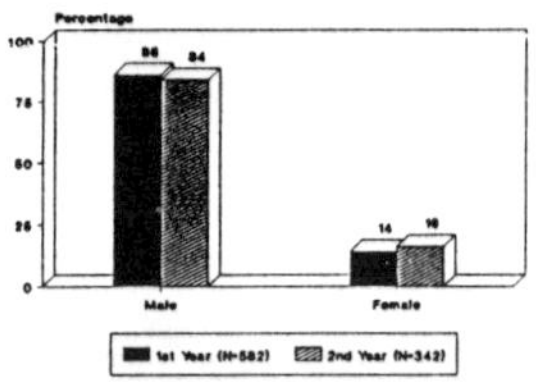

- In both years, about 80% had a history of incarceration. Among these IDUs, reporting of needle sharing while in custody remained unchanged.

Figure 3:

Needle use in jail/prison

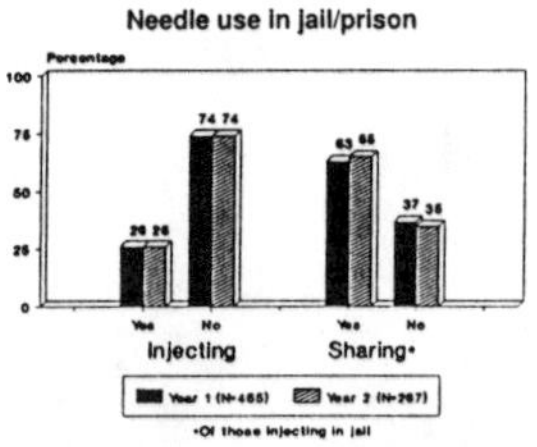

- Between the periods, needle sharing dropped from 45% to 35% for taking used needles and 42% to 33% for giving needles to others (p<0.05 for both).

Figure 4:

Taking used needles

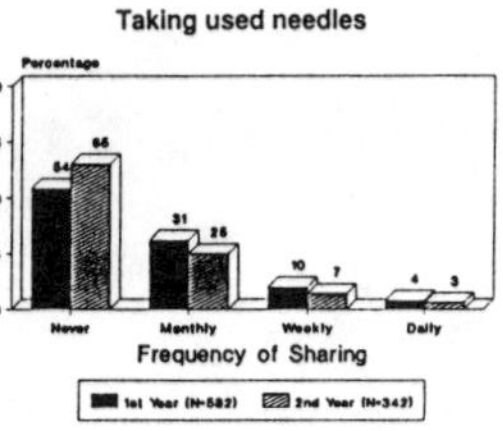

Figure 5:

Giving used needles

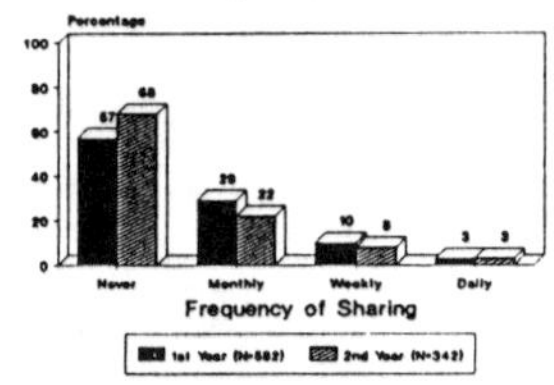

- Among those who took used needles, 59.5% reported always cleaning in the first period; 63.6% in the second.

Figure 6:

Cleaning used needles

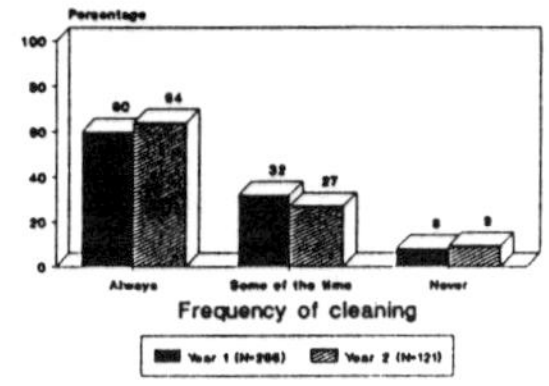

Figure 7:

Methods of cleaning used needles

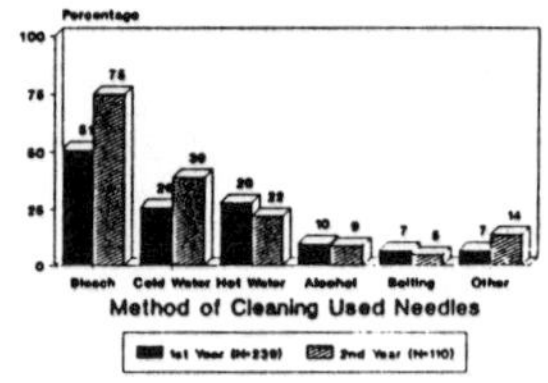

- IDUs reporting obtaining needles from a needle exchange increased as did those reporting the needle exchange as the most important source of needles.

Table 1:

Source of new, sterile needles

Source of Needles		Year 1 (N=582) N (%)	Year 2 (N=342) N (%)
Source:	Pharmacy	368 (63.3)	234 (68.6)
	Friends	214 (36.9)	85 (24.9)
	Needle Exchange	176 (30.3)	214 (62.8)
	Black Market	31 (5.3)	9 (2.6)
	"Other"	25 (4.3)	5 (1.5)
	Doctor	19 (3.3)	5 (1.5)
Most Important Source:			
	Pharmacy	253 (47.4)	121 (35.8)
	Needle Exchange	95 (17.8)	157 (46.4)
	Friends	111 (20.8)	40 (11.8)

- Overall, use of condoms did not improve significantly.

Figure 8:

Condom use with partners of opposite sex - Males

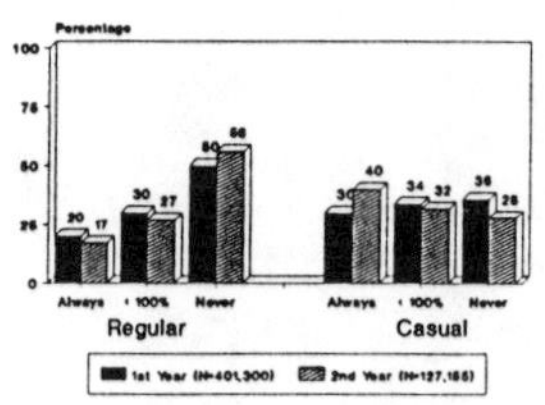

Figure 9:

Condom use with partners of opposite sex - Females

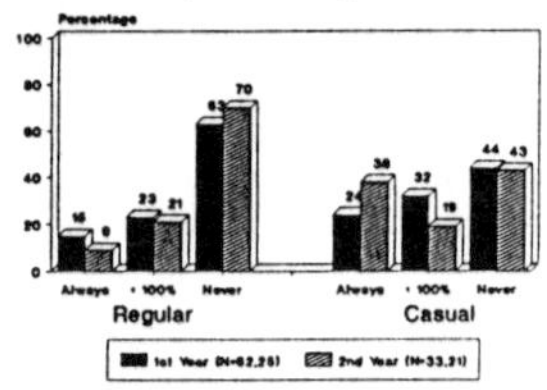

Figure 10:

Condom use with clients of opposite sex - Males

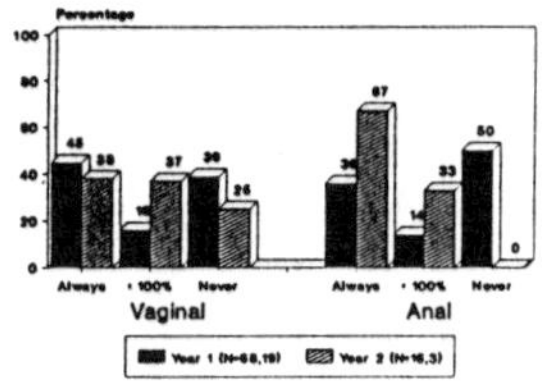

Figure 11:

Condom use with clients of opposite sex - Females

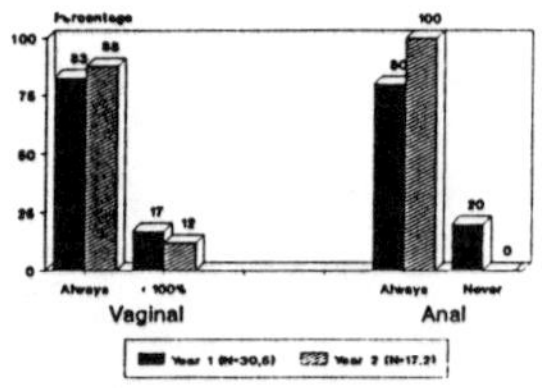

- The HIV prevalence did not significantly differ between the first year (4.3% ; 95% C.I. 3-6) and the second year (5.7% ; 95% C.I. 3-10).

Table 2:

HIV Prevalence data

Lab HIV Antibody Testing		Year 1 (N=582) N (%)	Year 2 (N=342) N (%)
Samples Given			
	Both dbs & saliva	441 (75.8)	316 (92.4)
	dbs only	20 (3.4)	4 (1.2)
	Saliva only	74 (12.7)	17 (5.0)
	Neither	47 (8.1)	5 (1.5)
Results: **			
	Positive	23 (4.3)	19 (5.7)
	Negative	510 (95.7)	315 (94.3)

CONCLUSIONS

- Needle-sharing declined significantly among out-of treatment IDUs recruited from the downtown core of Toronto between 1989 and 1992.
- Seroprevalence appears not to have increased significantly during the same time period.
- Although condom use with casual partners did increase somewhat for both sexes, this was not statistically significant.
- Needle sharing while in custody continued to be of serious concern in this population.
- Although we cannot be certain of a cause and effect relationship, this evidence of a decline in risky needle use, in the City of Toronto, concurrent with intensive prevention efforts, including needle exchange, is encouraging.

Funding Agency

National Health Research and Development Programme, Health and Welfare Canada.

EVALUATING MONTRÉAL'S NEEDLE EXCHANGE CACTUS-MONTRÉAL

Catherine Hankins and Sylvie Gendron, Centre for AIDS Studies,
Montréal-Centre Regional Public Health Team, Canada;
Julie Bruneau, Detoxification Unit, St.-Luc Hospital, Montréal, Canada;
and Élise Roy, Centre for AIDS Studies,
Montréal-Centre Regional Public Health Team, Canada

INTRODUCTION

Several criteria can theoretically be used to evaluate the success of needle exchange programmes. Among them are measures of awareness of the service in the target population of injection drug users (IDU), utilization rates, and satisfaction with the overall service among the clientele. Changes in injecting behaviour can be documented cross-sectionally or, better yet, followed over time in a cohort of IDU to provide a measure of the behavioural impact of prevention-education activities in the injecting drug using population. Once a baseline HIV prevalence proportions has been established, it can be followed prospectively to assess the stability of prevalence and document any increases or declines. The gold standard criterion for success, which has appears to have achieved general consensus, is the estimation of baseline HIV incidence with subsequent documented declines in incidence among injection drug users who are attending a needle exchange programme regularly.

From a more general perspective, the implementation and maintenance of needle exchange activities should ideally have positive influences on policy and programme development, both at the local and national level. Since the opening of CACTUS-Montréal *(Centre d'Action Communautaire auprès des Toxicomanes Utilisateurs de Seringues)*, there have been eight other projects initiated across the province of Québec in both urban and semi-urban settings. Among them is a project for pharmacy exchange currently in the pilot phase in Montréal and two projects involving community clinic and hospital-based exchange services in semi-urban areas. Finally, needle exchange programmes are perceived to have the potential to increase demand for methadone maintenance, detoxification services and rehabilitation programmes and therefore should result in expansion of these services although such an expansion has not been documented thus far in Québec.

The CACTUS-Montréal fixed site is located at 1209 Saint-Dominique Street in downtown Montréal. It has been operating seven nights a week from 21:15 to 04:00 since July 9, 1989. Clients enter the site directly from the street. There is no exterior sign identifying the building as a needle-exchange site other than several cactus plants in the window. Two teams, each composed of a male and female nurse, alternate to provide seven day coverage. In addition to disseminating information on AIDS and the prevention of HIV transmission, the nurses distribute condoms, alcohol swabs, lubricant, gloves and travel size bottles containing bleach or distilled water. They also exchange sterile needles and syringes for used ones. First time clients receive a pamphlet which demonstrates how to clean needles and how to use condoms. Additional print materials regarding AIDS and other STD as well as business cards which indicate resources and the range of treatment options available in Montréal for drug users are available on site. Anonymous testing for HIV antibodies accompanied by pre and post-test counselling is also offered at scheduled times in a closed private room.

The exchange policy is a one-for-one exchange to a maximum of 15 needles with one extra needle always provided. Individuals who arrive with no needle are provided with one needle with no examination for needle tracks. The exchange rate has averaged a relatively stable rate of 75-80% over the period 1991 to 1993. The total number of visits per week stabilized by one year of operation at approximately 1200 visits per week.

Two components of the CACTUS-Montréal evaluation will be discussed in this paper. The first concerns the findings of the awareness, utilization, and satisfaction study conducted in the first two years of operation and the second concerns data from the prevalence-incidence study underway at the CACTUS-Montréal fixed site.

AWARENESS, UTILISATION, SATISFACTION

To determine the degree of awareness, utilisation, and satisfaction with the services offered at the exchange's fixed site, injection drug using CACTUS-Montréal attenders were approached in three correctional medium security institutions and at a detox unit drop-in clinic for individual interviews of five to ten minutes duration[1]. Injection drug users from the correctional setting were study volunteers for an ongoing research project on risk factors for HIV infection among inmates in medium security correctional institutions[2]. This study involved a standardized nurse-administered interview, as well as personalized counselling and HIV antibody testing[3]. At the drop-in clinic the first five IDU presenting to the clinic per week were asked to participate. A preliminary plan to administer the questionnaire at the fixed site was abandoned because the physical setting was inappropriate and because the validity of data collected in the presence of service providers was questionable.

Most information (70%) concerning levels of awareness, utilisation, and satisfaction with the services offered at the CACTUS-Montréal fixed site was obtained from incarcerated IDU, the remainder being provided by IDU attending the detox unit drop-in clinic near the fixed site. Comparing the prison subjects with the detox clinic clients, a greater proportion of women ($p=.001$), exclusive cocaine users ($p=.0005$), and people who had attended CACTUS-Montréal more than 15 times ($p=.03$) were represented among prison subjects. Overall, seventy-three per cent (73%) of those interviewed had heard about CACTUS-Montréal and respondents readily identified that needle-exchange services and free condoms were available at CACTUS-Montréal. Publicity for the fixed site mainly occurred by word of mouth, with 57% of aware respondents having heard about the programme from another IDU. Fifty-five per cent (55%) of those who were aware of the existence of CACTUS-Montréal had visited the fixed site, and 76% of these had actually been to CACTUS-Montréal more than five times. Attenders generally expressed satisfaction with the fixed site personnel (88% liked the staff) and 98% of attending IDU indicated that they had received the services they asked for when they visited the site. Location and opening hours did not appear to suit everyone however. When asked what they liked about CACTUS-Montréal, the most frequent responses were "the staff" and "it's free." None of the respondents suggested that CACTUS-Montréal dispense or exchange more needles than current quotas.

Within the context of a seroepidemiological study conducted in the three correctional institutions, an analysis of seroprevalence levels in injection drug users by attender or non-attender status was conducted. One hundred and sixty-three (163) men and 130 women participated in the study. Among male injection drug users, 8.6% (14/163) were seropositive with a marked discrepancy noted between rates in attenders and non-attenders. Among male attenders of CACTUS-Montréal, 20.5% (8/29) were positive versus 4.8% (6/124) of non-attenders ($p=0.002$). This contrast was not observed among the 130 women, 15 of whom were seropositive (11.5%). The rate among female attenders was 11.6% (8/69) and among non-attenders it was 11.5% (7/61). Comparing all attenders and non-attenders, attenders were twice as likely to be HIV-positive with 14.8% of attenders (16/108) and 7% of non-attenders (13/185) found to be infected ($p=0.05$). With respect to the behavioural profiles of male inmates, attenders ($n=39$) and non-attenders ($n=126$) were equally likely in the six months prior to incarceration to have injected with a syringe from a dealer ($p=0.24$) and to have given, shared or sold a used syringe to close friends ($p=0.23$) or to people in shooting galleries ($p=0.97$). In prison, attenders and non-attenders were equally likely to have injected drugs ($p=0.35$). However, attenders were significantly more likely to have had bleach in their possession ($p<0.0005$) and to have injected with a needle from someone they did not know well ($p=0.001$). This preliminary analysis suggests that CACTUS-Montréal may be attracting a particularly high risk population, at least with respect to male participants.

HIV ANTIBODY SEROPREVALENCE AND SEROINCIDENCE

Volunteers were enlisted at the fixed site of CACTUS-Montréal to provide anonymous samples for HIV antibody detection. On one randomly chosen evening per week during a three-hour period IDU were approached as they were leaving the site and asked to provide a blood specimen obtained via fingerprick or a saliva specimen collected in a sputum collector or Omni-sal. The sensitivity of saliva testing using the dried blood spot testing as a gold standard was 92.7% with a specificity of 100%[4]. Since no false positive results were detected, data from individuals with only saliva specimens were combined with data from individuals with dried blood spot specimen results for analysis. Filter paper and saliva specimens were identified by a random bar code number, ensuring complete anonymity for all samples at the laboratory. This code was also affixed to a service delivery/behavioural form to permit the linkage of serology results to information concerning behaviours in the previous 7 days as well as to basic information on age and sex found in the CACTUS-Montréal client code. Such a link allowed for the characterization of participants and refusers and served to identify repeat samples for the estimation of overall seroprevalence and seroincidence. No information was collected which could be used to personally identify any one individual. Participants who desired knowledge of their HIV status were referred to clinical testing services at CACTUS-Montréal or at anonymous testing sites.

Overall, 25% of individuals who were approached agreed to provide a specimen. Most refusers seemed to refuse because they were in a hurry. Seroprevalence data were culled by year so that each person was represented only once per twelve month period. Individuals who had never obtained or returned needles and who had never responded to questions concerning injection drug use practices were excluded from the analysis.

Analyses for the period January 1990 to January 1993 yielded the following seroprevalence proportions:

PREVALENCE IN IDU ATTENDERS				
	Seropositive	Total	Proportion	95% CI
Year 1	49	442	11.1%	(8.4-14.4)
Year 2	51	345	14.8%	(11.3-19.0)
Year 3	45	270	16.7%	(12.4-21.7)

*Chi-square for trend: 4.74, df=2 (p=.003)

Using the CACTUS-Montréal client code, repeat tests on the same individual were identified to assess seroconversions and to calculate estimates of incidence for the same 36 month period. The date of seroconversion was calculated as the mid-point between the last negative and first positive result. Incidence was calculated as a proportion (%) and as a rate in person-years (incidence density).

In 36,805 person-days of observation, 13 of 136 (9.6%) individuals, for whom at least two test results were available, seroconverted. The overall incidence rate was 12.9 per 100 person-years of observation (95% CI: 6.9; 22.0). Preliminary analyses revealed that factors such as age, gender, cocaine use, condom use, and the sexual orientation of males were not significantly associated with seroconversion. Among those who had borrowed needles in the previous seven days, the incidence rate was 18.7 per 100 person-years versus 2.5 for those who had not (p=.02). Likewise, among those who had loaned needles in the previous seven days, the incidence rate was 20.3 per 100 person-years versus 2.2 for those who had not (p=.01). Further analyses are being conducted to examine these and other sociodemographic and behavioural factors which may be associated with seronconversion and higher incidence rates.

CONCLUSION

The challenge in evaluating any prevention programme lies in the attempt to determine direct programme effect by measuring the gap between what would have likely happened had there been no programme and what actually has occurred in terms of behaviour change and seroprevalence/seroincidence. With respect to CACTUS-Montréal, this challenge is heightened by the finding that the programme, which has a greater than 2 to 1 ratio of male to female attenders, appears to be attracting a higher risk male clientele. This may account for the fact that prevalence has not yet completely stabilized in this population and that incidence rates remain unacceptably high. However, findings from behavioural studies at CACTUS-Montréal[5] have revealed that the loaning of needles has declined from 31% to 20% since the beginning of operation and that 62% of those who inject with a used needle do so after having cleaned with bleach, in combination with another method or alone, compared with 30% in the first two months of operation[6]. This suggests that this core group of injection drug users may possibly be contributing less now to HIV transmission among injection drug users that they were two years ago. The fact that these individuals are attracted to the site and are participating in risk reduction activities should be viewed as having positive implications for the eventual reduction of HIV transmission in Montréal's injection drug using community.

ACKNOWLEDGMENT

This study was supported by grant #6605-3463-AIDS from the National Health Research and Development Program, Department of Health, Canada.

REFERENCES

1. Hankins C, Gendron S, Bruneau J, Rouah F, Paquette N, Jalbert M, Prévost F, Gomez B. Consumer awareness, utilization, and satisfaction with CACTUS-Montréal's needle exchange. Eighth International Conference on AIDS, Amsterdam, July 19-24, 1992.

2. Hankins C, Gendron S, Handley M, Rouah F, O'Shaughnessy M. HIV-1 Infection Among Incarcerated Men - Québec. *CDWR* 1991;17-43:233-5.

3. Hankins C, Gendron S, Richard C, O'Shaughnessy M. HIV-1 Infection in a Medium Security Prison for Women - Québec. *CDWR* 1989;15-33:168-70.

4. Hankins C, Gendron S, Rouah F, Godbout C, Mayr I, Lepine D. Rising prevalence? Declining incidence? Montréal's needle exchange: A successful verdict or is the jury still out?. IXth International Conference on AIDS, Berlin, June 6-11, 1993.

5. Hankins CA, Gendron S, Rouah F, Cyr D, Lai-Tung MT, Racine L, Charlebois AM, Handley M. Le programme d'échange de seringues de CACTUS-Montréal: Description du service et profil comportemental de la clientèle. *Revue sexologique* 1993;1:57-75.

6. Hankins CA, Gendron S, Roy É, Bruneau J. Evaluation of CACTUS-Montréal: A pilot intervention programme for injection drug users (July 1989 - July 1991). Report submitted to the National Health Research and Development Program, April 1993.

Rising Prevalence? Declining Incidence? Montreal's Needle Exchange: A Successful Verdict or Is the Jury Still Out?

Hankins C, Gendron S*, Rouah F*, Lepine D***

*Centre for AIDS Studies, Public Health Unit, Montreal General Hospital, Canada; **Health and Welfare Canada, Ottawa, Canada

OBJECTIVE

To assess trends in the seroprevalence and seroincidence of HIV-1 among injection drug users who attend the CACTUS-Montréal fixed-site needle exchange in dowtown Montreal, Quebec.

METHODS

- One 3-hour randomly chosen period weekly
- IDU are approached as they are leaving the fixed site and asked to participate
- Dried blood spot specimen obtained by fingerprick or saliva specimen (sputum collector or Omni-sal)
- 36 months: January 1990 to January 1993
- Bar codes link behavioural questionnaire to serology and/or saliva results
- Date of seroconversion calculated as the mid-point between last negative and first seropositive result
- Incidence calculated as a proportion (%) and as a rate in person-years (incidence density)

RESULTS

PREVALENCE IN IDU ATTENDERS*

	Seropositive	*Total*	*Proportion*	*95% CI*
Year 1	49	442	11.1%	(8.4-14.4)
Year 2	51	345	14.8%	(11.3-19.0)
Year 3	45	270	16.7%	(12.4-21.7)

**Chi-square for trend: 4.74, df=2 (p=.003)*

INCIDENCE IN IDU ATTENDERS

	Year 1	*Year 2*	*Year 3*	*Total*
Number converting	6/111	7/85	0/19	13/136
Percent (%)	(5.4%)	(8.2%)	—	(9.6%)
Person-time (days)	16,510	16,707	3,588	36,805
Incidence/100 person-years	13.3	15.3	—	12.9
95% CI	(4.9-28.9)	(6.1-31.5)	—	(6.9-22.0)

SALIVA SENSITIVITY

		Dried blood spot +	Dried blood spot −	
Saliva	+	51	0	51
	−	4	429	433
		55	429	484

Sensitivity: 92.7%; Specificity: 100%

FACTORS ASSOCIATED WITH SEROCONVERSION AMONG IDU*

Age:	*Below median*	*Above median*		Male sexual orientation:	*Homo/Bi*	*Hetero*	
	16.5/100 p-y	9.6/100 p-y	p=.24		17.4/100 p-y	8.3/100 p-y	p=.30
Sex:	*Male*	*Female*		Needle borrowing:	*None*	*Any*	
	14.8/100 p-y	7.7/100 p-y	p=.25		2.5/100 p-y	18.7/100 p-y	p=.02
Cocaine use:	*None*	*Any*		Needle lending:	*None*	*Any*	
	14.2/100 p-y	12.5/100 p-y	p=.72		2.2/100 p-y	20.3/100 p-y	p=.01
Condom use:	*None*	*Any*					
	13.1/100 p-y	12.8/100 p-y	p=.66	*p values calculated assuming exact binomial distribution			

DISCUSSION

- Participation rates: 25% with most seemingly refusing because they were in a hurry
- Demographic profiles of participants and non-participants are similar, however, generalizability to all attenders or to all IDU in Montreal is not justified
- Variable intervals between testing dates means exact timing of seroconversion not known
- Sensitivity of saliva testing may be improved if samples are adequate, are correctly stored, and are tested within 1 month. Borderline results should undergo confirmatory testing.

CONCLUSION

- Seroprevalence has risen over the 36 months from 11.1% to 16.7%
- Needle borrowing and lending practices are significantly associated with seroconversion among IDU attending CACTUS-Montréal
- We are unable to detect changes in seroincidence
- Whether needle exchange attendance has a demonstrable protective effect remains to be determined

Dr. Catherine Hankins • Centre for AIDS studies, Public Health Unit, Montreal General Hospital • 980 rue Guy, Suite 300A • Montreal, Quebec H3H 2K3 • Tel: (514) 932-3055 Fax: (514) 932-1502

Research supported by the National Health Research and Development Program, Health and Welfare Canada

CONSUMER AWARENESS, UTILIZATION, AND SATISFACTION WITH CACTUS-MONTRÉAL'S NEEDLE EXCHANGE

Hankins Catherine A,* Gendron S,* Bruneau J,** Rouah F,* Paquette N,* Jalbert M,* Prévost F,** Gomez B.*

** Centre for AIDS Studies, DSC – Montreal General Hospital; ** Hôpital Saint-Luc; Montréal, Québec, Canada*

OBJECTIVES

- To ascertain the extent of awareness among injection drug users of the existence of Montréal's needle exchange service
- To determine utilization rates and patterns
- To measure levels of satisfaction among injection drug users (IDU) who have visited the site

BACKGROUND

CACTUS-Montréal's Fixed Site for Needle Exchange

- Open 2100 to 0400 hours since July 9, 1989
- Provides needles, condoms, water, bleach, lubricant, gloves, and kits
- Exchange policy: 1 for 1, to a maximum of 15 with 1 extra needle
- Exchange rate: 74%
- Average visits per week in 1991: 1204

METHODOLOGY

- Subjects: injection drug user volunteers
- Location: drop-in clinic in a detox unit (n=173) and three medium-security correctional institutions (n=319)
- Methods: individual confidential interviews
- Timeframe: 20-month period starting in November 1989

RESULTS

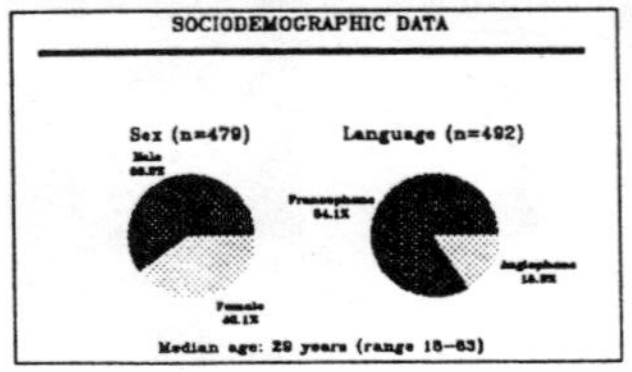

CACTUS AWARENESS

Overall, 73% of the study subjects had heard of CACTUS and sources* of information (n=345) were:

· IDU friends and other IDU	190	55%
· Posters in prison	33	10%
· Television and newspapers	44	13%
· Non-IDU friends (15), other inmates (13), pamphlets (11), radio (9), or drug counsellors (6)		each <5%

* *More than one response was possible*

CACTUS UTILIZATION

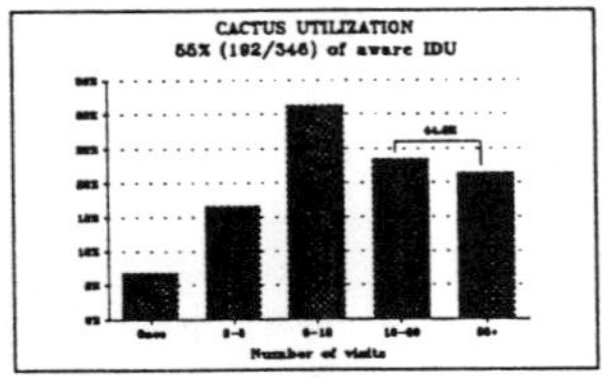

REASONS* FOR NON-ATTENDANCE AMONG IDU (n=154) WHO HAVE HEARD ABOUT CACTUS

- 60 or 39% can get clean needles elsewhere
- 34 or 22% no longer inject drugs or wish to stop
- 28 or 18% unaware of the services offered
- 17 or 11% were not interested

* *More than one response was possble*

SATISFACTION AMONG ATTENDERS

· Received the services asked for	187/190	98%
· Likes the staff	165/188	88%
· CACTUS is in a good location†	130/191	68%
· Operating hours suit her/him	90/191	47%

† *Prison subjects were more satisfied with location* (p<.0005)

ASPECTS* ATTENDERS LIKE (n=174)

· The staff	33	20%
· Services are free	29	17%
· Service is fast	19	11%
· Locale is clean	17	10%
· The idea, the concept	16	9%
· No questions are asked	13	7%

* *More than one response was possible*

ASPECTS* ATTENDERS DON'T LIKE (n=170)

· Nothing	78	46%
· Operating hours	38	22%
· Site too far/bad location	16	9%
· Questionnaire	13	8%
· Not enough condoms	6	4%
· A lot of police in that neighbourhood	4	2%

* *More than one response was possible*

When asked what else CACTUS ought to offer, clients indicated methadone, a detox programme, medical examinations, more information, toilets and chairs, legalized cocaine, and longer hours.

PLANS FOR A RETURN VISIT (n=188)

· Does not intend to return†	109	58%
· Intends to return	30	16%
· Maybe or doesn't know	49	26%
† *No longer injects or wishes to stop* (n=102)	63	62%

63/188 or 33.5% of those responding to this question no longer inject or wish to stop, a finding which can be explained by the choice of study sites (prison settings and a detox unit drop-in clinic).

COMPARISON OF SUBJECTS

Comparing prison subjects and detox clinic clients no significant differences were found for the variables median age, language, attended CACTUS at least once, and visited CACTUS only once.

Differences were found for the following variables:

	Prison subjects	Detox clinic clients	
· Women	45% (42/313)	30% (50/166)	p=.001 χ^2=10.5
· Exclusive cocaine users†	70% (190/270)	33% (47/142)	p<.0005 χ^2=19.2
· Heard about CACTUS through non-IDU source	116/224 (52%)	33/121 (27%)	p<.0005 χ^2=19.2
· Attended fewer than 16 times	58/119 (49%)	47/72 (65%)	p=.026 χ^2=5.0

† *6 months prior to incarceration versus past 7 days for detox*

SEROPREVALENCE RATES AMONG PRISON SUBJECTS

	Attenders	Non-Attenders	Total
· Men	20.5% (8/39)	4.8% (6/124)	8.6% (14/163)
· Women	11.6% (8/69)	11.5% (7/61)	11.5% (15/130)
· Total	14.8% (16/108)	7.0% (13/185)	10.0% (29/293)

All of the difference between attenders and non-attenders can be attributed to a striking difference between male attenders and male non-attenders, 20.5% versus 4.8%, p=.002. The apparent difference observed between men at 8.6% seropositive versus women at 11.5% seropositive was not statistically significant.

CONCLUSION

- Awareness (73%), utilization (55%), and satisfaction (47-98%) levels are high
- Main means of communication is by word of mouth from IDU to IDU
- Seroprevalence rates are unacceptably high
- Prison settings and clinical services for IDU are good sites to evaluate needle exchange programmes

Research supported by the National Health Research and Development Programme, Health and Welfare Canada

NEEDLE EXCHANGE AND BLEACH DISTRIBUTION PROGRAMS: THE AUSTRALIAN EXPERIENCE

ALEX WODAK, Alcohol and Drug Service, St. Vincent's Hospital, NSW, Australia

SUMMARY

There is a large and consistent body of HIV seroprevalence data from a variety of sources which indicates that HIV infection is still relatively uncommon (< 5 %) in Australian injecting drug users (IDUs). AIDS data are consistent with this. The epidemic thus appears to be well under control at present among IDUs. HIV infection is, however, prevalent among homosexual/bisexual males. Substantial overlap between these populations provides the preconditions for potential rapid spread of infection. National estimates of the number of IDUs range from 100,000 to 200,000.

The course of the HIV epidemic in Australia differs from that of many other western countries as an IDU component has not yet occurred. HIV infection now appears to be spreading slowly with the number of new cases of HIV infection nationally estimated to be about 600 per year.

AIDS was identified as a priority issue soon after the epidemic was first recognised. The role of prevention was given particular emphasis and there was no disagreement about the critical role of IDUs in the epidemic. It was accepted in the early 1980s that it would be necessary to implement a range of strategies including some sensitive measures to maintain control of HIV among IDUs in order to contain the epidemic in the general community. Consequently, prevention strategies relevant to IDUs were identified early, adopted with broad support and implemented vigorously. IDUs (and other high-risk groups) were involved in the identification and implementation of HIV prevention policies. Adoption of HIV prevention measures within prisons has however, been slow, difficult and incomplete. A national drug policy of minimisation of harm was declared in 1985 at a meeting of senior political leaders. This policy facilitated the adoption and later implementation of pragmatic HIV prevention strategies.

Sterile injecting equipment has been readily available in all major cities and large towns since 1988/1989 and in critical areas beginning in 1986. Drug store sales and needle and syringe exchange programmes (NSEPs) have played a major role in increasing the availability of injection equipment. Drug stores and NSEPs service different populations of IDUs. Several years were required for most needle and syringe exchange outlets to reach maximum throughput and begin to achieve efficiencies. Unit cost of exchange and distribution appears to be decreasing. After six years of NSEP, unintended negative consequences have been relatively minor and consisted of littering of public places with discarded equipment and two detected uses of NSEP facilities for drug dealing. Littering was quickly overcome by a series of measures including special collection arrangements, disposal bins and the marketing of specially developed plastic boxes ("Fitpack") which contain sterile equipment and a tamper resistant device for retaining used equipment. Approximately three to four million needles and syringes are distributed in Australia each year. Availability is still being expanded.

Explicit education campaigns directed to IDUs began in 1987. Expansion and improvement of drug treatment began in 1985. National methadone capacity increased more than six times between 1985 and 1993 and is now over 13,000. The national methadone guidelines have been revised and liberalised several times in recent years. Community bleach distribution programmes began in 1988. However, demand for bleach was never impressive. Decontamination practices with bleach were often deficient. Consequently, even if there was good evidence that bleach effectively destroyed HIV *in vitro*, there would be some doubt about the likelihood of this benefit being achieved *in vivo* because decontamination procedures are often deficient. Organisations of drug users began to be formed in 1985 but were established with government support in all jurisdictions by 1988. Research has played an important role in defining and evaluating strategies.

There is some evidence that high risk injecting practices are becoming less common in Australian IDUs. As in other countries, baseline levels of unsafe injecting practices were very high and unsafe sexual practices appear to have declined only slightly. HIV prevention policies are widely regarded in the community, among politicians and health policy makers as having successfully prevented spread of HIV among IDUs although rigorous proof of the effectiveness of strategies is unavailable, probably unobtainable and was wisely never regarded as a prerequisite for adoption and expansion of prevention programmes. HIV prevention policies for IDUs continues to have very strong community and political support. Community support for NSEP and methadone has been shown in a telephone poll to be 80-90%. Media coverage for AIDS and HIV prevention strategies for IDUs is (with very rare exceptions) understanding and supportive. Bleach programmes are still supported although their future appears somewhat uncertain following recent and accumulating evidence of lack of efficacy.

There is recent concern that the magnitude and consequences of IDU-related epidemics of other blood borne viruses including Hepatitis C (HCV) have been seriously underestimated. Continuing high incidence levels of HCV, especially among young IDUs, continuing high levels of risk behaviour and international spread of HIV among (and from) IDUs in an increasing number of countries suggest that complacency about the possibility of future spread of HIV related to IDU in Australia is unwarranted. There is some recent evidence that HIV spread in prisons has also been underestimated both in terms of documented seroconversions and public health impact. Evidence has emerged recently of an unofficial needle and syringe exchange programme successfully conducted for almost a year in several prisons in NSW.

The Australian experience with HIV prevention among IDUs has stimulated a more critical appraisal of prohibition. There is increasing support for the view that prohibition is expensive, ineffective, counter-productive and impairs the effectiveness of efforts to control the spread of HIV.

These conclusions may be of interest to other countries - especially those which share many similar characteristics such as the United States. However, the many major differences between Australia and the United States must also be borne in mind when attempting to extrapolate from the Australian experience to North America.

INTRODUCTION

HIV/AIDS presents a major challenge to the international community. There is much to be learnt from both positive and negative experiences of other countries. This paper describes the current state of the HIV epidemic among IDUs in Australia. The Australian response to the HIV epidemic has been deservedly praised. Favourable comments have been made by international experts as well as local, independent, public health practitioners. The aim of this paper is to present the Australian experience to an American audience to assist efforts to slow the spread of HIV infection among and from IDUs in the United States. Comparisons between the two countries have been drawn even if these may appear to be unflattering to the nation generously hosting this meeting. The temptation to echo anodyne and diplomatic platitudes has been resisted. It is hoped that critical comments will be accepted as being offered in good faith and in the interest of protecting public health.

There are at least two very important connections between Australia and the United States that are relevant to this paper. All of the earliest cases since the first case of AIDS was diagnosed in Australia in 1982 were homosexual/bisexual males who had lived for some time in the United States. Also, New York was the first city in the world to attribute a large proportion of AIDS cases to IDUs. From an Australian perspective, the response to this challenge seemed curiously minimal. The notion of "preventing another New York" occurring in an Australian city was often discussed when responses to the threat of an IDU related epidemic in Australia were being developed. Australia learnt from the negative US experience to the extent that Sydney has been included in a study of "prevented" HIV epidemics among IDUs together with Glasgow (Scotland), Lund (Sweden), and Tacoma (Washington State) (Des Jarlais, submitted for publication).

EPIDEMIOLOGY

HIV Infection

There is a large and consistent body of evidence which indicates that HIV infection is still relatively uncommon in Australian IDUs. These data include published and unpublished HIV seroprevalence surveys of IDUs. A recent review (Kaldor, 1993) of all published HIV seroprevalence surveys indicates that prevalences of less than 5% have been found consistently in female and heterosexual male IDUs although prevalences are far higher among homosexual/bisexual male IDUs. Seven studies published between 1985 and 1991 reported prevalences of HIV of 1%, 4%, 5%, 1%, 3%, 2% and 4% among IDUs after excluding homosexual/bisexual males (Kaldor, 1993).

These findings are supported by HIV test results of prison entrants in several jurisdictions which continue to be well under 1%. HIV seroprevalence among prison entrants in New South Wales was only 0.59% despite an AIDS incidence of 357.9 per million. In Victoria, HIV seroprevalence among prison entrants was 0.47%. It is generally assumed that more than 50% of prison inmates in Australia are serving time for drug-related offences and an even higher percentage are IDUs. Anecdotal information from testing laboratories is also consistent with a low prevalence of HIV infection among IDUs. A low prevalence of HIV infection has also been reported in a number of studies of prostitutes.

The number of new diagnoses of HIV infection nationally was estimated to be about 1,201 in the year to 31 March, 1992 and 1,031 in the year to 31 March, 1993 (National Centre in HIV Epidemiology and Clinical Research, 1993). Of cases with a documented known exposure category among the 17,068 new diagnoses of HIV infection cumulative to 31 March, 1993, 81.9% were attributed to male homosexual/bisexual contact, 2.8% to male homosexual/bisexual contact and IDU and 4.9% to IDU alone. It is estimated that there were only 600 new HIV infections nationally each year in the period 1989 - 90 (National Centre in HIV Epidemiology and Clinical Research, 1992). These trends are shown in Figure 1.

AIDS Data

A cumulative national total of 4,102 AIDS cases (including 4,073 persons over the age of thirteen) had been reported up to March 31, 1993 representing a case load of 23.6 per 100,000 (National Centre in HIV Epidemiology and Clinical Research, 1993). Of the cases in adults, 3,462 (84.4%) were homosexual/bisexual males, 128 (3.1%) were homosexual/bisexual male IDUs and only 78 (1.9%) were female or heterosexual male IDUs with an additional 405 (9.8%) consisting of heterosexuals, haemophiliacs, recipients of blood transfusions or blood products or undetermined. These data are consistent with seroprevalence data suggesting that HIV has not yet become established in heterosexual IDUs in Australia.

Comment

The low prevalence of HIV infection in IDUs in Australia allows multiple interpretations including late entry of HIV into the IDU population, limited pool of infection in other risk groups, limited overlap between risk groups, substantial spread remaining undetected and serendipity.

All of these possibilities can be effectively discounted except the last. HIV infection has been present in the heterosexual IDU population in Australia since at least 1985 when one of 200 Sydney IDUs in drug treatment, a heterosexual male from the United States (resident in Australia for about a decade), tested seropositive but several of his sexual and needle contacts were HIV infected (Blacker, 1986). The area most associated with drug use in Australia is in eastern Sydney and is also associated with a very large community of homosexual/bisexual males constituting the national epicentre of the HIV epidemic. The geographical overlap of these two populations makes the low prevalence of HIV among Australian IDUs all the more remarkable. The gay community in Sydney has long maintained close links with the gay community in San Francisco. Not surprisingly, HIV entered the gay population of Sydney relatively early.

A steep gradient of HIV infection has been observed in a study of 1,245 Sydney IDUs in 1989 (Ross, 1992, AIDS Care 139-48) with 3.2% of heterosexual male, 12.1% of homosexual/bisexual male and 35.4% of homosexual male IDUs infected with HIV suggesting that HIV entered the IDU population from homosexual/bisexual male IDUs. As 5.6% of male IDUs were homosexual and 13.1% were homosexual/bisexual (ANAIDUS, 1991), there was clearly considerable overlap with non-drug using homosexual populations.

The course of the HIV epidemic in Australia differs from that of many other western countries in that a significant IDU component has not yet occurred. The first case of AIDS was diagnosed in Australia in 1982. In the early 1980s, Australia had a high per capita incidence compared to other OECD countries. In 1983, Australia ranked fourth among developed countries in terms of AIDS cases per capita with 1.1 cases of AIDS per 100,000 population. By 1991, Australia had slipped to sixth place with 16.6 cases per 100,000 being overtaken by Spain (23.3) and Italy (17.2). Both Italy and Spain have experienced an explosive spread of HIV infection among IDUs who now represent over 60% of all AIDS cases in those countries. If Australia had still retained fourth highest ranking of AIDS cases per capita among developed countries, this would mean that instead of 4,073 cases of AIDS as of the March 31, 1993, 5,717 AIDS cases would have been expected. Of all known AIDS cases in Australia at present, 64% have died. There are therefore an estimated 1,052 Australians alive today because the epidemic appears to have run a different course in Australia than some other countries. The major difference has been the absence of an epidemic in IDUs. If the medical management of each AIDS case in Australia cost A$50,000, and a figure of A$100,000 is far more realistic, this represents a saving of 1,644 AIDS cases, 1,052 lives and A$53,000,000.

It is reasonable to conclude that HIV entered the Australian IDU population early, that substantial HIV infection is present in other risk groups, that there is substantial overlap between IDUs and other risk groups and that substantial undetected spread of HIV among IDUs can be discounted. Accordingly, the most parsimonious conclusion is that the course of the epidemic has been altered compared to other countries.

POLICY RESPONSE

AIDS was identified as a priority issue early in the epidemic. A National AIDS Task Force was established rapidly. A highly controversial national advertising campaign in 1987 on a "Grim Reaper" theme succeeded in its aim of raising awareness of AIDS as an issue. The Health Minister at the time described AIDS as "the greatest threat to public health in Australia since Federation" (i.e. 1901). The role of prevention was given particular emphasis and the need to maintain control of HIV among IDUs was well accepted (Wodak, 1992). Prevention strategies were identified early, adopted with broad support and implemented vigorously. IDUs (and other high-risk groups) were involved in the identification of prevention policies and their implementation. Parliamentary all-party AIDS committees were established at Federal and State levels with explicit agreement to refrain from party political conflict. A national drug policy of minimisation of harm had been declared in 1985 at a meeting of the Prime Minister and State Premiers and facilitated the adoption and implementation of sensitive HIV prevention strategies even though AIDS had not influenced consideration of the original drug policy. The Prime Minister's wife set a prominent example in the mid-1980s indicating that discrimination against persons with HIV infection was unacceptable.

The Prime Minister's wife also launched a "Never ever share needles" pamphlet in December, 1987. This campaign made no mention of abstinence from drug use. It was well known that one of her daughters had been an IDU and this endorsement of harm minimisation by such a prominent member of the community was a critical development in the nation's response to the impending threat of an epidemic. IDUs became aware of the hazards of needle sharing before HIV had gained a substantial foothold in this population.

In 1989, a National HIV/AIDS Strategy was agreed following lengthy consultation (Department of Community Services and Health, 1989). This document endorsed needle and syringe exchange and distribution programmes and resulted in policy and financial commitments covering a three year period. In 1991 it was noted that "programs for IDUs receive a larger share (37.4%) of total education and prevention funding ... than programs for any other target group. Funding grew substantially in all States and Territories from 1989-90 to 1990-91 with a 36% increase overall." (Inter Governmental Committee on AIDS, 1992)

Adoption of HIV prevention measures within prisons however, has been slow, difficult and incomplete. A communique covering strategies to prevent the spread of HIV in prisons was unanimously endorsed at a national conference in November 1990 (Douglas, 1991) but has had little effect.

NSEP PROGRAMMES

Development and Expansion

A vigorous and at times acrimonious debate about needle and syringe availability as a prevention strategy took place in 1985-6 with covert support for implementation coming from senior political and Health Department figures. A pilot (illegal) programme was established in Sydney in November, 1986. In December, 1986, the New South Wales Department of Health established a drug store based needle and syringe distribution scheme with NSEPs set up from 1987. All other jurisdictions (except one) rapidly established drug store schemes and NSEPs. The last jurisdiction to introduce needle and syringe exchange has permitted NSEPs to be established unofficially while waiting for some years for the appropriate legislation to be passed. Sterile injecting equipment has been readily available in all major cities and large towns in Australia since 1988/1989 (see Table 1). Providing NSEP services to rural IDU populations has often been difficult because of logistical problems and the more conservative nature of small towns.

Several years were required for most NSEPs to reach maximum through-put and begin to achieve efficiencies. For example, a NSEP in western Sydney recently increased its throughput more than ten times (from 3,000 to 40,000 units per month) over a two year period within a constant budget by building up a fixed outlet at the expense of a mobile unit. A survey in October, 1992 of 43 clients of this service found that 84% rated the service as excellent with the remaining 16 rating it as good (Duckett et al, 1993). The cost of distribution per unit declined from A$2.86 in 1991 to A$1.04 in 1992 and is expected to decline to A$0.96 in 1993/94. Similar trends are occurring elsewhere in the country. In some places, mobile units operate from cars with paging devices or portable telephones. This presents a difficult balance between the higher unit cost of providing mobile NSEPs and the need to service more vulnerable and less mobile populations. Mobile units were recently scrapped in one state as a cost cutting exercise.

It is difficult to estimate the quantity of injection equipment made available in Australia each year but it is likely that at least three to four million sterile needles and syringes are distributed or exchanged each year. In 1991, New South Wales (population 6.5 million) had 32 primary and 90 secondary outlets while Victoria had 102 outlets (Inter Governmental Committee on AIDS, 1992).

Unintended Negative Consequences

After six years of NSEP in Australia, there have been relatively few unintended negative consequences. Littering of public places with discarded used equipment was briefly an issue which threatened to jeopardise (then) fragile public support. This problem was overcome by a series of measures including specialised collection of used equipment, special disposal bins and the marketing of specially developed plastic boxes ("Fitpack") which contain sterile equipment and a tamper resistant device for retaining used equipment. The Fitpack was designed with the assistance of members of a government funded drug users organisation. Staff of NSEPs have been detected using these facilities to also distribute illicit drugs on two occasions. In one state, a NSEP was operated by a government funded organisation of drug users. Following allegations of embezzlement, the operation was handed over to a government agency (with subsequent decline in throughput). A study of urine analysis specimens obtained from two methadone units, one of which was immediately adjacent to a pilot NSEP, concluded that sterile needle and syringe availability did not appear to increase the frequency of drug use in patients of methadone programmes (Wolk, 1990).

The mean frequency that sterile needles and syringes where used by IDUs (n=2,451) when injecting drugs ranged in four cities in 1989 from 69.1% to 79.6% with the overall mean for respondents being 72.6% (ANAIDUS, 1991). Respondents were also asked "how easy do you think it is to obtain new (sterile) needles and syringes at the present time?" with answer options being that it was easy 0-25%, 26-50%, 51-75%, 76-98% or 99-100% of the time. The mean percentage of the time respondents in three cities in 1989 reported finding it easy to obtain new injecting equipment ranged from 72.0 to 84.3%.

The Queensland government introduced exchange and distribution schemes after the other states and thus availability in Brisbane lagged behind other cities in the study. Male respondents found it significantly easier to obtain equipment than female respondents (77.2 +/- 26.8; 73.5+/- 26.9; $p<0.01$) (ANAIDUS, 1991).

The importance of drug stores as outlets was emphasised in responses to the question "where do you get your new needles and syringes?" Drug stores, NSEPs and after hours drug stores were the most important sources (see Table 2).

The mean number of needles and syringes obtained in the most typical using month (n=2,422) in 1989 was 54.2 +/- 91.6. The most important time to obtain equipment was mid-afternoon to midnight with the period 9 pm to midnight being especially important (ANAIDUS, 1991). When asked to indicate how needles and syringes could be made more available, a range of responses was obtained but more drug stores selling needles and syringes, vending machines and special needle and syringe exchanges were the most common answers received (ANAIDUS, 1991).

Availability of injection equipment had further improved in two of the cities twelve months after the original data collection (ANAIDUS, 1992) with the mean number of respondents reporting that it was easy to obtain new equipment in Sydney increasing from 84.3 to 93.0% (see Table 3). Drug stores were still the major source of new equipment but NSEPs were nominated as a more important source than twelve months earlier.

Needle and syringe exchange schemes have broadened the scope of their activities without diminishing the enthusiasm of their staff. They now often prefer to be known as HIV prevention units and in some areas have become involved in AIDS coordination and HIV prevention advocacy. Vending machines have been introduced in small numbers but are still undergoing evaluation. Their introduction took much longer than anticipated. Vending machines are unlikely to ever replace NSEPs but are being used to provide an affordable 24 hour service in areas with a particularly high incidence of drug use.

IDUs who usually attended NSEPs or drug stores to obtain sterile injecting equipment were compared (Wodak, submitted for publication). Discriminant function analysis correctly allocated 75% of respondents. Those whose usual source of supply was NSEPs obtained more than twice as many needles and syringes per month, injected alone less frequently, were more likely to reside in the inner city than outer suburbs, injected with new needles and syringes more frequently than those whose usual source was drug stores, and were less likely to be in drug treatment. NSEP attenders reported that they found it more easy to obtain injection equipment a significantly greater percentage of the time, were younger, less likely to inject with a needle and syringe used by someone else, and spent more money on drugs per week than respondents whose usual source of supply was drug stores. Almost twice as many drug store as NSEP attenders were employed (although unemployment was common in both groups). NSEPs attracted a greater proportion of women. These data suggest that some IDUs were deterred from obtaining injection equipment from drug stores by modest prices, while others in drug treatment prefer to obtain their equipment from the (presumably) more anonymous setting of a drug store. Different kinds of IDUs appear to utilise different kinds of needle and syringe outlets

Legal impediments to HIV prevention have recently been comprehensively reviewed including obstacles to NSEP operation (Inter Governmental Committee on AIDS, 1992). The Legal Working Party made recommendations covering repeal of self administration and other offences, the need for more non-custodial sentencing options and supported further research including the investigation of drug policy reform.

NON NSEP PROGRAMMES

During the 1980s, considerable efforts were made to develop effective policies and review progress. In more recent years, the attitude that the epidemic of HIV among Australian IDUs has been prevented has become commonplace and is often accompanied by a sense of complacency.

Explicit education campaigns directed to IDUs began in 1987. A number of education campaigns have been conducted including mass campaigns which may have also contributed to the broad support existing for HIV prevention activities. Homosexual and homosexual/bisexual male IDUs have been specifically targeted in education campaigns. Social marketing approaches have been used to raise and maintain a high level of awareness about HIV/AIDS in sub-populations of IDUs. A low level campaign targeting homosexual male IDUs has been running in NSW for some years using the slogan "FIT FOR A QUEEN. NEW OR CLEAN."

Expansion and improvement of drug treatment began in 1985 with national methadone capacity increasing in the last eight years more than six times. The most rapid expansion of methadone capacity has occurred in NSW (Gaughwin, 1993) which has 34% of the national population and almost 60% of the nation's AIDS cases. The national methadone guidelines have been revised a number of times in recent years in an effort to liberalise programmes to increase their attractiveness, improve retention rates, reduce costs and assist national efforts to contain HIV infection in IDUs. The unit cost of providing methadone programmes has been falling in real terms and is now about A$1,200 per person per year. Other modalities of drug treatment have also been expanded and improved. AIDS research is regarded as a priority area and is still funded separately.

Organisations of IDUs have been established in all jurisdictions with government support and funding. The Australian Prostitutes' collective was established in 1985.

IDU representatives are invited to actively participate in policy development and implementation.

National efforts were made to increase bleach availability and utilisation. Many NSEPs had difficult distributing bleach to IDUs as sterile injection equipment was so available there was little interest in obtaining alternatives. Since the biological effectiveness of bleach as a decontamination agent began to be questioned publicly in the US in 1993 (National Institute on Drug Abuse. Community Alert Bulletin, March 1993), the wisdom of advocating bleach decontamination has been reviewed. Decontamination practices of IDUs in Australia fall far short of acceptable and are a further reason for reviewing exhortations to IDUs to use bleach.

EVALUATION

There is some evidence that high risk injecting practices are becoming less common but as in other counties, baseline levels of unsafe injecting practices were very high and unsafe sexual practices appear to have declined only slightly. HIV prevention policies are widely regarded as having successfully prevented the spread of HIV among IDUs although rigorous scientific proof of their effectiveness is unavailable, probably unobtainable and was wisely not regarded as a prerequisite for adoption and expansion of prevention programmes. HIV prevention policies for IDUs continue to have very strong community and political support.

In 1989, one sixth of a Sydney sample (17%) were at low risk of HIV infection as they had never shared injection equipment, cleaned injecting equipment effectively 100% of the time it was shared, and were celibate, monogamous, or had not had unsafe sex in the past six months (Wodak, in press). Half (51%) had either unsafe injecting or sexual behaviour, with the remaining third (33%) engaging in both unsafe injecting and sexual practices. Comparison of two large and consecutive (1989 and 1990) samples of Sydney IDUs recruited in non-treatment settings were consistent with major risk reduction (Ross, in press) (see Table 4).

These data are drawn from two cross-sectional samples and therefore the possibility that the differences observed were due to sampling cannot be discounted. Nevertheless, the strength and consistency of the behavioural differences, the similarities in demographic characteristics and drug use of the two samples, and the similarity of findings in comparable studies in other countries suggest that these behavioural differences are real. They are all the more remarkable when it is considered that the two samples were recruited less than twelve months apart.

Attributing benefit to any single intervention is impossible when multiple strategies have been implemented at about the same time, the intensity of implementation is difficult if not impossible to measure, and the effect of interventions is in all likelihood synergistic. In a categorical sense, these methodological problems can not be resolved without a controlled trial of communities randomly allocated to a single intervention or no intervention. The ethical, logistic, financial and public health problems of attempting such a study are such (Des Jarlais, 1993) that there is no alternative, especially given the urgency of the epidemic, to making a judgement on the grounds of plausibility, feasibility, cost and international experience. At issue is whether authorities in a particular country prefer to be roughly right or precisely wrong. Australian authorities, perhaps reflecting a characteristically pragmatic and non-ideological national approach, preferred the former option. So too did most other developed countries.

LOOMING PROBLEMS

Hepatitis C and Other Blood Borne Viruses

Continuing high levels of unsafe injecting practices and international spread of the HIV epidemic within and to an increasing number of countries suggest that complacency about the possibility of future spread of HIV among (and from) Australian IDUs is unwarranted. There is increasing concern in Australia that the magnitude of the Hepatitis C (HCV) epidemic and its consequences has been seriously underestimated.

High incidence levels of HCV in Australian IDUs, especially young IDUs, evidence of annual incidence rates for Hepatitis B and C of between 10 and 20 % in Victorian inmates with more than one occasion of prison entry (Crofts, 1993a), and recent estimates that there are five times more people in Australia infected with HCV than HIV and at least a fifteen times higher incidence of HCV than HIV (Crofts, 1993b) may lead to a reassessment of the public health threat of IDU-related blood borne viruses. Evidence of continuing high incidence levels of Hepatitis B and C among IDUs in Australia also indicates the potential for spread of other blood borne viruses including HIV.

Although the morbidity and mortality associated with HIV exceeds that of HCV, the much larger pool size and higher incidence of HCV in Australia suggests that far greater attention needs to be directed in the future to the containment of blood borne viruses in addition to HIV. It is estimated that at least 20% of HCV infected individuals will develop cirrhosis within 5-10 years with up to 5% developing a hepatocellular carcinoma.

Prisons

There is some evidence that HIV spread in prisons has been underestimated in terms of documented seroconversions. The relatively short mean duration of imprisonment in relation to the "window period" for seroconversion suggests that entry-exit testing of HIV infection underestimates the extent of the problem. A network of IDUs who became infected with HIV while in prison is currently being investigated with at least one of these cases being virtually certain (K. Dolan, personal communication). There are about a dozen published cases of HIV infection in prison world-wide but none of these cases can be regarded as definite.

IDUs enter correctional facilities from diverse geographic and social backgrounds. They usually remain within correctional facilities for relatively brief periods during which time they are often moved frequently mixing with many other prisoners. In contrast, unsafe injecting practices among IDUs in the community are increasingly restricted to small social networks. HIV infection within such a network has far less public health impact than infection of a prison inmate with the potential for wide dissemination of HIV within correctional facilities and subsequently following release.

Unsafe injecting practices in prison are less frequent than in the community but may be more hazardous for several reasons. Injecting equipment is less available in prison and is therefore likely to be shared between a larger number of partners. Bleach is also less available inside prison. Drug injecting and equipment decontamination is also likely to be more furtive with less opportunity to carefully decontaminate injecting equipment.

Evidence of an unofficial needle and syringe exchange programme successfully conducted for almost a year in several prisons in NSW has emerged recently and has been presented to a committee of inquiry. This unofficial strictly "one for one" trial involved over 100 prisoners and was conducted by an HIV infected prisoner with covert assistance of some health professionals and possibly with the knowledge of some correctional staff. The existence of a prison NSEP lasting almost twelve months raises the possibility of considering this intervention more widely at a time when the effectiveness of current decontamination strategies relying on bleach have been called into question.

In 1990, an HIV infected prisoner stabbed a NSW prison officer with a syringe filled with the inmate's blood. The prison officer seroconverted over the next months becoming the first documented case of occupational exposure of a prison warder. It is anticipated that recommendations to consider a pilot NSEP in an Australian prison will therefore meet much resistance and accordingly should not be supported at the risk of endangering more likely interventions.

PROHIBITION UNDER INCREASING SCRUTINY

The Australian experience with HIV prevention among IDUs has stimulated a more critical appraisal of prohibition. There has been increasing support for the view that prohibition is expensive, ineffective, counter-productive and impairs the effectiveness of efforts to control the spread of HIV. The number of influential members of the community calling for a review of drug policy in recent years has been steadily growing. The Australian Parliamentary Group for Drug Law Reform was established in 1993 and includes representatives of the major parties with members drawn from Commonwealth, State and local levels of government.

A debate about the fundamental nature of drug policy has been slowly intensifying with fundamental reform strongly supported by many leaders of the medical and legal professions and most doctors involved in delivering HIV prevention or treatment services. The National Centre for Epidemiology and Population Health, Canberra, is investigating the possibility of a trial of controlled availability of currently illicit drugs and was awarded a grant of A$0.5 million by the Australian National University to further this work. This trial followed from a recommendation made by an Australian Capital Territory Legislative Assembly official enquiry into HIV, illicit drugs and prostitution.

Whether a debate about drug policy reform would have developed in the absence of adoption of needle and syringe exchange programmes is arguable. However, the fact that liberalisation of availability of injection equipment has been so beneficial and virtually unaccompanied by unintended negative consequences has certainly drawn attention to the lack of evidence of effectiveness, high costs and major adverse consequences associated with prohibition.

Prohibition is seen by some to keep street drug prices high and purity of street drugs low and thus reduce the possibility of IDUs making a transition to non-parenteral modes of administration. Prohibition also delayed the adoption and slowed expansion of NSEPs and also impeded the implementation of many other programmes needed to control the HIV epidemic.

RELEVANCE TO OTHER COUNTRIES

These conclusions may be of interest to other countries especially those which share many similar characteristics such as the United States. However, the many major differences between Australia and the United States must also be borne in mind.

The United States and Australia were both colonised by Great Britain. When the United States declared independence, Great Britain lost a favoured storage site for surplus prisoners. The search for a new gulag lead to the establishment of a colony in Australia. The two countries have similar political systems and the curses and blessings of a federal system of government. The Australian political system is sometimes referred to as Washminster reflecting the debt to both Westminster and Washington. The United States and Australia have been parliamentary democracies without interruption. English is the main language spoken in both countries. The area of the continental United States is only fractionally larger then Australia. Both countries have populations drawn from diverse cultures. US drug policies have been a dominant influence on Australia drug policies since soon after the turn of the century. In both countries, the drug policy is essentially prohibition although this takes a kinder and gentler form in Australia.

However there are many differences between Australia and the United States. Australia only has about 6% of the population of the United States. Like most other western countries, Australia has a universal health care system. A policy of harm minimization for illicit drugs has been adopted at the highest political level in Australia. This policy states that the aim "is to minimize the harmful affects of drugs on Australian society". In contrast, US drug policies has been dominated (explicitly) by attempts to reduce drug use. Although poverty and severe social disadvantage exist in both countries, Australia has never had a large urban under-class as is seen in a number of major US cities. Furthermore, policy makers and injecting drug users in Australia come from the same racial group and speak the same language. Moreover, injecting drug users and policy makers in Australia are in contact with one another. In recent years, some injecting drug users have been employed on Government projects *because* they were currently injecting drug users.

Social policies are markedly different in Australia and the United States. In Australia, abortion is readily available and ceased to be an issue several decades ago. Capital punishment was last carried out decades ago. In 1992, it was decided that sexual orientation of male and female military recruits would no longer be taken into account (despite strenuous opposition of the military). All Australian jurisdictions have laws restricting the availability of guns which are much stricter than in the United States. Crime rates and rates of imprisonment are much lower in Australia than the United States.

In most western countries including Australia, the questions policy makers ask about the availability of sterile injection equipment for injecting drug users is not whether this is a legitimate strategy to prevent the spread of HIV infection or even whether this policy contributes to improved control of the epidemic. Improving the availability of sterile injection equipment is assumed to make a most important contribution to the control of the epidemic even in the absence of categorical proof. In Australia, the standard of proof required for evaluating the contribution of needle and syringe exchange programmes to improve control of the epidemic was commensurate with the speed of spread of the epidemic and the magnitude of the consequences of an uncontrolled epidemic.

The critical question for policy makers in Australia regarding needle and exchange is how needle and syringe availability can be implemented more effectively and at lower cost. There is a strong desire to focus on improving availability particularly for groups of major public health importance such as homosexual/bisexual male injecting drug users. After seven years of needle and syringe availability, political, bureaucratic and community support is still overwhelming.

REFERENCES

Australian National AIDS and Injecting Drug Use Study (1992). Not in a Fit. Third Report of the Australian National AIDS and Injecting Drug Use Study (ANAIDUS), 1990 Data collection. Sydney.

Australian National AIDS and Injecting Drug Use Study (ANAIDUS) (1991) Neither a borrower nor a lender be. First Report of the Australian National AIDS and Injecting Drug Use Study (ANAIDUS), 1989 Data collection. Sydney.

Blacker P, Tindall B, Wodak AD, and Cooper D. (1986) Exposure of Intravenous Drug Users to AIDS Retro Virus Sydney, 1985. *Aust and N. Z. Med J*: 686-690.

Crofts N, Hearne P, Stewart T, Breschkin AM, Locanini SA. (1993a). HCV Among Prison Entrants in Victoria. Abstract. National Symposium on Hepatitis C. St. Vincent's Hospital. Melbourne. October 8th.

Crofts N, Wodak A. (1993b). Prevalence, carriage and incidence of HCV among IDUs in Australia. Abstract. National Symposium on Hepatitis C. St. Vincent's Hospital.

Melbourne. October 8th.
Department of Community Services and Health, National HIV/AIDS Strategy. (1989) A policy information paper. Australian Government Publishing Service. Canberra.
Des Jarlais DC, Friedman SR. (1993) Research. Dimensions of HIV prevention: Needle Exchange. (eds) J. Stryker, MD Smith. pp 63-75.
Des Jarlais, DC, Hagan H, Friedman SR, Friedman P, Goldberg D, Frischer M, Green S, Tunving K, Ljunberg B, Wodak A, Ross M, Purchase D, Millson ME, Myers T. Maintaining low HIV seroprevalence in populations of injecting drug users. (submitted for publication)
Dolan, K, Hall W, Wodak A, Gaughwin M. (1994) (letter) Evidence of HIV transmission in an Australian prison. *Med J. Aust 160*: 734.
Douglas R. (1991) AIDS in Australian Prisons. What are the challenges? in "HIV/AIDS and Prisons". (eds) J. Norberry, M. Gaughwin, S-A. Gerull. Australian Institute of Criminology. Canberra. pp 23-30.
Duckett M, Moore T, Ramsay J, Wodak A. (1993) Review of Western Sydney HIV/AIDS prevention and Outreach Service. May, 1993.
Gaughwin M, Kliewer E, Ali R, Faulkner C, Wodak A, Anderson G. (1993) The prescription of methadone for opiate dependence in Australia, 1985-1991. *Med J Aust 159*: 107-108.
Inter Governmental Committee on AIDS. (1992) The final report of the legal working party of the Inter Governmental Committee on AIDS. Australian Government Publishing Service. Canberra.
Kaldor J, Elford J, Wodak A, Crofts JN, Kidd S. (1993) HIV prevalence among IDUs in Australia: a methodological review. *Drug and Alcohol Review. 12*: 175-184.
National Centre in HIV Epidemiology and Clinical Research, Australian HIV Surveillance Report. Volume 9, Number 3. July 1993
National Centre in HIV Epidemiology and Clinical Research. National Working Group on HIV projections; Estimates and Projections of the HIV Epidemic in Australia, 1981 - 1994. Internal Technical Report 1 April 1992.
National Institute on Drug Abuse. (1993) Community Alert Bulletin, March.
Inter Governmental Committee on AIDS. Report on HIV/AIDS in Australia 1990-91. (1992) Australian Government Publishing Service. Canberra.
Ross MW, Stowe A, Wodak A, Gold J. (1993) Changes in equipment sharing in injecting drug users in Sydney 1989-1990. *Drug and Alcohol Review 12*: 277-281.
Wodak A, Stowe A, Dolan K, Ross MW, Gold J. (1993) Comparison of characteristics and HIV risk behaviours of injecting drug users attending needle and syringe exchange programs and pharmacies. Submitted for publication.
Wodak A, Stowe A, Ross MW, Gold J, Miller ME. (in press) Extent of HIV risk exposure of injecting drug users in Sydney. *Drug and Alcohol Review.*
Wodak A. (1992) HIV infection and injecting drug use in Australia: responding to a crisis. *Journal of Drug Issues 22 (3)*: 547-560.
Wolk J, Wodak A, Guinan J, Macaskill P, Simpson JM. (1990) The Effect of a Needle and Syringe Exchange on a Methadone Maintenance Unit. *Brit J Addict 85*: 1445-1450.

TABLE 1

Percentage New Needles and Syringes Were Easily Obtained in Four Cities, 1989 (ANAIDUS, 1991)

	Median	Mean	SDD	n
Sydney	95.0	84.3	20.7	1,225
Brisbane	50.0	58.6	27.6	582
Perth	90.0	83.4	20.0	194
Melbourne	75.0	72.0	24.4	349

TABLE 2

Usual Source of New Needles and Syringes

(n=2,422)(ANAIDUS, 1991)

	Source (%)	Response (%)
Drug store	47.9	70.9
Needle exchange	22.0	32.6
After hours drug store	14.3	21.2
Using friends	9.21	3.6
Non-using friends	1.2	1.8
Hospitals	1.2	1.8
Dealers	1.1	1.6
Doctors	0.9	1.4
Veterinary surgeons	0.5	0.8
Other	1.7	2.5

TABLE 3

Percentage New Needles and Syringes Were Easily Obtained in Two Cities, 1990 (ANAIDUS, 1992)

	Median	Mean	SDD	n
Sydney	99.0	93.0	14.3	544
Perth	90.0	85.5	17.1	148

TABLE 4

Differences in Risk Behaviour
(Ross, 1993)

Variable	**1989**	**1990**
n	1,245	550
# of times N & S used	2.9 +/- 3.1	1.9 +/- 2.3**
% time use new N & S 73.5 +/- 26.284.8 +/ 21.8**		
% of times easy to get new N & S	84.3 +/- 20.7	93.0 +/- 14.3**
% of times N & S used after someone else	19.0 +/- 25.8	9.7 +/- 18.5**
# of people accepted used N & S from in last 6 months	1.8 +/- 6.6	0.9 +/- 3.9*
# of people who use a N & S before being discarded	2.0 +/- 4.2	1.2 +/- 1.1**
share because withdrawal, intox.	5.1 +/- 1.7	6.0 +/- 1.6**
share because N & S unavailable	0.3 +/- 0.6	0.1 +/- 0.4**
share because risk low	0.5 +/- 0.7	0.2 +/- 0.5**
% new N & S from drug store	65.8	47.6**
% new N & S from after hours drug store	19.7	10.8**
% new N & S from NSEP	34.8	57.5**
% new N & S from IDU	9.9	11.9
	* $p < 0.01$	** $p < 0.001$

Figure 1: Estimated incidence of HIV infection in Australia, 1981 - 1990 for selected back-projection model

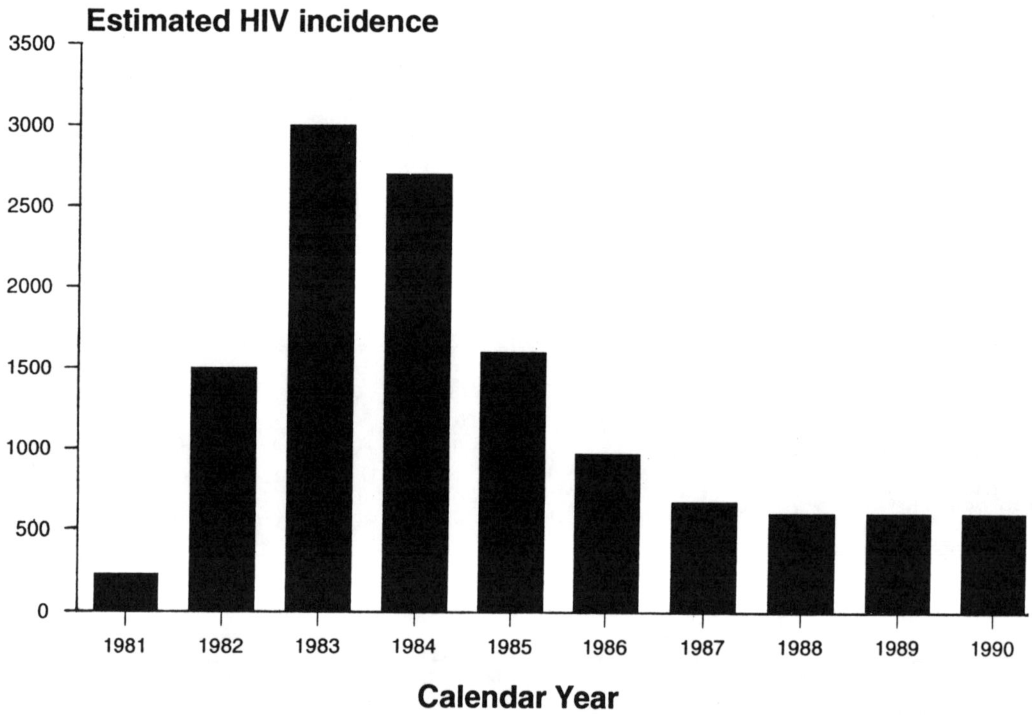

Source: National Centre in HIV Epidemiology and Clinical Research. National Working Group on HIV Projections: Estimates and Projections of the HIV Epidemic in Australia, 1981 - 1994. Internal Technical Report 1, April 1992, Figure 3, p. 26.

DISCUSSION: INTERNATIONAL EVALUATIONS OF NEEDLE EXCHANGE PROGRAMS

PETER SELWYN

Peter Selwyn noted that a large number of studies from the United States and many other countries throughout the world have provided generally consistent data about needle exchange programs. Nevertheless, underlying social and political dynamics in the United States seem to be requiring a standard of scientific proof for such programs that is much higher than that usually required of other preventive, or even clinical, interventions. The more important underlying dynamic appears to be the social context for policy concerning drug injection and related preventive interventions. The tendency to respond to drug injection within a criminal justice as opposed to a medical public health context inhibits responses that are truly preventive and educes instead responses that are more proscriptive and punitive. Thus, he observed, there is the irony that the United States, which is both heavily affected by injection drug use and by the AIDS epidemic, has served as an alarming negative example to other countries around the world. Other countries have gone on to develop comprehensive AIDS prevention programs targeted on drug users; in the United States, however, similar steps have not been taken in any systematic way, notwithstanding the many important steps undertaken in selected individual cities and communities.

He commented that it may be helpful to separate the issues that surround needle exchanges into three categories: (1) the data that exist, (2) the limitations of the data, and (3) the political, cultural, and often emotional issues that underlie the data. As for the data that exist, he said, it is clear that virtually all of the research that has looked at outcomes of needle exchange programs around the world points in the same direction--that is, toward no evidence of significantly increased use of drugs, initiation of drug use, or drug injection at an earlier age. There is also evidence of reductions in needle sharing among participants in needle exchange programs and lower or stable HIV seroprevalence. The importance of increased access to drug treatment and other medical interventions for active injectors is also a consistent finding.

Selwyn noted the methodological limitations of the data that have already been discussed--sampling frames, nonrandomized designs, inability to separate needle exchange effects from other program effects and secular changes over times, validity of self-report data, and so on. An important point that bears repeating is that use of HIV seroconversion as an outcome measure may not be feasible or even relevant to the evaluation of needle exchanges. In most of the studies that were presented, needle exchanges were being introduced into populations that were either already heavily saturated with HIV infection or still at a very low level of seroprevalence. Thus, statistically demonstrating a reduction in seroconversion would have been a priori difficult, just from the standpoint of sample size. Another important limitation is the inability to separate easily the effects of other behavioral factors, such as sexual risk behavior, from the effects of needle exchanges. Finally, not so much from a data standpoint, but perhaps more conceptually, there is the difficulty of proving that something did not happen. As the presentation on Australia's experience made clear, one cannot say that something would have happened otherwise had it not been for the programs that were implemented.

Turning to the underlying political and cultural framework, he noted, the social acceptability of a behavior, in general, lends itself proportionately to preventive, as opposed to punitive or proscriptive, approaches to that behavior. Thus, there has been less reluctance in the United States to introduce behavioral interventions aimed at reducing heterosexual transmission of HIV than transmission among homosexuals or bisexuals and injecting drug users.

In conclusion, Selwyn observed, based on the existing data and leaving aside the policy and underlying social dimensions for the moment, needle exchange programs do not make things any worse and there are some data--e.g., from Kaplan in New Haven--that they may make things better. They do not cause people to use drugs, they seem in many instances to promote positive behavioral change, they definitely help provide access to vulnerable and sometimes otherwise inaccessible populations, and they may reduce the risk of transmission of HIV. But, as all of the preceding presenters noted, needle exchange programs should not be looked at as a single or simple solution. The data from Amsterdam that were presented are an interesting reflection of this point. The fact that cocaine use, alcohol use, and homelessness were the factors that predicted HIV seroconversion, even among people who used the needle exchange, suggests that it is not simply a matter of handing out clean needles. The behavioral and social factors underlying drug use must also be addressed.

LEGAL ISSUES

AND DRUG PARAPHERNALIA

LAW AND POLICY

LAWRENCE GOSTIN, American Society of Law, Medicine, and Ethics, Boston, Massachusetts; and Georgetown University Law Center, Washington, D.C.*

Few issues at the intersection of law, policy, and public health are as fraught with conflict as the distribution of sterile injection equipment to impede the spread of infection with the human immunodeficiency virus (HIV) among intravenous drug users. At the heart of the controversy is a fundamental conflict between deeply entrenched drug-control policies and newly emerging public health policies.

Drug control policies are driven by the belief that if the supply of drugs and drug paraphernalia is aggressively cut off and if growers/manufacturers, sellers, and users are swiftly and severely punished, the result will be a reduction in drug abuse and the cycle of related violence.[1] The essence of drug control policy, therefore, is to create a scarcity of drugs and drug injection equipment, and to punish users.

The public health approach is markedly different from--and perhaps incompatible with--traditional drug control. Rather than creating a scarcity of sterile drug injection equipment, the public health approach makes it more readily available through bleach and syringe distribution programs. Rather than punishing users through the criminal justice system, the public health approach offers an array of educational and therapeutic interventions within the health system.[2]

Many people in government, criminal justice, and community groups believe that the public health approach cannot peacefully coexist with traditional drug control policies.[3] They think needle and bleach distribution programs deliver a mixed message that results in greater drug use. In their view, the drug control policy of "zero tolerance" is undermined when the state is asked to repeal, relax, or not enforce laws prohibiting distribution or possession of drug paraphernalia.

Public health officials, on the other hand, point to mounting evidence that bleach and needle distribution programs do not encourage people to begin or continue drug use, that such programs facilitate entry into drug treatment, and that the programs reduce transmission of HIV and other needle-borne infections.[4,5]

This paper, which is based on a continuing series of essays,[6,7,8,9] seeks to demonstrate the importance of a public health approach to controlling the dual epidemics of drug dependency and the acquired immune deficiency syndrome (AIDS) in the United States. It describes the body of law that prohibits the distribution or possession of drug paraphernalia, and proposes reforms that are consistent with the public health approach. The paper then examines prevailing legislative and litigation strategies to promote that approach.

---

* This paper was published in J. Stryker and M. D. Smith, eds., Needle Exchange. Menlo Park, Calif.: The Henry J. Kaiser Foundation, 1993. Reprinted by permission.

The public health approach does not require legalization of drugs, and this paper does not support such a proposal. Regardless of whether society ultimately decides to relax or repeal criminal prohibitions on drug use, the morbidity and mortality associated with the drug and AIDS epidemics will continue to require carefully crafted, public-health policies supported by adequate funding. Only those criminal prohibitions that impede public health efforts need to be reformed. If drug-control and public-health approaches are properly conceived, they can exist in harmony, and even synergy.

DRUG CONTROL POLICIES THAT LIMIT THE SUPPLY OF STERILE INJECTION EQUIPMENT

Researchers have identified powerful social and cultural forces that create an environment for the sharing of drug injection equipment. However, such sharing is not merely a learned response or a function of the culture and routines of drug users. It also is the direct result of a limited supply of needles and syringes, which can deny drug users realistic opportunities to engage in safer behavior.[10,11] Most drug users report that the scarcity of injection equipment is an important reason for sharing. Rather than obtaining sterile syringes and needles from pharmacists, health care professionals, or public health departments, they get their injection equipment from street sellers and shooting galleries.[12,13,14,15,16,17]

The limited supply of sterile injection equipment represents, in part, a conscious policy choice by the state. As long ago as 1921, the U.S. Supreme Court recognized the broad authority of the state to regulate the manufacture, sale, prescription, and use of dangerous drugs by exercising its police powers [Minnesota ex rel., *Whipple v. Martinson*, 256 U.S. 41 (1921)]. Later, the court made clear that the "range of valid choices which a state might make in this area is undoubtedly a wide one...." [*Robinson v. California*, 370 U.S. 660, 665 (1962)]. Pursuant to these broad powers, the states have long had a policy of limiting the supply of equipment needed for injecting illicit drugs. While the state cannot constitutionally penalize a person's drug-dependent status [*Robinson v. California*, 370 U.S. 660 (1962)], it undoubtedly has constitutional authority to control the instruments of drug use, even if the person has no control over his or her habit [*Powell v. Texas*, 392 U.S. 514, 532 (1968)].

Broadly speaking, two categories of legislation directly affect the supply of sterile drug injection equipment: drug paraphernalia laws and needle prescription laws.

Drug Paraphernalia Laws

At least forty-five states and the District of Columbia have drug paraphernalia laws. Most of these statutes are based on the Model Drug Paraphernalia Act formulated by the Drug Enforcement Administration in 1979. The act was designed as an amendment to the Uniform Controlled Substances Act.

The term "drug paraphernalia" is widely defined in these statues to include any equipment, product, or material of any kind that is primarily intended for use in introducing controlled substances into the human body. Clearly, hypodermic syringes and needles fall within this domain. Drug paraphernalia statues ban the manufacture, sale, distribution, or possession of a wide range of devices if the person knows that such devices may be used to introduce illicit substances into the body.

Therefore, drug paraphernalia laws require the presence of criminal intent to supply or use the equipment for an unlawful purpose. Under these statutes, it is not illegal to sell or distribute hypodermic needles and syringes when there is no knowledge that they will be used to inject illicit drugs. A pharmacist who sells hypodermic syringes and needles over the counter believing they will be used for a lawful purpose--for example, by a diabetic to inject insulin--does not commit an offense under drug paraphernalia laws.

The trend toward comprehensive drug paraphernalia laws was advanced by the U.S. Supreme Court's decision in *Village of Hoffman Estates v. Flipside, Hoffman Estates Inc.* [455 U.S. 489, rehearing den, 456 U.S. 950 (1982)]. The court held that broadly worded local laws not based on the Model Act were constitutionally valid. Many courts have followed *Flipside* and upheld statutes with broad definitions of drug paraphernalia [*Camile Corp. v. Phares*, 705 F.2d 223 (7th Cir. 1983); *Garner v. White*, 726 F.2d 1274 (8th Cir. 1984); *Stoianoff v. Montana*, 695 F.2d 1214 (9th Cir. 1983)].

In July 1984, the federal government further limited the supply of sterile injection equipment by enacting an umbrella statute to encompass any activity involving drug paraphernalia crossing interstate lines. The Mail Order Drug paraphernalia Control Act [Anti-Drug Abuse Act of 1986, ss. 1821-1823, PL 99-570, 21 U.S.C. 863 (Use of Postal Service for Sale of Drug Paraphernalia)] originally was designed to prohibit use of the U.S. Postal Service to send equipment to be used for drug injection [Cong. Rec. H6655-56 (daily ed. September 11, 1986)]. The plain language of the statute also covers "any offer for sale and transportation in interstate or foreign commerce," or import or export of drug paraphernalia [21 U.S.C. 857(a)]. Furthermore, it contains a similarly broad definition of drug paraphernalia [21 U.S.C. 857(d); the act also authorizes seizure and forfeiture of drug paraphernalia; 21 U.S.C. 857(c)], and has survived constitutional scrutiny [*United States v. Main Street Distributing Inc.*, 700 F. Supp. 655 (E.D.N.Y. 1988)]. The importance of the federal statute is its introduction of federal jurisdiction in an area traditionally reserved for the states.[18]

There is wide discretion in enforcement and prosecution under federal and state statutes. A state that chooses not to repeal its drug paraphernalia law could decide not to enforce it based on the public health imperatives of the HIV epidemic. If a state did this, federal authorities conceivably would take a different view and rigorously enforce the Mail Order Drug Paraphernalia Control Act. This means that the objectives of law-enforcement and public-health authorities, as well as those of federal and state agencies, must be harmonized.

Drug paraphernalia laws, including the federal Mail Order Drug Paraphernalia Control Act and comprehensive state statutes, present formidable obstacles for the injection drug user who complies with public health advice to use sterile injection equipment. Even if the user can buy a sterile hypodermic syringe over the counter, he or she still can be prosecuted for possessing it; the user must demonstrate a valid medical reason for possessing the equipment. Sometimes drug users are arrested for carrying syringes or even bottles of bleach.[19] To arrest the user who, in abiding by safer practices that the health department encouraged and aided, carries a syringe or bleach defeats the purpose of public health.

The impact of drug paraphernalia laws, therefore, is not simply the significant limit on the street supply of sterile injection equipment. The law also creates a marked disincentive for users to carry sterile equipment when they frequent a "copping place." Yet drug users need to be carrying sterile injection equipment precisely at this time, when they are buying and/or injecting heroin or cocaine.

PROPOSAL FOR REFORMING DRUG PARAPHERNALIA STATUTES

Drug paraphernalia laws, if they are to be consistent with public health objectives, should focus on prohibiting the illicit sale, rental, or distribution of drug injection equipment. Such prohibitions would affect the drug dealer or proprietor of a shooting gallery but not the health care professional, pharmacist, or public health official. The law would regulate the sale of hypodermic syringes and needles in much the same way it does currently--by ensuring that they are sold only in appropriate places (for example, in pharmacies, not in candy stores) by trained and experienced professionals, and that the equipment is in safe, sterile condition. There would not be any pretense that the authorized seller is unaware of the intent of the buyer. More importantly, the drug-dependent buyer would not be deterred by the threat of criminal sanctions for buying, possessing, or using the sterile injection equipment. Any unauthorized person who sold or distributed the equipment still would be subject to criminal penalties.

There are two justifications for these changes. First, the new law would focus its proscriptions precisely on those who endanger the public's health and well-being: illicit drug dealers and shooting-gallery or drug-hotel proprietors. These seller of hypodermics are unreliable distributors of sterile equipment, and are not subject to effective quality control or regulation. The probability that they will provide used, shared, and contaminated equipment justifies the criminal proscription. Second, just as society does not allow dealers to profit from the sale of drugs, so too should it forbid them to trade in drug paraphernalia. Drug paraphernalia laws applied to illicit sellers also would be an appropriate alternative for arrest or charge. If the police can demonstrate an intent to sell drug paraphernalia outside of a regulated pharmacy or other authorized location, that intent should be sufficient justification for prosecution, even if the dealer is not in possession of heroin or cocaine.

A new law focusing on the illicit sale of hypodermics, not on authorized sales and purchases, would allow drug users to possess sterile equipment, thus encouraging safer injection practices. It also would dampen the thriving black market in hypodermic syringes and needles, which poses a significant danger to public health.

Needle Prescription Laws

Drug paraphernalia laws do not prohibit or regulate the sale of hypodermics if the seller doesn't have any reason to believe that the equipment will be used for injecting illicit drugs. Accordingly, over-the-counter sales of hypodermic syringes and needles are permitted in most jurisdictions. Pharmacists are not obliged to question the buyer's intent when he or she purchases the equipment. Indeed, there aren't any professional guidelines for pharmacists in this respect. All of this leads in part to wide variations in sales practices.[20]

Racial and other biases can potentially limit the opportunities for drug users to purchase hypodermic syringes and needles at pharmacies.[21] Some pharmacists sell to all buyers, while others do not sell to those who show visible signs of injection drug use or cannot offer a plausible medical justification.[22,23,24]

Over-the-counter sale of hypodermic needles and syringes is significantly restricted in ten states (California, Delaware, Illinois, Maine, Massachusetts, New Hampshire, New Jersey, New York, Pennsylvania, and Rhode Island) and Puerto Rico[25] (Table). These jurisdictions have needle prescription laws. Such laws date back to the New York Boylan Act of 1914 [*People v. Gordon*, 336 N.Y.S.2d 753 (1972)].[26] The modern statutes prohibit the sale, distribution, or possession of hypodermic syringes or needles without a valid medical prescription. [See, for example, New York Consol. Laws, c. 40, para. 1747-d(3) and LSA-RS 40: 962 Subd. B; Massachusetts G.L.C. 94C, para. 27. Authority to possess hypodermics can be granted under several of these laws by the state commissioner of health, as occurred in New York City.] Needle prescription laws are more onerous than drug paraphernalia laws because they do not require criminal intent. Needle prescription laws that are regulatory and do not impose criminal liability on the buyer have been upheld by the courts [*People v. Bellfield*, 230 N.Y.S.2D 79, *aff*, 183 N.E.2d 230 (1962); also see *State v. Birdsell*, 104 So.2d 148 (1958)].

Under needle prescription laws, physicians may write prescriptions for hypodermic syringes and needles for patients under their care only if there is a legitimate medical purpose. A pharmacist must keep careful records of the sale of syringes and needles. If an injection drug user is charged with illegal possession of paraphernalia, the user must prove that he or she has sufficient authority to possess them [*Commonwealth v. Jefferson*, 377 Mass. 716, 387 N.E.2d 579 (1979)].

The "legitimate medical purposes" doctrine strengthens the regulatory effect of needle prescription laws. The doctrine is intended to hold a prescription invalid unless it is prescribed in good faith for a therapeutic purpose. Physicians have had their licenses withdrawn or have been convicted for improperly prescribing drugs or drug paraphernalia [Minnesota ex.re. *Whipple v. Martinson*, 256 U.S. 41 (1921)].

It is not clear if a physician could be successfully prosecuted today for prescribing sterile injection equipment for a drug user. Faced with the exigencies of the HIV epidemic, physicians could claim a good-faith intention to prevent the patient from contracting or transmitting HIV infection. Prescribing a sterile needle and syringe in this situation would not necessarily comport with prevailing medical practice. Yet the consensus of public health opinion is that intravenous drug users should have access to sterile injection equipment to impede the needle-borne transmission of disease.[27] So courts might well sustain the legitimacy of a medical prescription for sterile injection equipment to safeguard the health of the patient and the patient's needle-sharing and sexual partners.

Proposal for Repeal of Needle Prescription Statutes

Repeal of needle prescription laws is supported by many respected public-health and bar associations.[27,28,29,30] In effect, a repeal would allow pharmacists and other authorized retailers to sell hypodermics over the counter and without a medical prescription. Syringes and needles could be sold the same as other nonprescription medications and health materials. Because the state would not be instrumental in distributing drug injection equipment, the state would not be tacitly approving its use. Furthermore, repeal of these laws would not have a revenue impact on state legislatures. The only effect would be removal of the state as an obstacle to providing the sterile equipment that injection drug users need in order to comply with public health advice about protecting themselves and others from the needle-borne spread of HIV.

Most states and virtually all of Western Europe do not have needle prescription laws. These and many other jurisdictions permit over-the-counter sales of hypodermic syringes and needles.[31] Their experience has not shown any obvious adverse effects. They generally have a lower prevalence of HIV infection among drug users, and lower rates of drug use than states that do have such laws.[26,28] Though broad data of this kind do not provide scientific proof of a causal effect, they do supplement reports from drug users and researchers who say that sharing is related to the inaccessibility of sterile equipment.[32]

If a state were to repeal its needle prescription statutes, it would not necessarily have to abandon attempts to regulate the sale of hypodermic needles and syringes. Legislators concerned about the sensitivity of communities can require that sales take place only in certain locations, such as pharmacies, and that these items not be in view of customers. Social science research indicates that behavioral change is enhanced when people have full and accurate health information and the means to act on that information.[33]

In 1992, Connecticut gave policy makers and researchers their first opportunity to evaluate such proposals for reforming drug paraphernalia and needle prescription statutes. The legislature enacted a statute relaxing criminal prohibitions on the purchase and sale of hypodermic needles and syringes [Connecticut Public Act No. 92-185, as amended by May session, Public Act No. 92-11)]. The statute authorizes licensed manufacturers, wholesalers, and pharmacists to sell--and individuals to buy--ten or fewer hypodermic needles or syringes. The Centers for Disease Control plan to evaluate the impact of this law.

LEGAL BASIS OF SYRINGE EXCHANGE PROGRAMS

Drug paraphernalia and needle prescription statutes not only enhance the scarcity of sterile injection equipment but also may pose a legal barrier to public health programs designed to promote safer injection behavior. Such statutes render needle-and-syringe exchange programs prima facie unlawful in many jurisdictions. Because these laws proscribe the distribution and possession of injection equipment with knowledge that those who receive the equipment intend to use it for drug injection and don't have a valid medical prescription, exchange programs can be challenged as unlawful. Moreover, clients risk criminal prosecution for participating in such exchanges. Even if police do not enforce these statutes, the laws may have a chilling effect on drug users' participation in public health programs.

The hostility of legislators to needle and syringe exchanges is illustrated by a series of congressional bans on the use of federal funds for exchange programs. Since 1988, Congress has passed at least seven statutes that contain provisions prohibiting or restricting the use of federal funds for needle exchange programs and activities.[34] For example, the Alcohol, Drug Abuse, and Mental Health Administration Reorganization Act of 1992 stipulates that:

> None of the funds provided under [the Public Health Service Act] shall be used to provide individuals with hypodermic needles or syringes so that such individuals may use illegal drugs, unless the Surgeon General of the Public Health Service determines that a demonstration project would be effective in reducing drug abuse and the risk that the public will become infected [with HIV]. [U.S.C.A. 300ee-5 (West 1991)]

The ban applies regardless of the lawfulness of syringe programs in the states. The surgeon general has not yet decided whether to authorize federal funding. However, the U.S. General Accounting Office has found that exchange projects do provide possible public-health benefits; it may be only a short time before the Clinton Administration repeals or loosens the ban.

Because of the federal law, needle-and-syringe exchange programs must operate by means of state, municipal, or charitable funding. More importantly, these programs may have to defend their legal authority if they are challenged under state law. As of January 1993, more than thirty needle exchange programs in the United States and many more internationally were in some stage of implementation.[31]

Harmonizing the Objectives of Law Enforcement and Public Health

In November 1988, a pilot needle and syringe exchange was established in New York City after two years of political debate.[35] The mayor, acquiescing to pressure from neighborhood groups, declared that any exchange site within 1,000 feet of a school or day care center would be unsuitable. The program, therefore, was established on only one site--at the city health department itself. The department is adjacent to a city jail, the courts, and central policy headquarters.[5] The new mayor, David Dinkins, aborted the experimental program in early 1990 after only two years of operation because it had too few enrollees. (Another program has since been established.) This was not surprising, given the program's inaccessibility to most drug users and their fear of arrest and prosecution for possession of drug paraphernalia. Drug users, after all, would not have been expected to know that the state health commissioner had granted a waiver from the state needle-prescription law for the program.

The failure of New York City's exchange program to recruit a significant number of clients illustrates the importance of harmonizing the objectives of law enforcement and public health. The probability of success of needle and syringe exchanges also depends on the cooperation of city and state law-enforcement officials. If a city of state attorney general challenges the legality of a program, as occurred in Washington state, or if police arrest clients or even visible survey a program, prospective clients are certain to be discouraged from using it. Clients have been arrested for violation of a municipal drug-loitering ordinance at exchanges, such as the one in Seattle, Wash., that are government sanctioned. In San Francisco, Calif., such arrests have taken place under drug paraphernalia laws despite a directive by the chief of police to make enforcement of these laws a low priority when it comes to exchange clients.[36]

Criminal justice officials have discretion not to arrest and prosecute persons who violate criminal laws. Officials might exercise their prosecutorial discretion to overlook violation of drug paraphernalia laws when public health officials are operating needle exchange programs, but this discretion is an imperfect tool at best. It can be revoked at any time, it may not prevent street arrests (as the experience in San Francisco illustrates), and drug users have no way of knowing they won't be prosecuted, so they are reluctant to carry sterile equipment.

There needs to be a social contract among government departments that explicitly favors public health goals over law enforcement goals. This is justified by the seriousness of the needle-borne HIV epidemic. Law enforcement officers should not engage in surveillance or arrest any client of a needle-and-syringe exchange program sponsored or sanctioned by the public health department. The raison d'etre of drug control policies is to protect the health of the user and the public. When public health officials determine that exchange programs may serve as a bridge to treatment and reduce the spread of needle-based infection, the programs should take precedence over traditional law enforcement strategies. Drug control policies that fail to promote the health and safety of the community defeat their own purpose and lose legitimacy.

Establishing Authority for Needle and Syringe Exchanges

When legislators, public health officials, or community-based organizations set up needle and syringe exchanges, they may need to establish the legal authority for such programs. There are several legal strategies for bringing needle and syringe exchanges within the law:

- By establishing a specific statutory authority for the program.
- By obtaining a judicial declaration of lawfulness.
- By presenting a "necessity" defense against criminal prosecutions on a case-by-case basis.

Statutory Authority for Exchanges

Prior statutory authorization provides the most favorable legal environment for needle and syringe exchanges. It has been employed in Hawaii and Connecticut, which retained their state drug-paraphernalia laws but authorized the establishment of exchange projects.

In 1990, Hawaii enacted the first state-endorsed, needle-and-syringe exchange program in the United States [Hawaii Sess. Law 602 (Relating to a Pilot Program to Reduce the Transmission of Infectious and Communicable Diseases)]. The program is privately funded and operated by The Life Foundation, a nonprofit AIDS group. The statute required that state director of health to establish a pilot exchange program that would:

- Be designed to prevent transmission of HIV and hepatitis.
- Provide maximum security for sites and equipment.
- Provide a one-for-one exchange.
- Screen out noninjection drug users.
- Provide drug treatment, counseling, and education to all participants.
- Assess behavioral changes and enrollment in treatment.

The law does not give clients immunity from prosecution for violating the state drug paraphernalia law. However, to date, no arrests have been reported.

Also in 1990, the Connecticut General Assembly enacted legislation authorizing a demonstration needle-and-syringe exchange program in New Haven [Conn. Gen. Stat. section 19a-124 (An Act Concerning a Demonstration Needle and Syringe Program)]. Mayor John C. Daniels agreed to implement the program in August of that year, saying, "Needle exchanges may not work. But when you have a serious problem, you try to find serious solutions."[37] Notably, the statute added the demonstration project to a list of exceptions to Connecticut's needle-prescription and drug-paraphernalia statutes. The exchanges cannot operate within 1,000 feet of schools, in deference to the state statute pertaining to illicit drug sale or use around school perimeters. The exchanges offer a full range of prevention services: AIDS education, condoms and bleach packets, drug treatment, counseling and advocacy, and referrals for treatment of communicable and sexually transmitted diseases.[38] In January 1990, the New Haven Board of Health Commissioners passed a detailed resolution promoting a comprehensive strategy to curb the spread of HIV infection among intravenous drug users and their sexual partners and children [City of New Haven Board of Health Commissioners. A resolution in support of a comprehensive strategy to curb the spread of HIV among IVDUs, their sex partners, and children (January 17, 1990)].

The Connecticut Legislature expanded the statutory authority for needle and syringe exchanges beginning on July 1, 1992. The state department of health services was authorized to establish needle-and-syringe exchange programs in the three cities with the highest number of AIDS cases among injection drug users [Connecticut Public Act No. 92-3, as amended by May Session, Public Act No. 92-11)].

Similar bills to establish the lawfulness of needle-and-syringe exchange programs have been introduced in other jurisdictions. Gov. Pete Wilson vetoed legislation in California, saying, "Without clear and convincing evidence that these projects will successfully reduce the AIDS epidemic, we cannot afford to threaten the credibility of our ongoing antidrug efforts."

Judicial Declaration

Public health departments may have general authority to establish needle and syringe exchanges even in the absence of specific legislative approval. State and municipal public health statutes and regulations mandate that the spread of disease shall be impeded. These provisions may authorize or obligate state or city officers to create effective public health programs, including needle and syringe exchanges. Interesting jurisprudential issues emerge when public-health and criminal laws conflict. Public health laws may take precedence over criminal laws when the former provide more recent and more specific authority to protect community health. The National Lawyers Guild AIDS Network reasons that "acts which would be criminal if engaged in without legal authority, such as forced inoculations and quarantine, are lawful if ordered in accordance with public health laws."[36] In a sharp conflict between law enforcement and public health in Washington state, courts affirmed the power of health officials to set up exchanges. That experience demonstrates how litigation, by means of a judicial declaration, can facilitate needle and syringe exchanges.

In 1988, David Purchase, a former drug counselor, began a needle-and-syringe exchange program in Tacoma, Wash., in violation of state law but with the support of the chief of police. In January 1989, the Tacoma County Board of Health voted to institute the program formally and to pay Purchase a salary.[39] In July of that year, the state attorney general issued an opinion that the program violated the state's drug paraphernalia act. The county public health commissioner filed suit seeking a declaratory judgment that the exchange program was lawful. The court held that the program did not violate the act [*Allen v. City of Tacoma*, No. 89-2-09067-3 (Wash. Super.

Ct., Pierce County, May 9, 1990)], as that statute provides an exemption from liability for government officials who are engaged in the lawful performance of their duties. The court also noted that Washington's AIDS law [Wash. Rev. Code para. 70.24.400 (Supp. 1990)] authorizes locally developed public health programs that are designed to control the needle-borne spread of HIV.

In July 1990, the Spokane County Health District Board of Health, like the Tacoma board, adopted a resolution directing its health officer to set up a needle-and-syringe exchange program as part of an overall intervention to slow the spread of needle-borne infection. The board directed that the program be included in the Regional AIDS Network Plan authorized by the State Omnibus AIDS Act [RCW 70.24]. However, Washington's prosecuting attorney stated that, given the attorney general's opinion, he would authorize the arrest and prosecution of clients of the Spokane program. The board of health then brought action in Spokane County Superior Court seeking a declaratory judgment that the exchange program was lawful. The court issued a declaratory judgment in favor of the public health department, and the case was appealed to the Supreme Court of Washington.

In November 1992, the Supreme Court unanimously declared that the state's exchange programs were lawful:

> The Legislature has not explicitly directed regional AIDS services networks to develop needle exchange programs. However, the allowances for "needle sterilization" and "the use of appropriate materials" to combat the spread of AIDS can and should be liberally construed to include needle exchange. Moreover, we are persuaded that the broad powers given local health boards and officers under [the state Constitution] authorize them to institute needle exchange programs in an effort to stop the spread of HIV and AIDS. [*Spokane County Health District and Beare v. Brockett*, 1992. Wash. LEXIS 257, November 5, 1992).]

The Necessity Defense

Like Purchase, many community-based organizers and activities have distributed sterile injection equipment in the absence of a government-sanctioned program. They act in the good-faith belief that a public health emergency exists and that their efforts are necessary to save human life. More than twenty prosecutions have been brought against such individuals for violating state drug-paraphernalia and/or needle-prescription laws. In one case, prosecution was based on the state's business and professional code.[40] Many more volunteers have been arrested but not prosecuted. A volunteer in Worcester, Mass., and one in Peabody, Mass., are the only persons known to have been convicted; their cases are on appeal.

Some acquittals of exchange volunteers have been based on the fact that defendants lacked the requisite intent under a state's drug paraphernalia statute. More often, the acquittals have been based on the necessity defense, which has evolved under common law and varies among jurisdictions. Necessity is founded on the theory that conduct that would otherwise constitute a criminal offense is justified in extraordinary circumstances. The necessity defense applies to circumstances in which:

- The conduct was, through no fault of the defendant, necessary to avoid an imminent harm to a person or the public.

- No adequate alternative to avert the harm was available.

- The harm caused by the act was not disproportionate to the harm avoided.

- The defendant entertained a good-faith belief that the act was necessary to prevent a greater harm.

- The defendant believed that his or her behavior was reasonable in all circumstances.

The defense in needle exchange prosecutions usually has relied on a mass of public health evidence and testimony on each element of necessity: the rapid spread of needle-borne infection locally, the absence of government-sanctioned exchanges, the scarcity of treatment, and research data showing the effect that official exchanges in other jurisdiction have on seroprevalence and drug use.

Most acquittals, particularly in the following cases, suggest that courts are likely to be sympathetic to this defense.

The Criminal Court of the City of New York acquitted eight syringe-exchange volunteers on June 25, 1991. It noted: "The distinction, in broadest terms, during this age of the AIDS crisis is death by using dirty needles versus drug addiction by using clean needles. The defendants' actions sought to avoid the greater harm" [Decision and Order, *New York v. Bordowitz*, Criminal Ct. of City and County of New York, No. 90N028423 (June 25, 1991)].

The drafters of the New York necessity statute specifically referred to the "forcible confinement of a person ill with a highly contagious disease for the purpose of preventing him from going to a city and possibly starting an epidemic" [Commission staff notes, proposed N.Y. penal law (1964), para. 65.00, p. 317]. In *Doe v. Bolton*, the U.S. Supreme Court recognized that the right to protect a person's body could outweigh the interest of the government in guarding the health and morals of the public. "The significance of these decisions," said the court, "lies in the revelation of how far-reaching is the right of an individual to preserve his (or her) health and bodily integrity" [*Doe v. Bolton*, 410 U.S. 179 (1973)].

In *Commonwealth v. Parker* [Order and Findings, Boston Municipal Criminal Court, No. 89-0123 (January 23, 1991); Bench Ruling No. 89-01213, January 9, 1990)], the Boston Municipal Court acquitted Jon C. Parker because he lacked the intent needed under the state drug paraphernalia law and because he acted out of necessity.

In *Commonwealth v. Corbett*, the Massachusetts Supreme Judicial Court relied on the necessity defense in an analogous case from 1940. The court did not find that there had been a violation of a statute prohibiting the sale of contraceptives when the defendant sold condoms for the purposed of preventing the spread of sexually transmitted disease. The court stated that the public policy of the Commonwealth was to prevent the use of contraception but not "to permit venereal disease to spread unchecked" [*Commonwealth v. Corbett*, 307 Mass. 7 (1940)].

The *Parker* court found that the value protected by the law prohibiting possession of hypodermic needles and syringes is "as a matter of public policy eclipsed by a superseding value"--namely, AIDS prevention.

The Massachusetts Supreme Judicial Court was the first state supreme court to consider whether necessity could be raised as a defense to a charge of violating state criminal proscriptions against distributing drug injection equipment. In *Commonwealth v. Leno and Ingalls*, two men were convicted of possessing and distributing needles and syringes in an unofficial exchange program. The trial judge refused to give the jury an instruction that the defendants could be found not guilty if they had presented evidence on each element of the necessity defense. The defendants testified that they had conducted the exchange program solely for the purpose of saving lives.

One of the central elements of the necessity defense is that there was not an adequate alternative to avert the harm. In *Leno and Ingalls*, the Commonwealth of Massachusetts argued in its brief that sterilization with bleach was a viable alternative to distributing sterile injection equipment. However, a recent Community Alert Bulletin issued by the National Institute on Drug Abuse pointed out that bleach may not be as effective against HIV in blood (particularly clotted blood) as it is in a cell-free state. In a six-second cleaning, a 10% dilution of household bleach was not routinely effective in removing blood from syringes. These data reinforce the reasonable belief of the defendants that a distribution program was necessary to preserve the health and lives of two injection drug users.

Balancing Governmental Interests

The systematic refusal of courts to convict needle-and-syringe exchange volunteers under drug-paraphernalia or needle-prescription laws raises the question of the validity of these statutes. If the judicial system remains largely unconvinced that prosecution under these laws creates a greater public good than the breach thereof, can their continuation be justified as a matter of public policy? The reasoning of courts that public health exigencies of the needle-borne HIV epidemic outweigh the value of restricting the availability of drug injection equipment warrants consideration by legislatures. Legislative responses could include authorization of needle-and-syringe exchange programs, together with specific exemptions under existing criminal laws, or reform or repeal of drug-paraphernalia and needle-prescription statutes.

State-authorized exchanges have clear advantages over underground programs. Official exchanges can be designed to promote the public health and be established under carefully defined circumstances. These circumstances might include:

- Restricting exchanges to particular pilot sites.

- Requiring one-for-one exchanges.

- Mandating the provision of a full array of services and referrals, including diagnosis and treatment for drug dependency, HIV disease, sexually transmitted disease, and tuberculosis.

- Bleach and condom distribution.

- Carefully designed research.

CONCLUSION

Continued reliance on unofficial programs risks escalating the nonproductive struggle between public-health and drug-control objectives. Exchange volunteers and clients should not have to worry about informal arrangements whereby law enforcement officials don't arrest, district attorneys don't prosecute, and courts don't convict. A New Jersey Municipal Court judge, like the judges in the New York and Boston cases, said each ease has its own set of facts, that the court would not allow its decision to be viewed as "a license for other well-meaning groups or individuals to canvass this community and engage in a needle exchange program" [*State of New Jersey v. Carl Sigmon, Rodney Sorge, Brad Taylor, and Jon Parker*, Municipal Court, Hudson County, Jersey City, N.J., Docket No. V70 to V81, November 6, 1991].

After years of experience and sound research involving needle-and-syringe exchange programs in the United States and abroad, it is time for federal, state, and local governments to create their own programs to combat the dual epidemics of drug abuse and HIV infection. If policy makers view the growing body of data with objectivity and without attaching any political symbolism to it, they will conclude that well-designed exchange programs should be part of a comprehensive range of health and social services for drug users. Merely distributing injection equipment to drug users is not an inspiring public health goal, and no careful observer should be surprised by the intensity of political and community resistance to such distribution. However, if those programs can foster a measure of trust among drug users, promote greater use of sterile injection equipment and less sharing, provide counseling and education about safer drug injection and safer sexual intercourse,[41] and provide a bridge to an array of treatment services for drug dependency, HIV disease, sexually transmitted disease, and tuberculosis, then American society would be short-sighted if it rejected this potentially effective public health strategy.

REFERENCES

1. The White House. *National Drug Control Strategy.* Washington, D.C.: Government Printing Office, 1989.

2. National Commission on AIDS. *The Twin Epidemics of Substance Use and HIV.* Washington, D.C.: National Commission on AIDS, 1991.

3. Executive Office of the President, Office of National Drug Control Policy. *Needle Exchange Programs: Are they Effective? ONDCP Bulletin* 1992;7:1-9.

4. Kaplan E. H., O'Keefe, E. Let the needles do the talking! Evaluating the New Haven needle exchange. *Interfaces* 1993. In press.

5. New York City Department of Health. *The Pilot Needle Exchange Study in New York City: A Bridge to Treatment. A Report on the First Ten Months of Operation.* New York, N.Y.: New York City Department of Health, 1989.

6. Gostin, L. The interconnected epidemics of drug dependency and AIDS. *Harvard Civil Rights-Civil Liberties Law Review* 1991;26:113-184.

7. Gostin, L. An alternative public health vision for a national drug control strategy: "Treatment works." *University of Houston Law Review* 1991;28:285-308.

8. Gostin, L. The needle-borne HIV epidemic: Causes and public health responses. *Behavioral Sciences and the Law* 1991;9:287-304.

9. Gostin, L. Compulsory treatment for drug-dependent persons: Justification for a public health approach to drug dependency. *Milbank Quarterly* 1992;69:561-593.

10. National Institute on Drug Abuse. *Needle Sharing Among Intravenous Drug Abusers: National and International Perspectives.* Monograph No. 80. Washington, D.C.: NIDA, 1988.

11. Nelson, K.E., Vlahov, D., Cohn, S., et al. Human immunodeficiency virus infection in diabetic intravenous drug users. *Journal of the American Medical Association* 1991;266-2259-2261.

12. O'Keefe, E., Kaplan, E., Khoshnood, K. *Preliminary Report: City of New Haven Needle Exchange Program.* New Haven, Conn: New Haven Health Department, 1991.

13. D'Aguila, R. T., Williams, A. B. Epidemic of human immunodeficiency virus (HIV) infection among intravenous drug users. *Yale Journal of Biology and Medicine* 1987;60:545-567.

14. Murphy, S. Intravenous drug use and AIDS: Notes on the social economy of needle sharing. *Contemporary Drug Problems* 1987;14:373-396.

15. Des Jarlais, D. C., Friedman, S., Hopkins, W. Risk reduction for acquired immune deficiency syndrome among intravenous drug users. *Annals of Internal Medicine* 1985;103:755.

16. Des Jarlais, D. C., Hopkins, W. Free needles for intravenous drug users at risk for AIDS: Current developments in New York City. *New England Journal of Medicine* 1985;313:23.

17. Chitwood, D. D., McCoy, C. B., Inciardi, J. A., et al. HIV seropositivity of needles from shooting galleries in South Florida. *American Journal of Public Health* 1990;80:150-152.

18. Pascal, C. "Intravenous Drug Abuse and AIDS Transmission: Federal and State Laws Regulating Needle Availability." In *Needle Sharing Among Intravenous Drug Abusers: National and International Perspectives*, edited by R. J. Battjes, R. W. Pickens. Rockville, Md.: National Institute on Drug Abuse, 1988.

19. Stryker, J. IV drug use and AIDS: Public policies and dirty needles. *Journal of Health Policy, Politics and Law* 1989;14:719-740.

20. Ettelson, R. Sell needles & syringes to IV drug abusers? *Pharmacy Times* 1991;57:107-114.

21. Compton III, W. M, Cottler, L. B., Decker, S. H., et al. Legal needle buying in St. Louis. *American Journal of Public Health* 1992;82:595-596.

22. Goldberg, D. J. AIDS and intravenous drug use. *British Medical Journal* 1987;294:906.

23. Croatto, J. P., Ewart, F. J., Hage, B. H., et al. The role of the pharmacist in preventing a 'second wave' of the HIV epidemic among IV drug users. *Australian Journal of Pharmacy* 1987;68:602-604.

24. Glantz, A., Byrne, C., Jackson, P. Role of community pharmacies in prevention of AIDS among injecting drug misusers: Findings of a survey in England and Wales. *British Medical Journal* 1989;299:1076-1079.

25. National Association of Boards of Pharmacy. *1991-92 National Association of Boards of Pharmacy Survey of Pharmacy Law.* Park Ridge, Ill.: National Association of Boards of Pharmacy, 1991.

26. The Association of the Bar of the City of New York. Committee on Law and Medicine. Legalization of non-prescription sale of hypodermic needles: A response to the AIDS crisis. *The Record* 1986;41:809, 811.

27. Friedman, S. R., Des Jarlais, D. C., Sterk, D. E., et al. AIDS and the social relations of intravenous drug users. *Milbank Quarterly* 1990;68 (suppl 1):85-110.

28. The New York County Lawyers Association. Committee on Law and Reform. *Report of Drug-Related AIDS and the Legal Ban on Over-the-Counter Hypodermic Needle Sales*, 1988.

29. American Bar Association. AIDS Coordinating Committee. *AIDS: The Legal Issues*, 1988.

30. Des Jarlais, D. C., Friedman, S R. AIDS and legal access to sterile drug injection equipment. *Annals of the American Academy of Political and Social Science* 1992;521:42-65.

31. Porter, L., Gostin, L. *Legal Environment Surrounding the Availability of Sterile Needles and Syringes to Injecting Drug Users*. Geneva, Switzerland: World Health Organization. In press.

32. Des Jarlais, D. C. The first and second decades of AIDS among injecting drug users. *British Journal of Addiction* 1992;87:347-353.

33. Becker, M., Joseph, J. AIDS and behavioral change to reduce risk: A review. *American Journal of Public Health* 1988; 78:403.

34. U.S. General Accounting Office. *Needle Exchange Programs: Research Suggests Promise as an AIDS Strategy*. Washington, D.C.: U.S. General Accounting Office, 1993.

35. Anderson, W. The New York needle trial: The politics of public health in the age of AIDS. *American Journal of Public Health* 1991;81:1506-1517.

36. Keller, I. Needle exchange: HIV prevention takes on the law. *The Exchange* [National Lawyers Guild AIDS Network] 1992;17:1-7.

37. Jackson, P. Ugly reality convinces mayor to try needle exchange. *New Haven Register* August 1, 1990.

38. New Haven Health Department. *Needle Exchange Program Protocol: Executive Summary*, 1990.

39. Gross, J. Needle exchange for addicts wins foothold against AIDS in Tacoma. *New York Times* January 23, 1988:A8.

40. Trachina, J. *Forcing Needle Exchange Through the Courts: A Citizen's Approach to Syringe Exchange*. San Mateo, Calif.: AIDS Prevention Action Network, 1991.

41. Van den Hoek, A. J, Van Haastrecht, H. J., Coutinho, R. A. Little change in sexual behavior in injecting users in Amsterdam. *Journal of AIDS* 1992;5:518-522.

Table. States that Require a Prescription to Buy Syringes/Needles

California*	New Hampshire
Connecticut**	New Jersey
Delaware	New York
Illinois	Pennsylvania
Maine	Puerto Rico***
Massachusetts	Rhode Island

* Prescription not necessary if the equipment is to be used to inject insulin or adrenaline, and if the seller can identify the buyer and records the purchase.

** Necessary only if the transaction involves more than ten needles/syringes.

*** If the pharmacist knows the buyer, insulin syringes may be sold.

Source: *1991-92 National Association of Boards of Pharmacy Survey of Pharmacy Law*

NEW CONNECTICUT LAWS TO IMPROVE ACCESS TO NEEDLES AND SYRINGES: WHAT IS THEIR IMPACT?

Samuel L. Groseclose and Linda A. Valleroy, Centers for Disease Control and Prevention, Atlanta, Georgia; B. Weinstein, Connecticut Department of Public Health and Addiction Services, Hartford, CT; and T. Stephen Jones, W. J. Kassler, L. J. Fehrs, and R. T. Rolfs, Centers for Disease Control and Prevention, Atlanta, GA

INTRODUCTION

Human immunodeficiency virus (HIV) can be transmitted among injecting-drug users (IDUs) through the multi-person use (sharing) of HIV-contaminated needles and syringes. Increasing IDUs' access to and use of sterile needles and syringes may reduce HIV transmission. To help reduce IDUs' use of HIV-contaminated needles and syringes, Connecticut enacted new laws that took effect on July 1, 1992. One of the new laws permits, but does not require, pharmacists to sell up to 10 needles and syringes to individuals who do not have medical prescriptions. Another new law makes it legal for individuals to possess up to 10 clean needles and syringes. Prior to this, purchase and possession of needles and syringes without a prescription had been illegal in Connecticut. From July 1, 1992 through June 30, 1993, we conducted an evaluation to determine whether the changes in the needle prescription and drug paraphernalia laws were associated with changes in pharmacies' needle and syringe sales practices and needle and syringe sales, IDUs' needle and syringe-related purchasing and usage, and police officers' practices and risk of needlestick injuries.

EVALUATION FINDINGS

- Through a surveillance system monitoring needle and syringe sales at selected Connecticut pharmacies, we found that most, but not all, pharmacies sold nonprescription needles and syringes after the new laws.

- In pharmacies in neighborhoods where there was a high prevalence of injecting drug use, numbers of nonprescription needles and syringes sold and needle and syringe transactions increased steadily from July 1992 through June 1993.

- The percentage of IDUs who were aware of both new laws increased during the first 12 months after the new laws. Nine to 12 months after the new laws, over two-thirds of the IDUs interviewed knew about both new laws.

- After the new laws went into effect, IDUs reported more pharmacy purchasing of needles and syringes and less street purchasing. And, there was a shift from street purchasing to pharmacy purchasing as the most frequently reported source of needles and syringes.

- The percentage of IDUs who reported sharing needles and syringes decreased after the new laws.

- While law enforcement officers in Hartford were less likely to arrest persons for paraphernalia possession after the new laws were enacted, there was no difference in the percentage of IDUs who reported that they were hassled by police for possession of clean needles and syringes.

- And, while IDUs reported changes in needle and syringe possession, Occupational Safety and Health Administration reports of needlestick injuries among Hartford police decreased after the new laws.

POLICY RECOMMENDATIONS

As a first step, state and local public health officials, in collaboration with law enforcement officers, addiction services personnel, pharmacy and medical associations, and members of affected communities should review the laws limiting access to sterile needles and syringes in their jurisdictions.

Our data suggest that once legal restrictions on the purchase and possession of needles and syringes are removed, pharmacies will sell nonprescription needles and syringes, and IDUs will shift their needle and syringe purchasing from illegal "street" sources to pharmacies and reduce their needle sharing behaviors.

Therefore, policy-makers should consider:

- the repeal of needle prescription laws -- allowing increased availability of sterile needles and syringes, and

- the modification of drug paraphernalia laws -- specifically, decriminalizing the possession of needles and syringes.

The pivotal role of pharmacists and police officers in increased sterile needle and syringe availability for IDUs who will not or cannot stop injecting must be emphasized. Pharmacists and police officers should be brought into the discussions of this public health action and should be encouraged to take a more active public health role.

Public health officials should work with IDUs, pharmacists, and police officers to determine their needs and concerns related to HIV infection, addictions, and access to sterile needles and syringes and should educate them as necessary.

Knowledge of the new laws among IDUs was not complete. We would recommend that IDUs be given more information about what the new laws allow in practical terms.

COMMENT

We recognize that increasing sterile needle and syringe availability for IDUs who cannot or will not enter drug treatment programs requires the consideration of a variety of options including increased pharmacy sales and needle exchange programs. However, among these options, pharmacy sale of sterile needles and syringes offers an intervention that can be implemented with minimal, or no, public funding.

We recognize that HIV prevention efforts directed toward injecting-drug users must be comprehensive and should include drug treatment, and addiction and risk reduction counseling, in addition to the specific interventions to increase IDUs' access to and ability to possess sterile needles and syringes.

CANADIAN PHARMACIES' RESPONSE TO HIV AND HARM REDUCTION STRATEGIES: A REPORT FROM THE NATIONAL SURVEY ON COMMUNITY PHARMACIES AND HIV/AIDS PREVENTION

TED MYERS, Department of Health Administration, University of Toronto, and Department of Public Health, City of Toronto, Canada; RHONDA COCKERILL, Department of Health Administration, University of Toronto; MARGARET MILLSON, Department of Public Health, City of Toronto, and Department of Preventive Medicine and Biostatistics, University of Toronto, Canada; JAMES RANKIN, Addiction Research Foundation, and Department of Preventive Medicine and Biostatistics, University of Toronto, Canada; and CATHERINE WORTHINGTON, Department of Health Administration, University of Toronto, Canada

INTRODUCTION

This paper is a brief report on the Canadian Survey of Community Pharmacies and HIV/AIDS Prevention. It will focus on the policies and practices related to HIV of community pharmacies in order to (a) highlight this group's response to harm reduction strategies and its potential role in HIV prevention, and to (b) explore ethical issues that surround harm reduction for pharmacies.

BACKGROUND

Prior to describing the study results some background information for Canada will be provided in order to highlight possible differences from the United States with regard to the epidemiology of HIV/AIDS, the national response to injection drug use in relation to HIV/AIDS and factors that may influence this response.

Epidemiology of AIDS/HIV

Canada's first case of AIDS was diagnosed in 1979. Adult males comprise 93.8% of the 8,148 AIDS cases reported to date. Of the adult cases, injection drug use is known to be a possible factor in the risk of transmission in 5.9%.[1] (For males the rate is 5.6% and for females 9.4%.)

Eighty-nine percent of all AIDS cases (adult and pediatric) reported to date occur in three provinces, (British Columbia ,18%, Ontario, 41%, and Quebec, 30%), as may be seen in the Figure 1. Across Canada, there is variation in the known risk factors associated with HIV transmission. For example, injection drug use as a known risk factor ranges from 5% of cases in Quebec to 8% of cases in Alberta.

As in most countries, true estimates of the incidence of the HIV antibody in Canada's population are not possible because of difficulties in conducting broad-based HIV serostatus studies. For estimates of incidence of the HIV antibody in the Canadian population we rely predominantly on reports compiled from voluntary testing. These are incomplete because of variation across the country in methods of recording cases. It is assumed that the sharing of needles as a potential risk factor is underreported because injection drug users have fear of exposing this illegal activity. Some of the best estimates for HIV prevalence come from studies of convenience samples of injection drug users. In the period between 1985 and 1992 such studies report that between 1% to 25% are infected, depending upon the year, region of the country and target population.[2]

Canadian Response to HIV and Injection Drug Use

Prior to 1988, in response to concern about the spread of HIV among injection drug users, it was reported that a number of physicians across the country provided needles and syringes to their drug injecting patients. The need for greater action was highlighted at the Fourth International Conference on AIDS in Stockholm, in 1988. Simultaneously, Health and Welfare Canada and NAC-AIDS (National Advisory Committee on AIDS) subcommittee on injection drug use assumed leadership in response to the evidence for potential spread of HIV through injection drug use. The concern led to the establishment of a number of Injection Drug Use Pilot Outreach Programmes. The first outreach programme/needle and syringe exchange was reportedly established in 1989.[3] This programme, and others soon to follow, were multifaceted projects with various components including: risk and risk reduction education; provision of condoms, bleach kits, needle exchange; and addiction treatment referrals. Within the communities where these projects were successful extensive community-development work was undertaken. Further, there was general endorsement by three levels of government (Federal, Provincial and Municipal or City). To date, approximately 37 such community outreach programmes for injection drug users are in operation across the country. They operate out of a variety of locations including community social service agencies, street outreach agencies, departments of public health, hospital outpatient clinics and community-based AIDS organizations. The programmes that exist include mobile unit, ambassador outreach and fixed site models (and others). Variation also is found in the management and funding. Many are under the direction of medical and public health services, others are directly managed by community social service agencies and networks. Programmes continue to develop at a fairly rapid rate and there is a trend to more focussed programmes for specific population groups such as First Nations People (aboriginal) and sex trade workers, as only two examples.

Factors Influencing Canada's Response

Several organizational and policy aspects have influenced Canada's response to HIV in relation to the Injection Drug User.

Canada's Health Case System: Its Funding and Organization

The Canada Health Act of 1984 set out an agreement between the provinces and the federal government that emphasized five basic principles for health services: universality, comprehensiveness, portability, public administration and accessibility.[4] This may be seen to have influenced Canada's response in two ways. First, in principle, injection drug users are linked into the Health Care System. Second, in Canada there is a will and an interest in protccting this system, and prevention of hospitalizations is a major component. This is seen further in a general trend to conceptualize drug problems in terms of lifestyle rather than as a disease.

Canada's Drug Strategy

In 1987 Canada's Drug Strategy was inaugurated with new funding allocated in roughly equal amounts to a wide variety of enforcement, treatment and prevention activities. Although the overall predominant focus on illicit drugs might have been criminal prohibition, in fact, the philosophy behind the Canadian Drug strategy represented a tentative first step toward a harm minimization approach, and an increase in emphasis on demand (the user) versus supply reduction (the seller) strategies.[5] The national focus provided a catalyst for programme action at the provincial level where the expertise and jurisdictional authority exist. While the Canadian Drug strategy was influenced by the American "War on Drugs", it attempts to achieve a balance between the supply and the demand sides. Although smaller in scope, the Canadian strategy was more comprehensive than the American in terms of substances targeted (i.e. alcohol is included), and further, placed greater emphasis on prevention and treatment.[5]

Canadian Drug Laws

In Canada the most important legislation dealing with illicit drugs are within the federal governments' jurisdiction, namely, *The Narcotic Control Act* and *The Food and Drugs Act*. In brief, these acts deal with possession, trafficking, importing and exporting and "prescription shopping." Further, in 1989 amendments were made to the Criminal Code to make it illegal to knowingly import, export, manufacture, promote, or sell illicit drug *paraphernalia* or literature. (*Bill-264*, September, 1988). The provision or distribution of needles by the medical profession as a "medical device" as opposed to an "instrument for use" is <u>not</u> an offence under the criminal code. Interestingly, the amendment is generally interpreted to suggest that the supplying of needles and syringes for safer injection is <u>not</u> illegal.[6,7]

Canada's National AIDS Strategy (1990)

In 1990 the Federal government provided funding and a comprehensive statement of need and directions that should be taken which encompassed AIDS prevention, treatment and research. This National AIDS Strategy committed to support research initiatives to address the issue of HIV infection among people who use injection drugs[8]. It is through these initiatives that many of the early outreach programmes for injection drug users were funded.

Pharmacy Accreditations and Pharmacists Licensing

In the absence of paraphernalia laws, provincial pharmaceutical associations and colleges (regulatory and licensing bodies) have been largely responsible for setting policies that govern the actions of the pharmacists and the operations of pharmacies in their jurisdictions. For the most part, the sale of needles and syringes for illicit drug use has been discouraged by licensing bodies and in the professional education of pharmacists until recently. Yet, individual pharmacists in some jurisdictions have for some time sold needles and syringes in packages of one to non-diabetic drug users. During the AIDS epidemic the "no sale" policy has been repeatedly examined and an incremental change in policy has occurred. For example in the Province of Ontario in 1987 the sale of needles and syringes to injection drug users was opposed (although recognized as both a moral and public health issue), in 1988 sales were permitted with "professional discretion" because it was seen to be a public health issue and in 1992 the policy was further changed to promote sales of needles by permitting the open display and self selection of needles and syringes, with professional discretion.[9] In all provinces except British Columbia there has been movement towards more liberal practices. In British Columbia a policy was embedded in Bylaw B19(9) which indicates "*that no pharmacist shall (a) store hypodermic syringes and needles in an area of the pharmacy accessible to the public, (b) sell hypodermic syringes and needles unless he has established to his reasonable satisfaction that they are required for a lawful purpose, and (c) advertise, by any means, hypodermic syringes and needles.*" In 1988 the British Columbia Council of the College of Pharmacists recommended to the Provincial Ministry of Health that this bylaw be amended by the deletion of paragraph (b). However, the amendment has never been promulgated.

To summarize for the purposes of this paper, the current provincial regulatory body policies regarding sale of needles and syringes to non-diabetic drug users fall into four categories:

(a) No Sale (Illegal)
(b) Sale with Professional Discretion
(c) Sale with Self-selection possible. (Open display with discretion)
(d) No written policy.

The current policies of the provinces/territories are shown in Figure 2.

Rationale for the Canadian Pharmacy Survey

This study was designed to describe the variations in current practice in pharmacies across Canada with respect to HIV prevention and to explore the factors that influence these. A related purpose was to assess whether the role of pharmacists might be expanded, and to determine what organizational, educational, or policy changes might be required to accompany any change in role. This study was modelled on an earlier study conducted as part of the evaluation of the City of Toronto's Injection Drug Use Programme. For the 1989 study the sampling unit was the pharmacist rather than the pharmacy. Results were difficult to analyze because of this sampling frame and inability to determine the denominator (number of pharmacists in full-time and part-time employment was unknown, and several pharmacists may have worked in several pharmacies). As well, a low response was obtained. The study responses received reflected that there was a potential role for pharmacies. Data from interviews with injection drug users, another aspect of the evaluation, suggest that 30% of injection drug users experienced difficulty obtaining needles and 47% indicated that pharmacies and drug stores were their most important source of needles and syringes.[10]

METHOD

To conduct this cross-sectional, nation-wide survey of community pharmacies a mailed questionnaire was directed to owner-managers in all Canadian provinces and Territories. A random sample of owner-managers was selected from mailing lists provided by the provincial regulatory bodies. To ensure the sample chosen was of sufficient size to permit the analysis to be preformed the minimum targeted size within each province/territory was 150 or a 25% sample of all community pharmacies, which ever was greater. Therefore, the sampling ratio varied from 25% in some provinces to 100% in others (e.g., Prince Edward Island). The survey was mailed to 2,017 pharmacies and an eventual 1,976 were assessed to be eligible for inclusion as a result of updating of addresses.

The survey strategy used was the Dillman Total Design Method.[11] Two full mailings and two reminder card mailings plus a final telephone call were used to boost response. Letters of endorsement were provided by the regulatory body in each province (except British Columbia) and the Canadian Pharmaceutical Association, (the professional association for pharmacists).

The survey instrument was based on one used for the City of Toronto Survey of Pharmacists and the format followed that used for the Ontario Pharmaceutical Enquiry.[12] The survey instrument was finalized after an extensive literature review, focus group discussion and pilot study. It included sections on (a) Current Practices in Pharmacies, (b) Professional Practice (willingness of individual pharmacists to provide specific services), (c) Information Needs, (d) Issues and Attitudes, and (e) Practice Characteristics. The instrument was available in both of Canada's Official languages.

Analysis

The analysis presented in this paper will be primarily descriptive. Although the number of pharmacies in some of the provinces are small, to reflect upon the provincial policy this report retains each province as a unit of analysis. To simplify several questions relating to (1) willingness and support for provision of specific services to non-diabetic injecting drug users, (2) attitudes regarding the prevention of HIV, (3) perceived cause of injection drug use and (4) future roles for pharmacies, factor analyses with orthogonal rotation were executed. In this paper the results of these factor analyses are not presented. However, group means for composite variables developed from each of the factors are presented in graphic form.

RESULTS

Response

The overall response rate to the survey was high (84.6%). As may be seen in Figure 3 this ranged from a low of 71.4% in Quebec to the high of 96.6% in Prince Edward Island. Only 12% refused to participate. This ranged from 3.7% in the Yukon and North West Territories to a high of 22.4% in Quebec.

Characteristics

The majority of pharmacies represented in the study were independently run businesses [(54.6%) were independently owned, 20.5% were chain, 20.5% were franchises and 3.4% were co-operatives]. These proportions varied across the country. The majority, 50.4%, of respondents were owner-managers, just under a third were non-owner managers, and 29.7% were franchisees. Further, the majority of respondents, 60.8%, had been in pharmacy practice for longer than 10 years.

Current Practices

Knowingly Served a Person with HIV

Nationally, 29.5% of the respondents indicated that they had served a client who was HIV antibody positive or who had AIDS. Twenty-two percent indicated that they did not know if they had served a person who had tested positive for the HIV antibody. Across the country this ranged from a high of 49.5% in British Columbia to a low of 14.8% in Saskatchewan as shown in Figure 4. The three provinces with the greatest proportion of respondents reporting that they had served an HIV positive individual were British Columbia, Quebec and Ontario which corresponds to the known prevalence of AIDS.

Requests to Sell Needles and Syringes

Nationally, 7.9% indicated that they had received no requests to sell needles or syringes (in the past year); 33.8% estimated that they received 20 or fewer requests a year, 18.9% reported receiving 21-100 requests and 21.9% reported more than 100 requests. These rates varied across the country as shown in Figure 5. The provinces receiving the greatest proportion of requests were British Columbia, Ontario, Prince Edward Island and the territories. (Note: As the number of respondents in the eastern provinces and territories are small the graph may misrepresent. Many of the community pharmacists in smaller communities may know their drug using clientele and be prepared to sell. A single user who regularly obtains needles or syringes may inflate this. Further, because of the knowledge a pharmacist may have of their customers in smaller communities they may be prepared to sell needles and syringes for many uses - from basting food to injecting earthworms to keep them buoyant for fishing!)

Comparison of Requests for Needles and Syringe Sales to Knowledge of Serving Persons Living With HIV

Comparison of the proportion of respondents within each province/territory who knowingly have served a person living with HIV as shown in Figure 4 with Figure 5 reflecting requests to sell needles and syringes, shows that there is considerable correspondence between these two variables, except in the provinces with smaller populations. The province of Quebec shows a further variation. This may be a result of the fact that in Quebec many of the pharmacy services may be provided through specific community pharmacies designated as serving injection drug users and through community health centres.

Comparison of "Pharmacy Response" with "Requests to Sell"

A comparison of the two graphs, requests to sell (Figure 5) and response to requests (Figure 6) does not show complete congruence between requests and response within all provincial jurisdictions. This comparison suggests that the decision to sell may relate to both policy and to discretionary factors. To assist in the interpretation of these data two analyses were conducted; one relating provincial/territorial policy to sale of needles and syringes, and another examining factors considered by pharmacists when exercising discretion.

Pharmacy's Response to Requests to Purchase

Nationally, 17.0% of the owner-managers indicated that they would not sell needles and syringes to non-diabetic drug users, 29.1% would sell in some cases, 29.2% would sell in most cases and 24.6% indicated that they would sell in all cases.

Figure 7 shows the proportion of pharmacies within each province/territory agreeing to sell. The highest proportion reporting that they would not sell was 30.5% in British Columbia where sales are illegal. In that same province 31.4% would sell in some cases, 21% in most cases and 17.1% in all cases. The second highest proportion not selling was in Newfoundland (25.9%) where there was no policy. The highest proportion selling in all cases was in the Yukon and Northwest Territories (42.9%), followed by Manitoba (28.4%) and New Brunswick (27.1%).

Provincial/Territorial Policy and Sale of Needles

A significant association was found with needle and syringe sales and the actual provincial/territorial policy toward sales, shown in Figure 8 ($\chi^2=100.2$ df=9 p=0.000). The lowest sales were reported in the province where sales are illegal. There was little difference between provinces with discretionary policies and those with self-selection. (An analysis not reported here suggests in fact that pharmacists know whether a policy exists but are not always clear what the policy is. The self-selection policy was instituted in Ontario, the province with the largest sample of respondents, only weeks before the study was conducted). A further analysis was conducted comparing actual provincial policy with availability of bleach kits and needle disposal. The availability of bleach kits and needle disposal were not significantly associated with the current provincial/territorial policy.

Discretion in Sales

Of the pharmacies that indicated that they would sell, 69.8% indicated that they would use some discretion in their decision to sell (i.e. would sell in some or most cases).

This subgroup were asked whether various aspects relating to the client and practice influenced their decision to sell. Figure 9 presents the proportion indicating each of five aspects to be a "very important" reason. In order of importance these were the sobriety of the client, characteristics of the client, familiarity with the client, presence of other customers and time of day.

Professional Thinking and Potential Role for Pharmacies

A number of questions were asked in order to examine the current thinking and roles that pharmacies might assume. Specifically these deal with willingness to provide and support services to injection drug users, perception of those factors that cause injection drug use, agreement with strategies for preventing the spread of HIV and future preventive interventions. As indicated earlier in this paper factor analyses were used to develop composite variables. The group mean scores for these composite variables are presented in the next four graphs.

Pharmacy-Based Services for Injection Drug Users

Figure 10 reflects the respondents' willingness and support for specific pharmacy-based services for injection drug users. The respondents were most willing to provide counselling and literature (including information on safer needle use) followed by sale of needle and syringes. They were least supportive of being part of a needle and syringe programme based in their pharmacy.

Agreement with Interventions to Prevent the Spread of HIV

With regard to various measures to prevent the spread of HIV, the respondents were most prepared to endorse control and compulsory measures (e.g., Compulsory HIV antibody testing), followed by punitive measures (e.g., abstinence should be goal of treatment, and possession of needles should be made a criminal offence) (see Figure 11). They were least likely to endorse to more relaxed legislation regarding drug use.

Perceptions of Factors Contributing to Injection Drug Use

The respondents perceived peer pressure to be the greatest contributing factor to injection drug use, followed by personal and social values and personal traits, as shown in Figure 12.

Endorsement of Future Preventive Interventions

In order of preference respondents were prepared to endorse first, environmental and technological measures (e.g., disposal units in parks and non-reusable needle and syringe technologies); second, exchanges in selected pharmacies; third, mobile drug needle exchange units; and finally, the legalization (prescription) of illicit drugs and methadone (see Figure 13).

Change in Professional Thinking About Non-Diabetic Injection of Drugs

Figure 14 summarizes the respondents' subjective opinion about injection drug use since the threat of AIDS. Slightly over one quarter (27.3%) indicated that there was no change in their opinion. Almost half, 47.6%, indicated that they were more tolerant, 12.4% indicated that they were less tolerant, 9.7% indicated that they were confused, and 2.3% gave other explanations.

SUMMARY AND CONCLUSIONS

The high response to this survey reflects the professional interest in issues presented by HIV. HIV/AIDS has presented pharmacists with one of the largest challenges to their professional training, ethics and practice. In response to HIV there have been dramatic changes in pharmacy practices. In view of the recent introduction of many of these it is likely that change will continue to occur.

Survey respondents were in general very comfortable with an expanded role involving counselling, health promotion and disease prevention consistent with an expanded role that has been advocated in recent years[13]. Safer needle use, as a part of a health promotion approach, is divergent from traditional practices. While major changes have occurred it also appears that there has been some polarization of attitudes and response. Explanation for this is not simple and in fact further analysis is required to determine the full impact from several ethical perspectives including: professional, business and public health.

The study highlights the role that policy and education have in moving toward a harm reduction approach. From a policy perspective this study has borne out that government, regulatory body and professional association support may be an important catalyst to pharmacies' participation in programmes[14]. Further, it does not appear to be possible to implement such policies without continuing education. Data on knowledge and educational need, not included in this report, suggests that the study population's lowest levels of information related to such areas as the role of methadone in HIV prevention, and availability of needle exchange programmes. As with other health promotion campaigns additional skills training may be important.[15]

Movement forward with harm reduction strategies by pharmacies will require careful planning. Incremental introduction of services into pharmacies appears to be necessary. It is understandable that not all pharmacies, because of individual circumstance, may be expected to participate in a comprehensive needle sales or exchange programme. Successful implementation will require extensive community development and collaboration with other health professionals, public health officials, police, groups representing injection drug users, and Persons Living with HIV. Careful monitoring and evaluation of these programmes will be necessary to enhance their effectiveness.

ACKNOWLEDGMENTS

This project was funded by the AIDS Education and Prevention Unit, through the National AIDS Contribution Programme under the National AIDS Strategy, Health Canada. Appreciation is expressed to the Advisory Committee and to the Provincial Licensing Bodies.

REFERENCES

1. HIV/AIDS Division, Laboratory Centre for Disease Control.(1993) *Quarterly Surveillance Update: AIDS in Canada* Ottawa: Health and Welfare Canada, July

2. Remis RS, Sutherland WD. (1993) The epidemiology of HIV and AIDS in Canada: current perspectives and future needs. *CJPH*; 84 (Suppl): 34-38.

3. Bardsley J, Turvey J, Blatherwick J. (1990) Vancouver's Needle Exchange Program *CJPH* 81 (1) 39 - 45.

4. Crichton A, Hsu D and Tsang S. (1990) *Canada's Health Care System: It's Funding and Organization* Ottawa: Canadian Hospital Association Press.

5. Single E, Erikson P, Skirrow J, and Solomon R. (1991) Policy Developments in Canada Paper presented at " The Window of Opportunity" congress Adelaide, Australia, December.

6. Usprich SJ and Solomon R (1990) Notes on the Potential Criminal Liability of a Needle Exchange Program *Health Law in Canada*. 42 - 48.

7. Riley D. (1990) *The legality of syringe exchanges in Ontario: Report to the City of Toronto Board of Health* October 4, 1990.

8. Health and Welfare Canada (1990) *Building an Effective Partnership: the Federal Government's Commitment to Fighting AIDS*. Ottawa: Ministry of Supply and Services Canada

9. Ontario College of Pharmacists Newsletters (June 22, 1987; April 18, 1988; April 1989; June 1992)

10. Millson M, Coates R, Rankin J, Myers T, McLaughlin B, Major C and Mindell W. *The Evaluation of a Program to Prevent Human Immunodeficiency Virus in Injection Drug Users in Toronto*. Final report presented to the City of Toronto Board of Health, September 1991.

11. Dillman DA. (1978) *Mail and telephone surveys: the Total Design method*. New York: Wiley and Sons.

12. Cockerill R and Williams P. (1989) *Report on the 1989 survey of the dispensing practices and attitudes toward prescription drugs*. Prepared for Pharmaceutical Inquiry of Ontario.

13. Fincham JE, Smith MC. (1988) Pharmacists' Views About Health Promotion Practices. *Journal of Community Health* 13 (2) 155-33.

14. Zulaica D, Menoyo C, Zubia I, Urcelay A, Linaza I and Elizada B. (1991) *The anti-AIDS kit: a year's experience*. VIIth International Conference of AIDS Florence, June.

15. Smith FJ, Salkind MR and Jolly BC (1990) Community Pharmacy: a Method for Assessing Quality of Care. *Social Science and Medicine*. 31 (5) 603 - 607.

Proportion of Reported AIDS Cases by Province/Territory in Canada

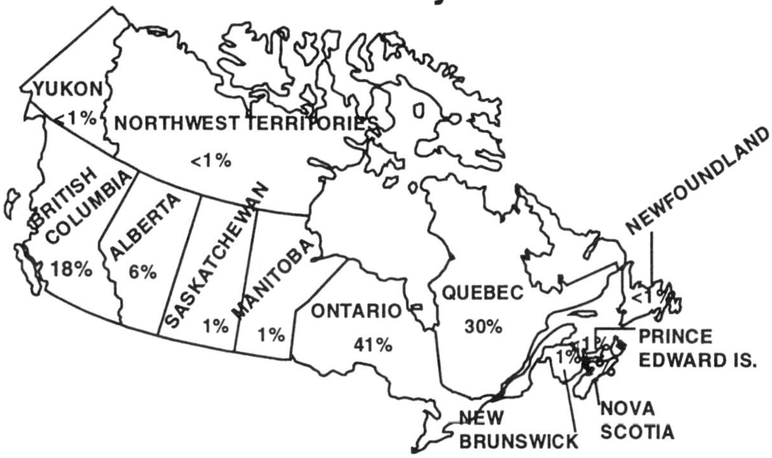

Current Policy by Province/Territory to Sale of Needles and Syringes in Canada

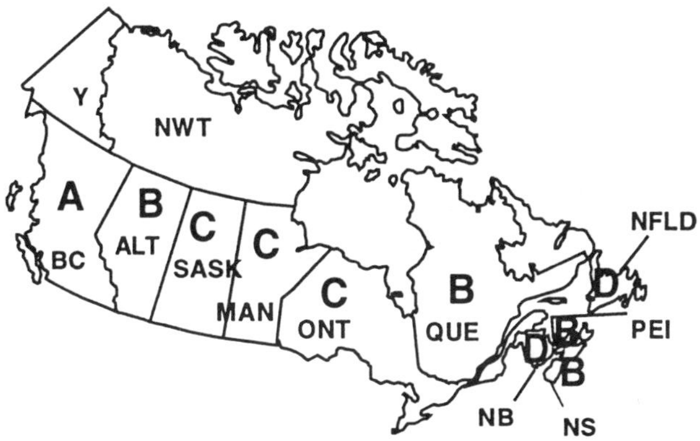

A=No sale B=Discretion C=Self-selection D=No Policy

Response by Province/Territory to Survey

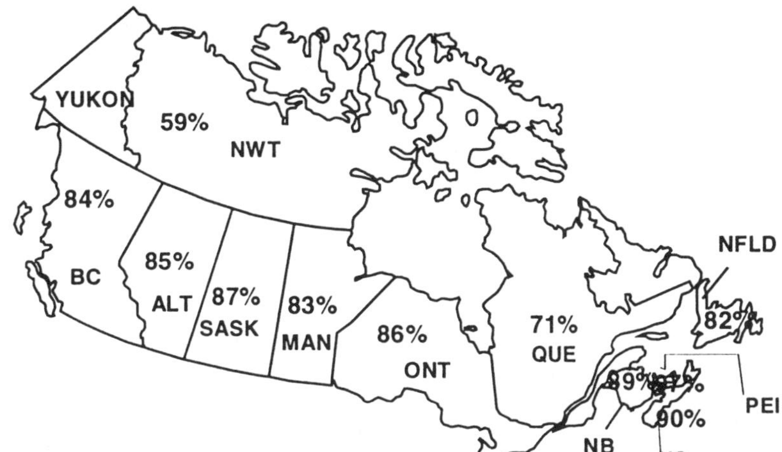

Proportion of Respondents Who Knew They Had Served A Person Living With HIV By Province/Territory

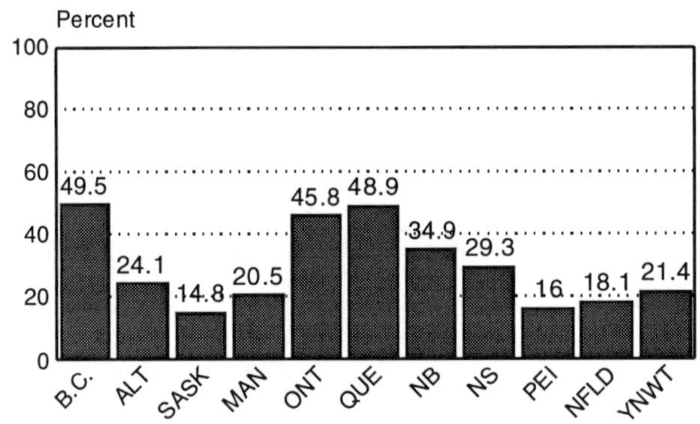

REQUESTS FOR NEEDLES AND SYRINGE SALES BY PROVINCE/TERRITORY

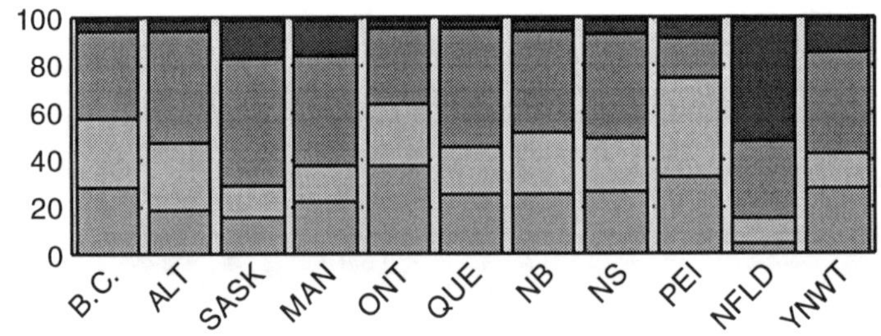

None	4.8	5.3	16.5	15	3.6	3.8	4.9	6.3	8.3	51.6	14.3
20 -	37.1	46.6	53.9	46.7	32.2	50	43.1	43.5	16.7	33.3	42.9
21-100	28.6	29	13.9	15.9	25.8	20.7	26.5	23.2	41.7	10.8	14.3
100+	29.5	19.1	15.7	22.4	38.4	25.5	25.5	26.8	33.3	4.3	28.5

Pharmacies' Response to Requests to Purchase Needles and Syringes

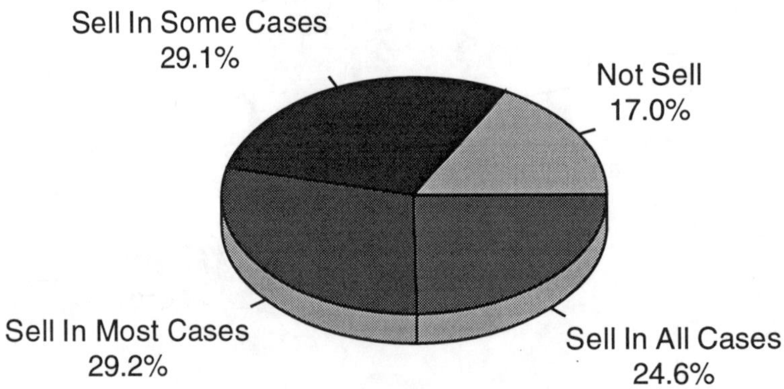

RESPONSE TO REQUESTS TO PURCHASE BY PROVINCE/TERRITORY

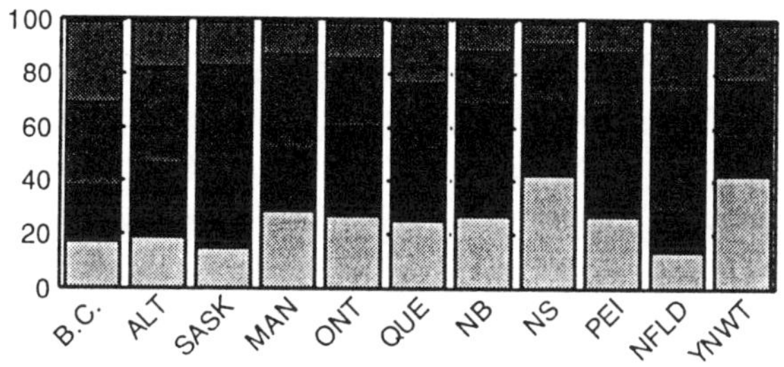

	B.C.	ALT	SASK	MAN	ONT	QUE	NB	NS	PEI	NFLD	YNWT
Not Sell	30.5	17.6	16.8	12.8	13.6	23.4	11.2	8.7	11.5	25.9	21.4
Sell some cases	31.4	35.9	39.8	34.9	25.3	25	19.6	20.9	19.2	44.7	21.4
Sell most cases	21	27.5	28.3	23.9	34.2	26.1	42.1	27.8	42.3	15.3	14.3
Sell all cases	17.1	19.1	15	28.4	26.8	25.5	27.1	42.6	26.9	14.1	42.9

Percent Who Sell Needles and Syringes by Provincial/Territorial Regulatory Policy

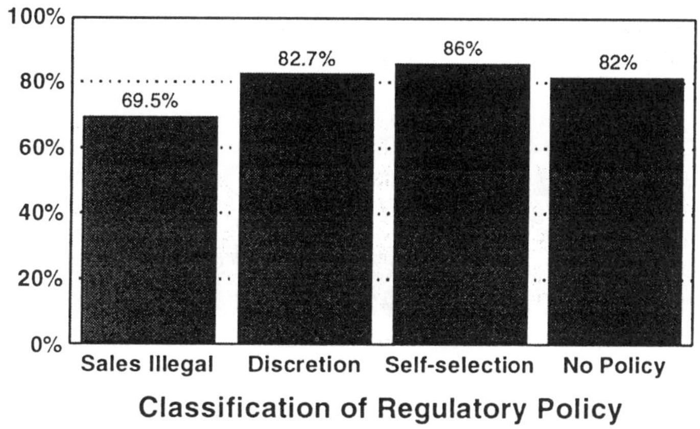

% Using Discretion Who Consider Specific Aspects "Very Important" in Decision to Sell Needles and Syringes

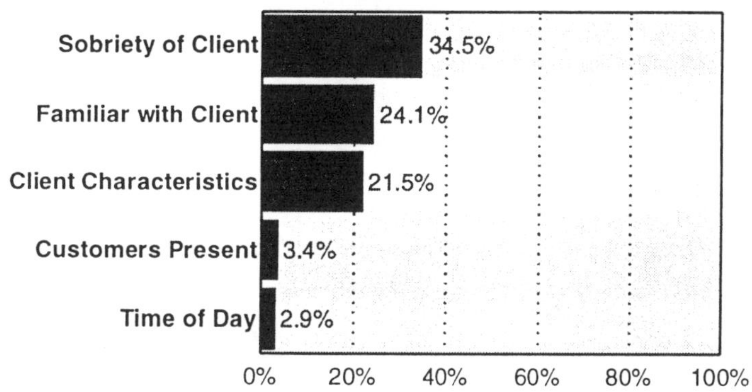

"Willingness and Support" for Provision of Pharmacy-Based Services to Injection Drug Users

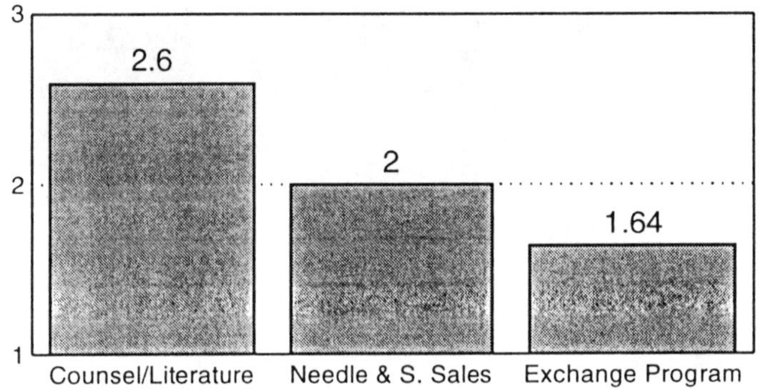

Group mean for composite variables developed from factor analysis)
(1 = Not at all willing/supportive, 3= Very willing/supportive)

Agreement with Interventions to Prevent the Spread of HIV

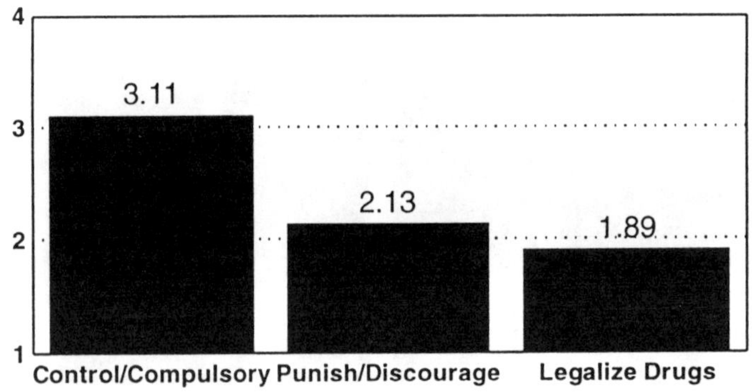

Group mean for composite variables developed from factor analysis)
(1 = Strongly Disagree, 4=Strongly Agree)

Factors Perceived to Contribute to Injection Drug Use.

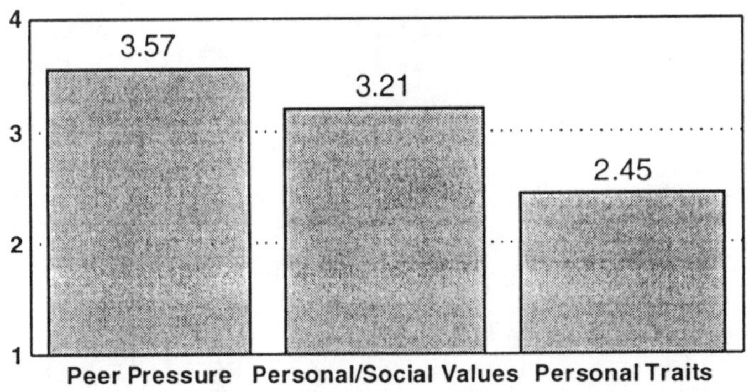

Group mean for composite variables developed from factor analysis)
(1 = Strongly Disagree, 4=Strongly Agree)

Endorsement of Future Preventive Interventions

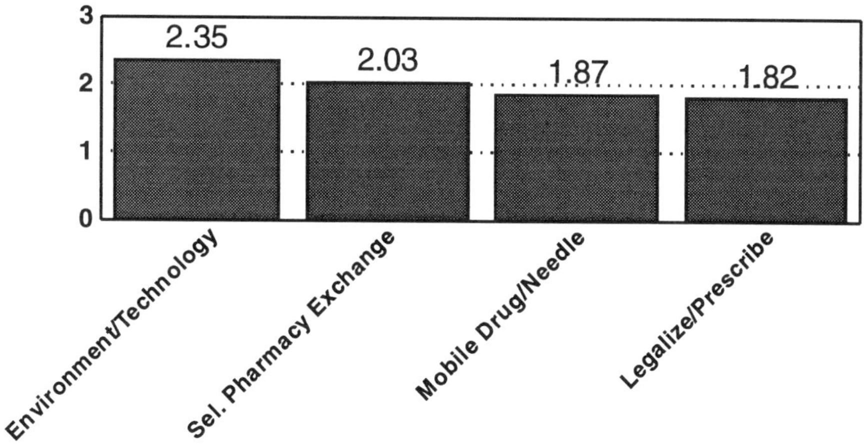

Group mean for composite variables developed from factor analysis)
(1 = Bad Idea, 2=Neither Good nor Bad, 3=Good Idea)

Change in Professional Thinking About Non-Diabetic Injection Drug Use Since AIDS

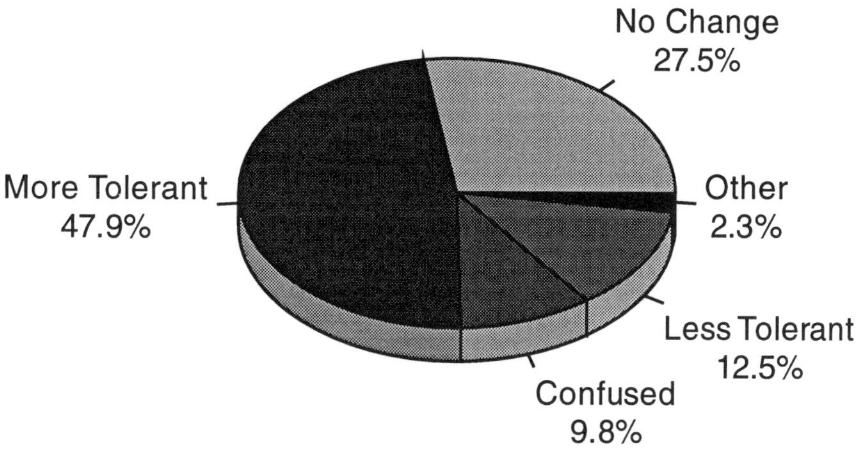

DISCUSSION: LEGAL ISSUES AND DRUG PARAPHERNALIA

LANE PORTER

Lane Porter commented on a number of major points brought out in the presentations. First, he observed, drug paraphernalia and needle prescription laws are often confused with one another, and it is important to understand the specific elements of each and how they can affect needle exchange programs. Second, in considering changes in drug paraphernalia laws, one must be clear about the objective being sought. There may well be some question as to whether such laws should be repealed or whether some modification of them is needed. Third, the presentation on the change in Connecticut's drug laws suggests that, once legal restrictions on the nonprescription purchase and possession of needles are removed, pharmacies will sell nonprescription needles to drug injectors. Fourth, the presentations on Connecticut and Canada point to the opportunities for pharmacists and other outlets to undertake other activities besides the selling of needles, for example, counseling, education, and providing a bridge to other social services.

During much of the workshop, Porter observed, there has been considerable discussion about the conflict between drug control strategies and efforts at harmonizing drug control and public health objectives. He said that consideration should be given to how the legal community can work with program planners in fashioning or enabling needle exchange programs that will be effective, well managed, and lawfully operated. In places in which needle exchange programs and pharmacy sale of needles are legal, it is important to consider experience in regard to the arrest of persons who supply needles on the grounds of aiding and abetting criminal activity. In New South Wales, for example, individuals must be affirmatively authorized to work in needle exchange programs, and such authorized persons are expressly exempt from the aiding and abetting provisions of the law.

Porter observed that zoning laws may also have an impact on the potential for needle exchange programs. The zoning requirements of local jurisdictions will definitely affect whether certain types of outlets will be permitted in a community. Finally, accreditation and licensing bodies also have a role to play. For example, he said, they should be considered in any establishment of training requirements for personnel involved in the distribution or sale of needles.

EVALUATION METHODS

ASSESSING THE EFFICACY OF NEEDLE EXCHANGE PROGRAMS: AN EPIDEMIOLOGICAL PERSPECTIVE

NOREEN V. HARRIS and JAMES P. MCGOUGH,
King County Department of Public Health, Seattle, Washington;
and NOEL S. WEISS, Department of Epidemiology, University of Washington

INTRODUCTION

In order to evaluate the efficacy of needle exchange programs, we must examine what they attempt to accomplish, and how they go about accomplishing it. Needle exchange programs have as their goal reducing the transmission of HIV (and other pathogens) among injection drug users. Such programs typically attempt to achieve their aims through three different kinds of interventions: first, the provision of materials such as sterile needles, bleach for syringe cleaning, and condoms; second, by providing education and information; and third, by referring clients to other interventions, such as drug treatment programs, social services, and medical care.

The success of all of these interventions may be achieved through behavior change. Freer access to sterile needles, bleach, and condoms may offer participants the materials necessary to adopt new, less-risky injection and sexual practices, and education may provide them with the motivation and skills necessary to make those changes. Drug treatment and access to social and medical services may decrease a drug-user's need to inject drugs, and so the number of times needles are shared.

It is also possible, however, that needle exchanges may be successful at reducing the transmission of HIV independently of changes in sharing patterns, if they reduce the likelihood that the needles that are shared are contaminated with HIV. In the absence of behavior change, such a reduction would take place if exchange programs either replaced a supply of contaminated needles with sterile ones or reduced "the number of people each needle shared" by shortening the circulation time of the average needle before it is replaced by a sterile one (Kaplan 1993). If a needle exchange program succeeded only in supplanting an existing supply of sterile needles, then there would be no reduction in the likelihood of their contamination with HIV.

CAUSAL INFERENCE

The evaluation of needle exchange programs involves a quest for evidence that needle exchanges caused a particular outcome of interest.

The development of causal hypotheses relies on an inductive approach which is commonly guided by a set of criteria (Hill 1965):

- Presence of an association, especially one that is consistent across studies.

- Presence of a strong association (i.e., a large relative risk). Weak associations may be causal, but are more likely than strong ones to be wholly the result of non-causal factors.

- A temporal relationship in which the putative cause precedes the effect.

- A gradient in the strength of the association that accords with predictions based on our biological, social, or psychological understandings of the issue (Weiss 1981).

- The plausibility of a causal relationship on other, non-epidemiological, grounds.

After the development of causal hypotheses, a deductive approach is followed in which predictions arising from those hypotheses are subjected to empirical tests. While we cannot "prove" causal hypotheses, we can (in principle) refute them. Hypotheses not falsified by the data at hand are "confirmed" in that they remain reasonably good explanations until they are falsified by new data, and are replaced by other hypotheses that better explain the observations (Popper 1965; Rothman 1986).

OUTCOMES OF INTEREST

Outcomes Related to Reducing Risk of HIV Transmission

In order to determine if needle exchange programs succeed in their aim of reducing the parenteral and sexual risk of HIV transmission among injection drug users, one could measure the prevalence or incidence of HIV, the behavioral predictors of HIV transmission, surrogate measures of those behaviors, or the number of different persons sharing individual needles.

HIV

There are two means of determining whether or not an individual has acquired HIV or any other parenterally or sexually transmitted infection during a specific time period. One could establish whether or not seroconversion occurred between baseline and follow-up testing <u>or</u>, when only one test is done, the presence of short-lived antibodies or antigens can in principle serve as markers of recent infection (Hart et al. 1989; van den Hoek et al. 1989; Nelson et al. 1991; Kaplan et al. 1991; van Ameijden et al. 1992).

Behavior

Some of the parenteral behaviors associated with HIV infection which could be measured include: "sharing" of injection equipment (the word here meaning injecting with needles after their use by others); sharing of injection equipment without effective cleaning; sharing with high-risk individuals; and the frequency of injection with uncleaned shared equipment (Donoghoe et al. 1989; van Ameijden et al. 1992; Guydish 1993).

Some of the sexual behaviors related to HIV infection which could be measured include: sex with multiple partners; sex without condoms; and sex with high-risk partners (Donoghoe et al. 1989; Stimson et al. 1989; Hart et al. 1989).

Surrogate Measures of HIV

Serological or other clinical evidence of recent acquisition of parenterally-transmitted or sexually-transmitted diseases other than HIV may serve to indicate that individuals were involved in high-risk activities that could also transmit HIV (van Haastrecht et al. 1991; Brettle 1991).

Number of Persons Sharing Each Syringe

Even in the absence of significant change in the propensity to share needles, a needle exchange might reduce the number of people who share the average needle. The fewer people sharing a needle, the smaller the chances of that needle becoming infected with HIV, and so the lower the risks of disease transmission. One could, in principle, measure the number of sharers directly, measure the average time that needles spend in circulation in a community (Donoghoe et al. 1989; Kaplan 1993), or measure syringe barrel wear as a surrogate of syringe use (Smith et al. 1981).

Outcomes Related to Injection Drug Use

It is possible that needle exchange programs promote drug use by "condoning" it, by making drug injection easier, or by fostering the initiation of new drug injectors. On the other hand, needle exchange programs might lead to a reduction in drug use by facilitating entry to drug treatment, or by supporting users in stopping or reducing injection. The mere presence of needle exchange programs might convince injectors of the seriousness of the HIV epidemic, and of the need to reduce or stop drug use to avoid AIDS.

Possible measures of drug use include initiation or cessation of injection, changes in the frequency of injection, and a shift to non-injection modes of drug use (U.S. General Accounting Office 1993).

POTENTIAL RELATIONSHIPS OF EXPOSURE TO OUTCOME

The impact of needle exchange might be related to the duration, recency, or directness of an individual's exposure to the exchange. Choice of a particular model or models of the possible relationship between exposure and outcome will have an important influence on the selection of appropriate measures of exposures and outcomes.

Duration Can Be Modelled in a Number of Different Ways

The One-Hit Model

Patrons of the exchange might achieve benefit after a single exposure. This model reflects what might happen if the very existence of the exchange alerted clients to the risk of AIDS, and convinced them to stop sharing needles or to stop using drugs. To assess such an impact, it would be necessary to classify participants in terms of past exchange use (ever *versus* never) and to measure the relevant outcomes after exposure to needle exchange (or in the cases of non-exchangers, during a comparable time period).

The Threshold Model

The effect of needle exchange might manifest itself only after a sufficient minimum number of repeated exposures. For example, it may be the case that outreach workers staffing the exchange table develop a rapport with clients, and earn their trust, only after a certain number of exchange encounters. It also might well be the case that the success of various risk-reduction educational and other interventions would be dependent on the development of that rapport and trust, and so require a certain number of needle exchange visits.

The Dose-Response Model

An effect of needle exchange might be related to the total amount of exposure; the effect might increase with increasing frequency, duration, or intensity of exposure, with no threshold level of exposure.

Recency of Exchange Might Also Be Modelled in Different Ways

Latency of Effects

In some cases the effects might be immediate, while in others a specified latent period might be required before benefit or harm accrues (Schlesselman 1982). If effects were immediate, a study that compared repeat exchangers to non-exchangers would not be able to detect any differences between them if the benefit from the exchange manifested itself right after the first visit.

Transience of Effects

The effects of needle exchange might be either permanent or transient. A change to lower-risk behavior might, for example, not persist as the novelty of the needle exchange intervention wanes, leading to "relapses" to higher-risk activity.

Directness of Effects

It is possible, particularly in communities with large-volume needle exchanges, that indirect effects might be of importance. Non-exchangers might derive "herd immunity" from needles and education provided them by those who are exchangers. In such circumstances, observational studies of individuals may not be able to tease out the effects of needle exchange without collecting data on sources of needles and information among both needle exchangers and non-exchangers. In this case it may also be more difficult to demonstrate an association between needle exchange and HIV risk. Direct and indirect effects might be in operation at the same time, of course, and they may have different impacts on different outcomes. As far as we know, all studies of individuals have looked only at direct effects.

STUDY DESIGN

There have been numerous attempts to glean information on the effect of needle exchange programs from surveys that do not include comparable, concurrently sampled, control groups (Donoghoe et al. 1989; Kaplan et al. 1991; Klee et al. 1991; Nelson et al. 1991; Guydish et al. 1993). Unfortunately, it is not possible on the basis of such surveys to assess whether or not the presence of a needle exchange is associated with the occurrence of HIV or the behaviors associated with HIV, let alone whether any presumed associations are <u>causal</u> in nature. Observations provided by these surveys can be suggestive of causation, but not conclusive.

Controlled epidemiological studies of the efficacy of exchange programs may consist of studies of populations or of individuals, and each type of study can be conduced as either an observational study or an experimental trial. No study design (epidemiological or otherwise) is without its strengths and potential shortcomings.

Observational Studies of Populations ("Ecologic Studies")

The unit of study in this design is a population or community of injection drug users. For example, the occurrence of HIV in communities with needle exchange programs might be compared with that in communities without needle exchanges. Such studies are relatively inexpensive, and often can be completed quickly when they rely on extant data. Differences observed, however, may not be due to the exposure of interest, but rather to differences in the populations or communities being compared. Because the number of communities under study is usually small, there is limited ability to examine other reasons for any differences in rates that are present in the different populations.

For example, Ljungberg et al. (1991) reported an HIV prevalence of 1% among injection drug users in Skäne, a southern province of Sweden which is served by needle exchange programs in the towns of Lund and Mälmo. By contrast, HIV prevalence among a injection drug users sampled in Copenhagen (a 45 minute ferry boat ride away from Lund) was 15%, among amphetamine injectors in Stockholm it was 4-6%, and among heroin injectors in Stockholm it was 45-60%. Neither Copenhagen or Stockholm are served by needle exchange programs. As the investigators acknowledged, there could well be differences other than the presence or absence of needle exchange programs which could account for the observed variation in HIV prevalence. Copenhagen is a large and cosmopolitan city, while Lund is a relatively small rural university town. Within Sweden, Stockholm has a concentration of heroin users (Käll 1992), many among whom are HIV-positive immigrants from high-incidence areas abroad (Kerstin Käll, Karolinska Institute, personal communication 1993).

The role of needle exchange in causing a reduction in HIV occurrence would be supported by large differences in HIV associated with needle exchange; demonstrated comparability between the exchange and non-exchange populations with respect to other predictors of HIV; and samples of communities large enough to enable statistical stability and the assessment of potential confounding.

For example, it would be difficult to interpret a comparison of HIV prevalence among injection drug users in Salt Lake City (which does not have a needle exchange program) with a population of injectors in New York City (which does have a needle exchange) because the two communities differ with respect to the timing of the epidemic and many demographic, sociologic, and cultural factors which may be predictors of HIV occurrence. However, comparisons of injection drug users among comparable New York City and New Jersey communities with and without exchanges, could possibly provide more valid evidence for a possible relationship of needle exchange programs to HIV transmission.

Experimental Trials of Populations (Community Intervention Trials)

Community intervention trials involve choosing a large number of communities, and then randomly or systematically assigning needle exchange programs to some number of the communities. No such trial has been attempted. If the number of communities were sufficiently large, random assignment of communities to needle exchange could achieve comparability with respect to the predictors of HIV. However, if a small number of communities are selected, the randomization process may not achieve such comparability. With an intervention as controversial as needle exchange, random assignment of communities may not be possible, and if it were, "contamination" of the comparison communities might be hard to prevent.

Observational Studies of Individuals

In these studies, the unit of study is the individual, and the sample size is the number of individuals who participated. There are three types of observational studies of individuals; cross-sectional, case-control, and cohort studies.

Cross-Sectional Studies

Many studies of needle exchange are essentially cross-sectional in nature. In such studies, the exposure (in this case needle exchange use) and the outcomes (e.g., HIV infection) are measured at the same point in time. Cross-sectional studies are usually less expensive than other observational studies, and can often be completed in relatively short time periods. The chief limitation of cross-sectional studies of needle exchange is the inability to determine which came first; the exposure (to needle exchange) or the outcome (for instance, HIV infection or behavior change).

For example, in prevalence surveys among injection drug users entering drug treatment programs, we found that HIV prevalence was higher among those who patronized the needle exchange than among those who did not (Harris et al., n.d.). From these data alone, it is not clear whether knowledge of HIV positivity led people to use the exchange, or exchange use led to acquisition of HIV infection.

Case-Control Studies

In a case-control study, the investigator compares a group with a particular outcome (for example, newly acquired HIV infections) with a comparable group of controls without the outcome (those free of HIV infection), to determine whether or not the groups differ with respect to exposure to needle exchange in the past (prior to acquiring HIV infection, or, in the case of controls, prior to a concurrent time period). Case-control studies, like cross-sectional studies, are less expensive and more quickly completed than are cohort studies. However, if the study requires asking subjects to recall past events, their inaccuracy in doing so may lead to a biased result. Also, in a case-control study it care must be taken to establish that the outcome truly followed exposure to needle exchange, and did not precede it.

For example, we conducted a case-control analysis in which we interviewed 2,500 drug injectors in Seattle, systematically recruited in a variety of settings. We defined as cases those who in the 12 months before interview either increased or maintained injecting with non-sterile needles, and we defined as controls those who either decreased or continued not to do so. We then compared the proportion of cases and of controls who had used a needle exchange prior to the 12 month period for which outcomes were measured, to clearly establish a temporal sequence between exposure to the exchange and injection behavior outcomes.

Cohort Studies

In a cohort study, the investigator classifies individuals with respect to exposure and follows them over time to assess subsequent outcomes. Cohort studies generally afford a greater opportunity to evaluate the temporal sequence between needle exchange use and the outcomes of interest than do other observational designs. Aside from the expense and the length of time it takes to complete them, a major consideration in conducting cohort studies, particularly of cohort studies of injection drug users, is the importance of maximizing follow-up.

A cohort study was conducted by Hartgers et al. (1989) in which they interviewed 72 injection drug users in Amsterdam who usually obtained their needles from an exchange, and 73 injection drug users who never or only irregularly used the exchange. A second interview was administered one year later.

If those who are successfully followed in a cohort study differ from those not followed, study findings may be distorted because observed differences in outcome between the exposed and the non-exposed might be due to factors connected with follow-up instead of, or in addition to, differences in the exposures of interest. The authors of the Amsterdam cohort study note that only 49% of exchangers, and even fewer non-exchangers (34%), returned for the follow-up interview, and that those successfully followed differed in important ways from those not followed. The differences between those followed and those not followed could conceivably account for the differences in outcome that they observed between exchangers and non-exchangers.

Experimental Trials of Individuals

In a randomized trial of the impact of a needle-exchange program, participants would be randomly assigned to either needle exchange or to no intervention (or to a different intervention). Subjects would be followed over time, just as in a cohort study, to determine subsequent outcomes. The advantage to such studies is that they avoid the distortion in results that might occur if those who self-select to attend a needle exchange program differ from those who don't with respect to risk behaviors. In fact, however, it may not be ethically, politically, or logistically feasible to assign some individuals to needle exchange and prevent others from attending, and as far as we know, no experimental trials have been carried out.

ISSUES OF METHODOLOGICAL BIAS

In epidemiologic studies, bias is present when the observed association between exposure and outcome does not accurately portray the (theoretical) true association. Although the lines between them are occasionally hard to draw, it is useful to consider three general categories of bias: confounding; selection; and information bias.

Confounding

Confounding is the distortion of the true association (or lack thereof) between an exposure and an outcome that is caused by the presence of another exposure or characteristic which also leads to the outcome of interest. In order for a factor to confound, it must be associated both with the outcome and with the exposure.

Sexual behavior (particularly male homosexual behavior) is an example of a potentially confounding factor which should be considered in studies of the impact of needle exchange on the risk of HIV. If men who have sex with men are either more or less likely than others to patronize needle exchange programs (that is, if male homosexuality is associated with the exposure), studies which fail to deal with this fact in design, sampling, or analysis could be confounded and so biased in their results. Nonetheless, few studies of needle exchange have controlled for such behavior.

An example of a study which did is that of Nelson et al. (1991), in which the investigators considered in the analysis the potential confounding effects of receptive anal intercourse in their study of the relationship of diabetes (who have access to sterile needles) to HIV prevalence among injection drug users.

There are a number of ways to deal with the problem of confounding.

- In design, one can match or stratify on potential confounders.

- In sampling, one can recruit index and comparison groups from the same underlying target populations in a representative (probabilistic) fashion.

- In analysis, one can conduct stratified, logistic regression, or other multivariate analyses which incorporate information on potential confounding factors and thus, permit assessment of, and adjustment for, bias resulting from confounding. Such analyses are possible, of course, only if relevant data on potential confounders have been collected.

Recently, investigators have begun to consider the effect of potential confounding factors in the evaluation of needle exchange programs.

For example, van Ameijden et al. (1992) investigated sex, date of intake visit, borrowing, intake site, and injection frequency as potential confounding factors and found it necessary to adjust for the latter variable when examining the effect of needle exchange.

Selection Bias

Rothman (1986; after Greenland 1977) states that selection bias occurs when "the relation between exposure and disease is different for those who participate and those who would be theoretically eligible for the study but do not participate".

We assessed HIV prevalence among STD clinic patients sampled in three ways: those who self-selected by requesting HIV counseling and testing; those who agreed to participate in a cross-sectional HIV prevalence survey offered to a systematic sample of patients; and the total STD clinic patient roster (through a "blinded" survey of leftover blood samples from all clients). As can been seen in Figure 1, which compares the findings from the three samples among gay and bisexual men, we found that the more the sample reflected self-selection, the lower the prevalence of HIV.

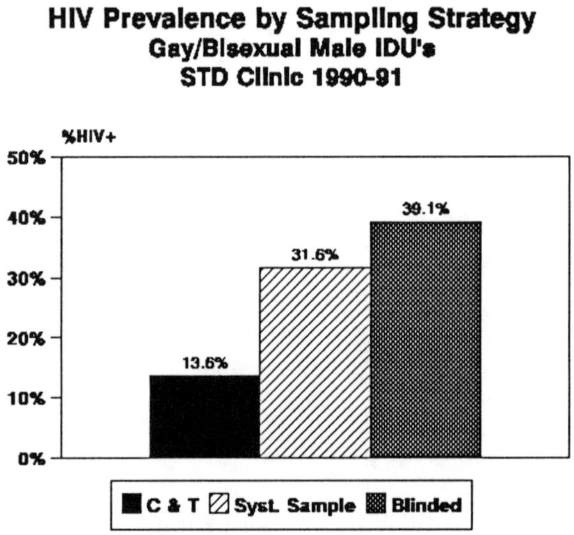

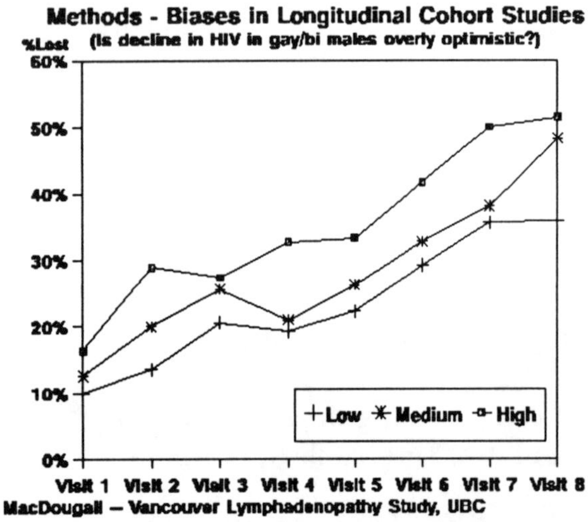

It is common in longitudinal studies that those who return for follow-up differ from those who don't. McDougall et al. (1991) followed gay and bisexual men over time, to measure HIV seroconversion. They divided the participants into high-risk, medium-risk, and low-risk groups based on behavior reported at baseline. By its end, only 50% of the high risk group remained in the study, compared to 70% of the low- risk group (see Figure 2). The investigators observed a declining HIV incidence among study participants, but note that the greater loss to follow-up of participants at greater risk may have biased the findings, possibly masking a true increase in HIV incidence.

As with confounding, there are strategies available for minimizing selection bias. One can:

- Define and represent the target population (or a sub-set of the population) for both index and comparison groups;

- Compare participants and non-participants on any baseline characteristics for which there are data; and

- Estimate the likely impact of non-participation on the findings.

As an example, Hart et al. (1989) compared study participants and non-participants on a number of relevant variables, and reported no substantial differences between them (although the study was small, and the statistical power to detect differences may have been limited). Another example of efforts to minimize selection bias can be found in van Ameijden et al. (1993).

Information Bias

Such error occurs when either exposure or outcomes are misclassified (when study information is incorrect). If such error occurs differentially across the index and comparison groups, the result would be either an exaggeration or an underestimation of the effect of needle exchange on the outcomes of interest.

For example, if exchangers were under greater pressure than non-exchangers to display socially desirable risk-reduction behavior (Kaplan et al. 1991), and so under-reported risky acts, the impact would be to overestimate the effect of needle exchange on risk behavior.

As another example, if exchangers were interviewed by one team of interviewers, and non-exchangers were interviewed by another team (as was done by Donoghoe et al. 1989), it is at least conceivable that team differences in training, style, attitude, or other factors might lead to differential misclassification error and so to bias.

If information error is non-differential across exposure or outcome categories the bias will be towards the null hypotheses (that is, towards the hypothesis that there is no effect of exposure on outcome).

For example, case-control studies often rely upon the ability of cases and controls to recall earlier experiences. If both have equal difficulty doing so, the misclassification error would be non-differential, and the resulting bias would be towards the null hypothesis.

An important source of measurement error is imprecision in the questions that are asked of study subjects.

For example, in a case-control analysis of the impact of needle exchange, using extant data from a number of different studies, we were limited to existing questions common to those studies. Such questions tended to be simple and imprecise. Knowing that respondents said "yes" to the question "In the past year, did you use bleach to clean needles before you shot up?" was not very helpful, because that answer didn't reveal whether they cleaned every time, half the time, most of the time, or every time they shot up.

Inadvertent measurement error may occur if, after data collection is complete, the investigators wish to consider a new and different model of the putative relationship between exposure and outcome.

Donoghoe et al. (1989) measured behavior change two to four months after initial exchange use. Measurement of outcomes over such short time frames would allow one to assess immediate effects, but would not allow assessment of a long-term effects.

Apart from striving for precision in measurement, one can attempt validation of self-reported exposure and outcome measures. It is also important to carefully consider models of the relationships between exposures and outcomes, and measure each in a manner appropriate to those models.

STATISTICAL POWER AND MEASURES OF PROBABILITY

Evaluation studies of needle exchange need statistical power sufficient to detect changes in outcomes that may be relatively modest in absolute terms, but are still of interest in terms of slowing the epidemic of HIV. For example, small studies that indicate only small, statistically insignificant differences in the frequency of drug use between persons who do and do not use a needle exchange may, because of their limited power, be missing a true effect of public health importance (Hart et al., 1989).

Other considerations affect power and sample size issues as well. Rare outcomes and rare exposures demand larger sample sizes, as may losses to follow-up and changes in exposure status in longitudinal studies (as when non-exchangers at baseline have become exchangers by follow-up). A larger sample size will also be required if one hopes to examine the possibility of modification of effect across subgroups.

In Seattle, for example, we have found that participation in the needle exchange and the risk of HIV infection both vary by drug of choice. If needle exchange had a different impact among heroin injectors than it did among amphetamine injectors, this modification of effect might be missed if the numbers of subjects in each group were too small, and missing it could result in under-estimation over-estimation of the efficacy of the exchange.

Measures of probability, especially p-values, have the narrow purpose of eliminating chance as an explanation for observed associations. A better approach to the analysis of association is to use estimates of relative risks (or odds ratios), and confidence intervals around those estimates. These measures provide an estimate of the strength and direction of the association, and the precision of the estimate.

GENERALIZABILITY

As noted above, when assessing a study of needle exchange, we can ask the following questions:

> Is there an association between needle exchange exposure and the outcomes of interest?
>
> Is the association likely to be due to chance, due to bias, or to causation?

If a causal interpretation is possible, we can ask ourselves about the extent to which the results might pertain to populations beyond the one studied. The results of a study of an officially-sanctioned needle exchange in a large metropolitan area on the east coast might not have much relevance to an un-sanctioned exchange operating in a small city in the midwest.

FUTURE NEEDS

We need to know just what effects needle exchange programs have, how they have their effects, and among which sub-groups they have their greatest effects. The best epidemiological evidence pertaining to these questions will be afforded by large, statistically powerful, well-designed, observational case-control or cohort studies. While randomized clinical trials might offer even stronger evidence of the impact of needle exchange programs, ethical, political, and logistic considerations weigh heavily against their ever being carried out.

This does not mean that we should wait until such studies are completed until we decide to support needle exchange programs in the face of the HIV epidemic. According to Bradford Hill:

> All scientific work is incomplete -- whether it be observational or experimental. All scientific work is liable to be upset or modified by advancing knowledge. That does not confer upon us a freedom to ignore the knowledge we already have, or to postpone the action that it appears to demand at a given time.

ACKNOWLEDGMENTS

The authors would like to thank Gail Hansen and Jan Fields (both of the Seattle - King County Department of Public Health) for their assistance, knowledge, and patience.

REFERENCES

van Ameijden ECJ et al., 1992, The Harm Reduction Approach and Risk Factors for Human Immunodeficiency Virus (HIV) Seroconversion in Injecting Drug Users, Amsterdam, *American Journal of Epidemiology*, 136(2):236-243.

van Ameijden ECJ et al., 1993, AA Major Decline in Risk Behavior Over 6 Years Among IDUs, IXth International Conference on AIDS, Berlin, WS-C21-2.

Brettle RP, 1991, HIV and harm reduction for injection drug users, *AIDS*, 5:125-136.

Donoghoe MC et al., 1989, Changes in HIV risk behavior in clients of syringe-exchange schemes in England and Scotland, *AIDS*, 3(5):267-272.

Greenland S, 1977, Response and follow-up bias in cohort studies *American Journal of Epidemiology* 106:184-187.

Guydish J et al., Evaluating needle exchange: are there negative effects? *AIDS*, 7(6):871-876.

van Haastrecht HJA et al., 1991, The Course of the HIV Epidemic among Intravenous Drug Users in Amsterdam, The Netherlands, *American Journal of Public Health*, 81(1):59-62.

Harris N et al., n.d. The impact of Seattle's needle exchange program in behaviors associated with HIV transmission. Unpublished manuscript.

Hart GJ et al., 1989, Evaluation of needle exchange in central London: behaviour change and anti-HIV status over one year, *AIDS*, 3(5):261-265.

Hartgers C et al., 1989, The impact of the needle and syringe-exchange programme in Amsterdam on injecting risk behaviour, *AIDS*, 3(9):571-576.

Hill AB, 1965, The environment and disease: Association or Causation? *Proceedings of the Royal Society of Medicine*, 58:295-300.

van den Hoek JAR et al., 1989, Risk Reduction among Intravenous Drug Users in Amsterdam under the Influence of AIDS, *American Journal of Public Health* 79(10):1355-1357.

Käll K, 1992, Effects of Amphetamine on Sexual Behavior of Male IV Drug Users in Stockholm--A Pilot Study, *AIDS Education and Prevention*, 4(1):6-17.

Kaplan EH, 1993, Let the Needles Do the Talking! Evaluating the New Haven Needle Exchange, *Interfaces*, 23.

Kaplan EH, 1991, Evaluating Needle-Exchange Programs via Syringe Tracking and Testing (STT), *AIDS & Public Policy J*, 6(3):109-115.

Klee H et al., 1991, The sharing of injecting equipment among drug users attending prescribing clinics and those using needle-exchanges, *British Journal of Addiction*, 86:217-223.

Ljungberg B et al., 1991, HIV Prevention Among Injecting Drug Users: Three Years of Experience from a Syringe Exchange Program in Sweden, *Journal of the Acquired Immune Deficiency Syndromes*, 4:890-895.

McDougall L et al., 1991, Bias in AIDS cohort studies and an empiric demonstration of Volunteer Bias in an Investigation of Homosexual Men, VII International Conference on AIDS, Florence, W.C. 95.

Nelson KE, 1991, Human Immunodeficiency Virus Infection in Diabetic Intravenous Drug Users, *Journal of the American Medical Association*, 266(16):2259-2261.

Office of National Drug Control Policy, 1992, Needle Exchange Programs: Are They Effective? *ONDCP Bulletin* No. 7.

Popper KR, 1965, *The Logic of Scientific Discovery*, New York, Harper & Row.
Rothman, KJ, 1986, *Modern Epidemiology*, Little, Boston/Toronto, Brown and Company.

Schlesselman JJ, 1982, *Case-Control Studies: Design, Conduct, Analysis*, Oxford University Press, New York, Oxford.

Smith A et al., 1991, Evaluation of the needle exchange program in Darwin, *Venereology*, 4(2):76.

Stimson GV et al., 1989, Syringe exchange schemes: a report and some commentaries, *British Journal of Addiction*, 84:1283-1290.

U.S. General Accounting Office, 1993, Needle Exchange Programs; Research Suggests Promise as an AIDS Prevention Strategy, Report to the Chairman, Select Committee on Narcotics Abuse and Control, House of Representatives, GAO/HRD-93-60.

Weiss NS, 1981, Inferring causal relationships; Elaboration of the criterion of "dose-response", *American Journal of Epidemiology*, 113:487-490.

AN EVALUATION OF NEEDLE AND SYRINGE EXCHANGE IN SAN FRANCISCO

John K. Watters, Urban Health Study, Institute for Health Policy Studies, and Department of Family and Community Medicine, School of Medicine, University of California, San Francisco;
Michelle J. Estilo, College of Physicians and Surgeons, Columbia University;
George L. Clark, Prevention Point Research Group, San Francisco, California; and
Jennifer Lorvick, Urban Health Study, Institute for Health Policy Studies, School of Medicine, University of California, San Francisco

INTRODUCTION

The sharing of contaminated injection paraphernalia is a major route for transmission of human immunodeficiency virus (HIV) in the United States (1-3) and is one of the principal means by which HIV infection has spread in Italy, Spain, and Thailand (1, 4). In the U.S., one quarter (24%) of the 310,780 AIDS cases diagnosed among adults and adolescents through June, 1993 occurred among heterosexual injection drug users (IDUs). An additional 3.5% (10,800) were adults whose sole risk factor was having a sexual partner who injected drugs. Over half (56.2%) of the pediatric AIDS cases diagnosed in the U.S. through June, 1993, were attributed to HIV transmission from mothers who injected drugs themselves or who engaged in sexual activity with injection drug users (5). It is estimated that there are 1.2 million IDUs in the United States, about 15% of whom are believed to be enrolled in drug treatment on any day (6). Successful prevention of further spread of HIV in this population is crucial to national infectious disease prevention objectives (7). An unknown number of Americans in these risk categories are infected with HIV.

In an effort to reduce the sharing of injection equipment, programs have been established which provide sterile needles and syringes to drug users in exchange for their used equipment. Previous studies have reported that syringe exchange programs have played a significant role in lowering rates of needle-sharing in Amsterdam, (8, 9); Sweden (10); Australia (11); the United Kingdom (12-14); Tacoma, Washington (15); New Haven, CT (16); and New York City (17, 18). Other studies have reported that syringe exchange programs have served as sources of referrals into social services, medical services and drug treatment (16, 19). In New Haven, researchers reported that new HIV infections among clients of a legal syringe exchange had been reduced by one-third (17).

Opponents of syringe exchange have claimed that these programs will facilitate and therefore increase illicit drug injection. We conducted a study to determine whether syringe exchange is harmful or beneficial as risk reduction for injection drug users. We evaluated an all-volunteer syringe exchange program in San Francisco, CA known as "Prevention Point." Estimates of the number of injection drug users in San Francisco, range from 13,000 to 16,000 in a city of approximately 740,000. The daily census in drug abuse treatment programs in San Francisco is approximately 1,500 individuals. Waiting lists for publicly supported drug treatment slots exist in virtually all clinics.

Three research questions relevant to the health policy debate regarding syringe exchange were used as evaluation criteria: (1) how readily and to what degree has the syringe exchange been used by IDUs; (2) to what degree has syringe exchange stimulated injection drug use through increased injection frequency and recruitment of new users; and (3) to what degree is the use of syringe exchange predictive of abstinence from syringe sharing?

METHODS

Data Sources and Sampling

Data for the study were derived from two sources: (1) the Urban Health Study, a semi-annual survey of IDUs in San Francisco; and (2) Prevention Point syringe exchange program records. The Urban Health Study is a semi-annual cross-sectional study of IDUs recruited in natural settings in three inner-city communities in San Francisco. During the 1987 through 1989 cross-sections, respondents were also sampled in two 21-day drug detoxification clinics. Communities chosen for study were selected for high densities of IDUs relative to other San Francisco neighborhoods as indicated by review of drug treatment program admissions, drug arrest data, and ethnographic studies. All respondents were screened for visible signs of repeated drug injection. After the purpose of the study was explained, and informed consent obtained, respondents were interviewed using a standard questionnaire dealing with AIDS knowledge; medical, drug use, and sexual histories; and known HIV/AIDS risk behaviors. Interviews were conducted by trained interviewers employed by the Urban Health Study. Respondents were paid for their participation, given pretest and posttest counseling, and given referrals to medical and social services by trained staff. In the present study, we used eleven semi-annual cross-sectional surveys collected as part of the Urban Health Study, between January 1987 and June 1992 (n=6216). Excluded from further analysis were 572 respondents who reported no current injection drug use. The number of interviews included for each of the cross-sections were as follows: Spring 1987, n=596; Fall 1987, n=576; Spring 1988, n=598; Fall 1988, n=607; Spring 1989, n=505; Fall 1989, n=503; Spring 1990, n=411; Fall 1990, n=460; Spring 1991, n=456; Fall 1991, n=459; Spring 1992, n=473.

"Prevention Point" is a volunteer-based syringe exchange program which began operating in November 1988 on a San Francisco street corner, and in a second neighborhood using a "mobile" team. The mobile team used a baby perambulator to deliver necessary supplies to a neighborhood that contained many homeless persons. Additional street corner sites were added in May, 1989; September, 1990; and December, 1991. In September, 1992, the original mobile team was reassigned to two different fixed locations. During the study period, all exchange sites operated during evening hours

(6:00 to 8:00 pm). While technically illegal, the Prevention Point program has operated without major disruption from police and with the tacit approval of two successive mayoral administrations. Program volunteers provide a strict one-for-one exchange in which a sterile, single-use, 27.5-gauge, 0.5 inch, 1 cc, U-100 insulin syringe is exchanged for each syringe deposited in a Sharps biohazardous waste container by the client. Limitations on the number of syringes program clients were permitted to exchange have changed over the course of the study. Prior to May, 1989 a ten syringes per client visit limit was in effect. Between May 1989 and August 1990, this limit was increased to twenty syringes per client visit. In August, 1990 all limits on the number of syringes that could be exchanged were abandoned. Volunteers also distribute one-ounce bottles of bleach, condoms, cotton, and alcohol wipes, and provide referrals to drug treatment, HIV testing and counseling and other social and medical services upon request. Prevention Point records used for this study extend from program implementation (November, 1988) through mid-1992. Client contacts were recorded on a standard form by program personnel each time an individual presented at a Prevention Point site and exchanged at least one syringe.

Outcome Measures

Utilization of syringe exchange program was assessed using three indicators: (1) the number of client contacts and syringes exchanged as reported in program records of Prevention Point syringe exchange program; (2) frequency of visits to syringe exchange as reported by participants in the Urban Health Study from 1989 to 1992; and (3) sources of syringes reported by Urban Health Study participants interviewed between 1987 and 1992. *Negative impacts* of the syringe exchange program were examined using three variables included in the Urban Health Study dataset: (1) changes in the self-reported frequency of injection over time (1987-1992); (2) changes in the age distribution of the cross-sections (1987-1992); and (3) proportion of respondents reporting first injection during previous year (1989[1] to 1992). *Syringe-sharing* was examined by assessing the relationship between reported syringe exchange use in the past year and reported needle-sharing based on self-reported number of needle-sharing partners in the 30 days prior to interview. The accuracy of the term "needle-sharing" has been questioned, since IDUs may use previously-used syringes that are not perceived as "shared" (20). Consequently, participants in the Spring 1992 cross-section (N=473), were asked if they injected during the past 30 days using syringes that they know had been used by someone else, including a close friend or lover. The Pearson product moment correlation coefficient between this variable and reported "needle-sharing" in the past 30 days was robust ($r=0.83$, $p<0.01$).

---

[1] Item added to survey questionnaire in Spring 1989.

Correlates of needle-sharing were identified using a pool of 752 unduplicated respondents from the most recent full year of data available (Fall 1991/Spring 1992). In instances of multiple interviews, only the first observation was used. Out of 932 interviews, 176 "duplicate" observations and 4 observations with missing data concerning syringe-sharing behaviors were dropped from this analysis. The demographic composition of this cross-section closely approximated the entire sample (data not shown).

Statistical Analysis

One-way analysis of variance with Scheffe's test for multiple comparisons was used to identify differences in the mean number of syringes exchanged and the reported frequency of injection over successive cross-sections. Differences in the proportion of IDUs utilizing the syringe exchange >25 times in the past year, and the proportion of new injectors over-time were assessed using the Mantel-Haenszel χ^2 test for trend. Differences in odds ratios between cross-sections were tested using Woolf's method, and summary odds ratios were calculated when appropriate (21). For univariate comparisons, two-tailed χ^2 tests or Fisher's exact tests were used to examine the relationship between categorical variables and needle-sharing in the past 30 days; Student's t-tests were used to examine the relationship of continuous variables. Odds ratios and 95% confidence intervals were computed for categorical variables. Multiple linear regression (for continuous outcomes) and logistic regression (for categorical outcomes) was used to control for possible cohort effects in comparisons made over multiple cross-sections. Factors predicting needle-sharing were identified using non-hierarchical logistic regression in a Fall 1991/Spring 1992 sub-sample (n=752). All possible interactions of main effects were tested. Statistical analysis was performed using the *Statistical Package for the Social Sciences*, Chicago, Illinois (22).

RESULTS

Table 1 presents selected demographic characteristics of the study population. Analyses of cross-sections were performed over the eleven cross-sections of data incorporated in the study. Changes in grant support forced the elimination of the 21-day drug detoxification clinics from the sampling frame in January, 1990. This resulted in two post-January 1990 changes in sample composition: (1) the proportion of IDUs enrolled in drug treatment programs decreased from 37% to 17%; and (2) the percentage of African Americans increased from 47% to 56%, the percentage of Hispanics decreased from 17% to 14%, and the percentage of Caucasians decreased from 36% to 30%. Among street-recruited IDUs, there was no significant change in proportion of respondents enrolled in drug treatment over the 11 study cross-sections. Changes in sampling frame occurred prior to the 1991-1992 cross-section used in our analysis of needle-sharing in Table 2 and Table 3.

Utilization of Syringe Exchange Program

Client contacts reported by Prevention Point rose steadily from program implementation in late Fall 1988 through Spring 1992, when client contacts peaked at 16,600 contacts over a six month period. During Spring 1989, 7,821 syringes were exchanged as compared with 343,883 syringes exchanged during Spring 1992. The ratio of syringes exchanged to clients who presented at the exchange sites increased from two syringes per client contact to 21 syringes per client contact between Fall 1988 and Spring 1992. There was a significant increase in the mean number of syringes exchanged for other people on the part of Urban Health Study respondents between Fall 1989 and Spring 1992 ($F=6.603; p<0.0001$). In Fall 1989, 50 respondents (9.9%) reported exchanging syringes for a mean of 4.3 others, while in the Spring 1992 cross section, 72 respondents (15.2%) reported exchanging syringes for a mean of 10.3 others. Between Fall 1989[2] and Spring 1992, reported utilization of syringe exchange at any time in the past year by respondents in the Urban Health Study increased from 50% to 61%. The proportion of respondents who reported using the syringe exchange at least 25 times in the past year doubled between 1989 and 1992, from 14% to 28% (Mantel Haenszel χ^2 test for trend = 40.26; df = 1; $p < 0.00001$).

We also found major shifts in the principal sources of syringes reported by Urban Health Study respondents between 1987 and 1992. An increase was observed in the proportion of respondents who reported syringe exchange as their usual source. By Fall 1990, syringe exchange had become the most frequently cited source of syringes and remained the major source of syringes throughout the observation period. In Spring 1992, 45% of respondents interviewed reported "usually" obtaining their injection equipment by exchanging at Prevention Point. Thirty-two percent reported that buying syringes on the street was their usual source, while 23% reported using other sources including friends, relatives, diabetics, pharmacies, dealers, shooting galleries, renting or stealing syringes see (see Figure 1).

Frequency of Injection

The median number of reported daily injections in the year prior to interview declined between 1987 and 1992 from a high of 1.9 per day in Fall 1987 to 0.7 in Spring 1992. Median daily injection frequencies in the past year peaked prior to implementation of syringe exchange. This decline in injection frequency over time was significant in analysis of variance over the eleven cross-sections ($F=16.17; p<0.0001$). Scheffe's test for multiple comparisons revealed a significant decline ($p< 0.05$) between the Spring 1987 to Fall 1988 cross-sections, and between the Fall 1990 and Spring 1992 cross-sections.

---

[2] Needle-exchange item first added in Fall 1989 survey.

Recruitment of New and Younger Users into Injection Drug Use

Over the five and one-half year study period, the mean age rose six years, from 35.8 years in Spring 1987 to 41.6 years in Spring 1992. Age was normally distributed, and the mean standard deviation for the eleven cross-sections was 8.3 years. Minimum age did not change significantly between cross-sections. The mean age of the youngest participant across samples was 19; minimum age ranged from 15 to 20. We found a significant progressive decline in the proportion of persons who reported first injecting drugs in the previous year, from 3.0% in Spring 1989[3] to 1.1% in Spring 1992 (Mantel-Haenszel χ^2 test for trend=9.65; df=1; $p<0.002$).

Syringe Sharing-Univariate Analysis

An overall decline in sharing behavior was observed throughout the observation period with 66.3% reporting sharing in Spring 1987 and 35.5% reporting sharing in Spring 1992. We found no remarkable differences in the proportion of non-users of the exchange who reported sharing needles over the three-year observation period (1989-1992) following program implementation. When all observations from 1989-1992 were considered, IDUs who reported syringe exchange use > 25 times in the past year were less likely to report needle-sharing in the past 30 days than those who used the exchange less frequently or not at all (Mantel-Haenszel summary odds ratio=0.71; 95% confidence interval= 0.59, 0.87).

The unduplicated Fall 1991/Spring 1992 sample (n=752) closely approximated the demographic composition of the total sample. Univariate relationships to needle-sharing in the past 30 days from variables in the Urban Health Study data-set may be found in Table 2. A smaller proportion of African-Americans reported needle-sharing in the past 30 days. Homelessness, reported injection of "speedballs" (concurrent injection of heroin and cocaine), heroin injected alone, injected-cocaine, and crack cocaine use in the past month, had significant associations with needle-sharing. Daily injection drug use (≥ 30 injections in past 30 days) and a history of drug treatment within the past five years were also associated with needle-sharing. Both older age and needle-exchange as primary syringe source had protective effects. Respondents who reported regular use of bleach within the past six months were less likely to share syringes, as were respondents who reported use of condoms 100% of the time during sexual activity.

---

[3] Age of first injection was introduced in the Spring 1989 questionnaire.

Syringe Sharing-Multivariate Analysis

In logistic regression, we found six main effects independently associated with needle-sharing in the past 30 days (see Table 3). Greater frequency of syringe exchange use in the past year was associated with not sharing syringes in the past 30 days. Other protective factors associated with sharing syringes were: increasing age, African American ethnicity, reported condom use 100% of the time during penetrative intercourse (anal, oral, vaginal); and having previously received a HIV antibody test result. Frequency of injection of cocaine in the previous month was a significant predictor of needle-sharing. We found a significant interaction between two continuous variables in the logistic regression model which improved the fit of our model to the data. This interaction adjusts for the difference in the effect of syringe exchange use on sharing behavior relative to years of age. The relationship between needle-sharing, age, and frequency of syringe exchange use is illustrated in Figure 2. Curves depict adjusted odds ratios for needle-sharing for selected age groups. The median age (40 years) for the Fall 1991/Spring 1992 subsample ($n=752$) was selected as the referent for calculating odds ratios to illustrate the interaction. Figure 2 shows a decline in the likelihood of needle-sharing among 20 and 30-year olds with increasing frequency of syringe exchange use when adjusted for factors in the model. There was no change in needle-sharing likelihood among 40 and 50 year olds with increasing use of syringe exchange.

DISCUSSION

Our findings confirm that IDUs will participate in syringe and needle exchange programs that can be easily approached and negotiated. In San Francisco, syringe exchange was readily adopted by IDUs, and appears to have quickly replaced the black market as a primary source of injection equipment. The ability of syringe exchange to recapture used and potentially infectious syringes for safe disposal should also not be underestimated. During October, 1992, the Prevention Point syringe exchange program collected and safely incinerated approximately 13,000 used syringes each week. In a recent study, investigators detected HIV-1 antibodies in 7% of a random sample of 83 syringes returned to the San Francisco syringe exchange program (23). By extrapolation, approximately 3,600 syringes contaminated with HIV were removed from the environment during the month of October, 1992 by the syringe exchange program. There was no support for the hypothesis that syringe and needle exchange contributes to drug abuse in our study population. The gradual but statistically significant decline in self-reported frequency of injection over the study period may reflect a historical artifact which mirrors growth in the popularity of "crack" cocaine (which is smoked, not injected), or other unmeasured factors. We found a decreasing level of initiation into drug injection over-time. Guydish et al. (24) noted similar declines in needle-sharing and initiation into injection drug use among persons admitted to drug-abuse treatment programs in San Francisco before and after implementation of the syringe exchange program. Fluctuations in drug use practices are common (25), and initiation into drug use (including the practice of injection) have been shown to be influenced by the interplay of a host of familial, social, psychological, cultural, and historical factors (26-31). Previous studies reported needle-sharing was lowered among non-exchangers as well as regular exchangers in the Netherlands and the United Kingdom (32, 33). However, in our study, we found no significant decline in needle-sharing over-time among respondents who reported no syringe exchange use in the year prior to interview. These differences in study outcomes may stem from different drug use patterns, exchange program structures, and/or social circumstances found among European IDUs and those studied in San Francisco.

We found syringe exchange use to be a strong, independent predictor of not sharing needles and syringes in the recent past when adjusted for age, ethnicity, previous HIV testing and counseling, frequency of injection of cocaine, and consistent use of condoms. Younger IDUs were more likely to report needle-sharing than their older counterparts overall, but were less likely to report needle-sharing with more frequent use of syringe exchange. This finding is reflected in the interaction of age and frequency of syringe exchange use in multivariate analysis. Thus, the San Francisco syringe exchange program appears to have had its greatest benefit among younger users. We speculate these younger persons depend more heavily upon syringe exchange as a source of clean injection equipment than do older IDUs with other established sources for needles and syringes.

Other factors with independent relationships to needle-sharing were race, condom use, and injection of cocaine. It is noteworthy that African American ethnicity was inversely related to syringe sharing. Other studies have found African American IDUs to be at elevated risk for HIV infection relative to IDUs who are members of other ethnic groups in San Francisco (34, 35) and elsewhere (36, 37). African American ethnicity has been found as an independent risk factor for HIV in multivariate models that include injection frequency (35, 38). Possible reasons for this include differential reporting bias and/or social factors related to social networks, sexual activity, and sharing practices that are neither well measured nor understood. IDUs who reported consistent use of condoms "all of the time" were less likely to share syringes. We have previously reported that changes in sexual behavior in response to AIDS prevention messages have trailed gains in needle-cleaning and not sharing (39). It is possible that those who are able to negotiate the use of condoms in the intensely personal and subjective domain of human sexual behavior, are likewise better able to adapt their behavior to avoid needle-sharing. Recent injection of cocaine predicted needle-sharing in multivariate analysis. This may reflect the subordination of health concerns to the drive to inject drugs with whatever equipment is available. Cocaine injectors, who typically inject many times during a "run" of one or several days, may have difficulty obtaining a sufficient supply of clean needles. We speculate that prevention programs, including syringe-exchange efforts, will need to reach into the environments where these individuals practice high-risk behavior in order to adequately support the adoption of lower risk alternatives to needle-sharing. We think it especially noteworthy that having received a previous HIV test result (which by California law are voluntary, confidential, and include both pre-test and post-test counseling), was a significant, independent predictor of not-sharing needles. This effect was independent of the outcome of the HIV antibody test (positive or negative). Our study is limited in that it identifies correlates of sharing syringes but not *causes* of reduced sharing. As is the case with virtually all survey research, we used self-reports of respondents recruited into the study from the population of interest; in this case IDUs. Consequently, these data may be subject to problems of recall, intoxication, socially desirable responses, and/or other sources of bias (40). However, high validity of self-reported drug use in a multi-site study using similar methods and instrumentation has been reported (41). The targeted samples used were not true random samples, therefore our findings may not generalize to other populations of IDUs. The short (30-day) time-frame used for some items is a limitation. However, the use of longer periods may amplify problems in accuracy of recall. Despite these limitations, the study contains useful information regarding a significant health technology and related policy issue: namely, the feasibility, and potential risks and benefits of syringe exchange as a method of HIV/AIDS prevention for IDUs.

In multivariate analysis, two inverse correlates of syringe-sharing appeared as promising health interventions. These were syringe exchange and voluntary, confidential HIV testing and counseling. While an independent factor associated with not sharing needles, syringe exchange should not be viewed as a substitute for a comprehensive approach to drug abuse treatment and prevention, nor as an infectious disease prevention nostrum. However, our findings are consistent with other studies that have suggested that increased availability of sterile syringes can play a useful and significant role in helping to attenuate the practice of needle-sharing, and the high rate of infectious disease transmission that accompanies this practice (8-18, 42). Our results suggest that syringe exchange programs and voluntary HIV testing and counseling help reduce needle-sharing. Such programs should be continued, expanded to meet existing needs, and implemented in areas where not currently available.

ACKNOWLEDGMENTS

A previous version of this paper was read at the VII International Conference on AIDS, Florence Italy, June, 1991. The authors are especially grateful for the support of the American Foundation for AIDS Research (Grant number 001037-7RG). Additional support for this study was derived from the San Francisco Department of Public Health, Office of AIDS (contract # 83-07069); the U.S. Centers for Disease Control (cooperative agreement # U62-CCU902017); and the National Institute on Drug Abuse (grant nos. RO1 DA04212 and UO1-DA06908). Acknowledged are the contributions of the study participants; and the staff of the following organizations: Prevention Point Needle Exchange Program; Haight-Ashbury Free Clinics, Inc.; San Francisco General Hospital Substance Abuse Services; the MidCity Consortium to Combat AIDS; and the Urban Health Study, School of Medicine, University of California, San Francisco. Acknowledged also are the contributions of Yu-Teh Cheng, M.A., Kyung Hee Choi, Ph.D., M.P.H., Brian Edlin, M.D., T. Stephen Jones, M.D., Walter Hauck, Ph.D., Alex Kral, M.S., Mark Segal, Ph.D., Starley B. Shade, B.A., and David Vlahov, Ph.D.

REFERENCES

1. Wodak A, Moss A. HIV and injecting drug users: from epidemiology to public health. *AIDS* 1990;4(suppl):S105-S109.

2. National Commission on AIDS. Report: The twin epidemics of substance abuse and HIV. National Commission on AIDS. Washington, DC; July, 1991.

3. Choopanya K, Vanichsensi S, Plangsringarm K, et al. Risk factors and HIV seropositivity among injecting drug users in Bangkok. *AIDS* 1991;5(12):1509-1514.

4. Chin J. Epidemiology keynote speech. VII International Conference on AIDS. Florence Italy: 1991.

5. CDC. Report: HIV/AIDS surveillance report, second quarter edition. U.S. Dept. of Health and Human Services, Public Health Service, Centers for Disease Control, National Center for Infectious Diseases, Division of HIV/AIDS. July, 1993.

6. Wiley JA, Samuel MC. The prevalence of HIV infection in the USA. *AIDS* 1989;3(Supplement 1):71-78.

7. US Department of Health and Human Services. *Healthy People 2000: National Health Promotion and Disease Prevention Objectives*. Washington, DC: U.S. Government Printing Office (DHHS publication number No. [PHS] 91-50212, 1991.

8. Hartgers C, Buning EC, van Santen GW, et al. The impact of the needle and syringe-exchange programme in Amsterdam in injecting risk behavior. *AIDS* 1989;3:571-576.

9. van den Hoek JA, van Haastrecht HJ, Coutinho RA. Risk reduction among intravenous drug users in Amsterdam under the influence of AIDS. *Am J Public Health* 1989;10:1355-1357.

10. Ljunberg B, Christensson B, Tuning K, et al. HIV prevention among injecting drug users: three years experience from a syringe exchange program in Sweden. *JAIDS* 1991;4:890-895.

11. Buzolic A. Report: Needle and syringe availability and AIDS prevention: Modifications of existing legislation. Australia Ministerial Task Force on Drug Strategy. Queensland, Australia; June, 1988.

12. Stimson GV. Syringe-exchange programmes for injecting drug users [Editorial Review]. *AIDS* 1989;3:253-260.

13. Pye M, Kapila M, Buckley G, Cunningham D. A comparative study of local AIDS programs in the United Kingdom. V International Conference on AIDS. Montreal, Canada: 1989.

14. Hart GJ, Carvell ALM, Woodward N, et al. Evaluation of needles exchange in central London: behaviour change and anti-HIV status over one year. *AIDS* 1989;3:261-265.

15. Purchase D, Hagan H, Des Jarlais DC, Reid T. Historical account of the Tacoma syringe exchange. V International Conference on AIDS. Montreal, Canada: 1989.

16. Kaplan EH, Heimer R. HIV prevalence among intravenous drug users: model-based estimates from New Haven's legal needle exchange. *JAIDS* 1992;5:163-169.

17. New York City Department of Health. Report: The pilot needle exchange study in New York City: A bridge to treatment. A report on the first ten months of operation. New York City Department of Public Health. New York; December, 1989.

18. Des Jarlais DC, Hagan H, Purchase D, et al. Safer injection among participants in the first North American syringe exchange program. V International Conference on AIDS. Montreal, Canada: 1989.

19. Carvell AM, Hart GJ. Help-seeking and referrals in a needle exchange: a comprehensive service to injecting drug users. *British Journal of Addictions* 1990;85:235-240.

20. Grund JP, Kaplan CD, Adriaans NF, et al. The limitations of the concept of needle sharing: the practice of front loading [letter]. *AIDS* 1990;4:819-821.

21. Schlesselman JJ. *Case-Control Studies: Design, Conduct,Analysis*. New York: Oxford University Press, 1982.

22. SPSS, Inc. *SPSS Reference Guide*. Chicago: SPSS Inc., 1990.

23. Guydish J, Clark G, Garcia D. Detecting HIV antibodies in needle exchange syringes (letter). *AIDS* 1992;6:739-740.

24. Guydish J, Bucardo J, Young M, et al. Evaluating needle exchange: are there negative effects? *AIDS* 1993;7(6):871-876.

25. Kozel NJ, Adams EH. Epidemiology of drug abuse: an overview. *Science* 1986;21:970-974.

26. Stimson G. Plenary. VII International Conference on AIDS. Barcelona, Spain: 1992.

27. Ellickson PL, Hays RD, Bell RM. Stepping through the drug use sequence: longitudinal scalogram analysis of initiation and regular use. *Journal of Abnormal Psychology* 1992;101:441-451.

28. Dinwiddie SH, Reich T, Cloniger CR. Patterns of lifetime drug use among intravenous drug users. *J Subst Abuse* 1992;4:1-11.

29. Dinwiddie SH, Reich T, Cloniger CR. Prediction of intravenous drug use. *Comprehensive Psychiatry* 1992;33:172-179.

30. Catalano RF, Morrison DM, Wells EA, et al. Ethnic differences in family factors related to early drug initiation. *Journal of Studies on Alcoholism* 1992;53:208-217.

31. Morrison V. Starting, switching, stopping: users' explanations of illicit drug use. *Drug and Alcohol Dependence* 1991;27 :213-217.

32. Donoghoe MC, Dolan KA, G. V. S. Changes in injectors' HIV risk behaviour and syringe supply in UK 1987-1990. *VII International Conference on AIDS* 1991;Book 2(abstract # TH.C.45):66.

33. Hartgers C, van Ameijden EJC, van den Hoek JAR, Coutinho RA. Needle sharing and participation in the Amsterdam syringe exchange program among HIV-seronegative injecting drug users. *Public Health Rep* 1992;107(6):675-681.

34. Watters JK, Cheng Y, Segal M, et al. Epidemiology and prevention of HIV in intravenous drug users in San Francisco, 1986-1989. VI International Conference on AIDS. San Francisco, CA: 1990.

35. Chaisson RE, Bachetti P, Osmond D, et al. Cocaine use and HIV infection in intravenous drug users in San Francisco. *JAMA* 1989;261:561-565.

36. Koblin BA, McCusker J, Lewis BF, Sullivan JL. Ethnic/ethnic differences in HIV-1 seroprevalence and risky behavior among intravenous drug users in a multisite study. *American Journal of Epidemiology* 1990;132:837-846.

37. D'Aquila RT, Peterson LR, Williams AB, Williams AE. Race/ethnicity as a risk factor for HIV-1 infection among Connecticut intravenous drug users. *Journal of Acquired Immunodeficiency Syndromes* 1989;2:503-513.

38. Schoenbaum EE, Hartel DH, Selwyn PA, et al. Risk factors for human immunodeficiency virus infection in intravenous drug users. *New Eng J Med* 1989;321:874-879.

39. Watters JK, Downing M, Case P, et al. AIDS prevention for intravenous drug users in the community: street-based education and risk behavior. *Am J Community Psychol* 1990;18(4):587-96.

40. Lampinen T, Wiebel WW, Watters JK. Intravenous drug users, HIV testing and counseling [Letter]. *JAMA* 1989;262:1331.

41. Watters JK, Needle R, Brown BS, et al. The self reporting of cocaine use [letter]. *JAMA* 1992;268:2374-2375.

42. Nelson KE, Vlahov D, Cohn S, et al. Human immunodeficiency virus infection in diabetic intravenous drug users. *JAMA* 1991;266:2259-2261.

Table 1: Selected Demographic Characteristics: IDUs in San Francisco, 1987-1992 (N=5,644)

	n	%
AGE[1]		
≤30	995	17.6
31-40	2753	48.8
41-50	1408	25.0
≥51	487	8.6
GENDER[1]		
Male	3893	69.0
Female	1750	31.0
RACE[1]		
African-American	2546	45.1
Caucasian	1941	34.4
Latino	795	14.1
Other	357	6.3
CURRENTLY IN DRUG TREATMENT[1]		
Yes	1529	27.1
No	4078	72.6
Other Answer	9	.2
EVER IN DRUG TREATMENT (past 5 years)[1]		
Yes	3008	53.4
No	2624	46.5
EMPLOYED[1]		
Yes	1179	20.9
No	4401	78.2
Other Answer	50	.9
CONSIDER YOURSELF HOMELESS[2]		
Yes	1445	32.4
No	2987	66.9
Other Answer	30	.7

[1] Missing Cases
[2] Question added in 1990 (n=4,462)

Table 2: Selected Characteristics and Reported Needle-Sharing in Past 30 Days - Fall 1991/Spring 1992 (N=752)

Characteristics	#/Share/n	%	Odds Ratio	95% Confidence Interval
RACE				
African-American	114/383	(29.8)	1.00	----------
Caucasian	91/215	(42.3)	1.73	1.20 - 2.49
Latino	40/94	(42.6)	1.75	1.07 - 2.85
Other	22/59	(37.3)	1.40	0.73 - 2.57
GENDER				
Male	181/532	(34.0)	0.80	0.58 - 1.11
Female	86/220	(39.1)		
AGE				
≤30	34/73	(46.6)	1.00	----------
31-40	129/314	(41.1)	0.80	0.46 - 1.38
41-50	84/277	(30.3)	0.50	0.29 - 0.87
≥51	20/88	(22.7)	0.34	0.16 - 0.70
EMPLOYED				
Yes	56/149	(37.6)	1.12	0.77 - 1.62
No	211/603	(35.0)		
CONSIDER YOURSELF HOMELESS				
Yes	121/300	(40.3)	1.42	1.05 - 1.93
No	141/438	(32.2)		
EVER IN TREATMENT (past 5 years)				
Yes	142/357	(39.8)	1.42	1.05 - 1.91
No	125/396	(31.8)		
CURRENTLY IN DRUG TREATMENT				
Yes	34/104	(32.7)	0.87	0.55 - 1.39
No	225/630	(35.7)		
≥30 INJECTIONS (past 30 days)				
Yes	141/356	(39.6)	1.41	1.04 - 1.90
No	126/396	(31.8)		
INJECTED HEROIN (past 30 days)				
Yes	208/546	(38.1)	1.53	1.08 - 2.17
No	59/206	(28.6)		
INJECTED SPEEDBALL (past 30 days)				
Yes	135/333	(40.5)	1.48	1.10 - 2.00
No	132/419	(31.5)		
INJECTED COCAINE (past 30 days)				
Yes	144/333	(43.2)	1.83	1.36 - 2.48
No	123/419	(29.4)		
INJECTED AMPHETAMINES (past 30 days)				
Yes	61/155	(39.4)	1.23	0.86 - 1.77
No	206/597	(34.5)		
SMOKED CRACK COCAINE (past 30 days)				
Yes	162/401	(40.4)	1.59	1.17 - 2.15
No	105/351	(29.9)		
PRIMARY SOURCE OF SYRINGE=EXCHANGE				
Yes	94/317	(29.7)	0.64	0.47 - 0.87
No	173/435	(39.8)		
ALWAYS USE BLEACH (past 6 months)				
Yes	101/329	(30.7)	0.69	0.51 - 0.93
No	166/423	(39.2)		
ALWAYS USE CONDOMS (past year)				
Yes	10/89	(11.2)	0.20	0.10 - 0.39
No	257/663	(38.8)		
EVER GIVEN PREVIOUS HIV RESULTS				
Yes	172/555	(31.0)	0.48	0.34 - 0.68
No	95/197	(48.2)		

Table 3: Logistic Regression Analysis of Needle Sharing in Past 30 Days - Fall 1991/Spring 1992 (N=752)

Variable	Adjusted Odds Ratio	95% Confidence Interval	*p*=
SYRINGE EXCHANGE USE[1] (10 use increment)	0.54	0.35 - 0.84	.0064
AGE (10 year increment)	0.59	0.45 - 0.78	.0001
AFRICAN-AMERICAN (vs others)	0.58	0.42 - 0.81	.0012
ALWAYS USE CONDOMS[2]	0.17	0.08 - 0.35	.0001
PREVIOUS HIV TEST RESULT[3]	0.48	0.34 - 0.69	.0001
INJECTION COCAINE USE[2] (10 use increment)	1.05	1.01 - 1.08	.0072
INTERACTION[4] (age by frequency of syringe exchange use)	---	---	.0210

[1] past year
[2] past 30 days
[3] ever
[4] see Figure 2

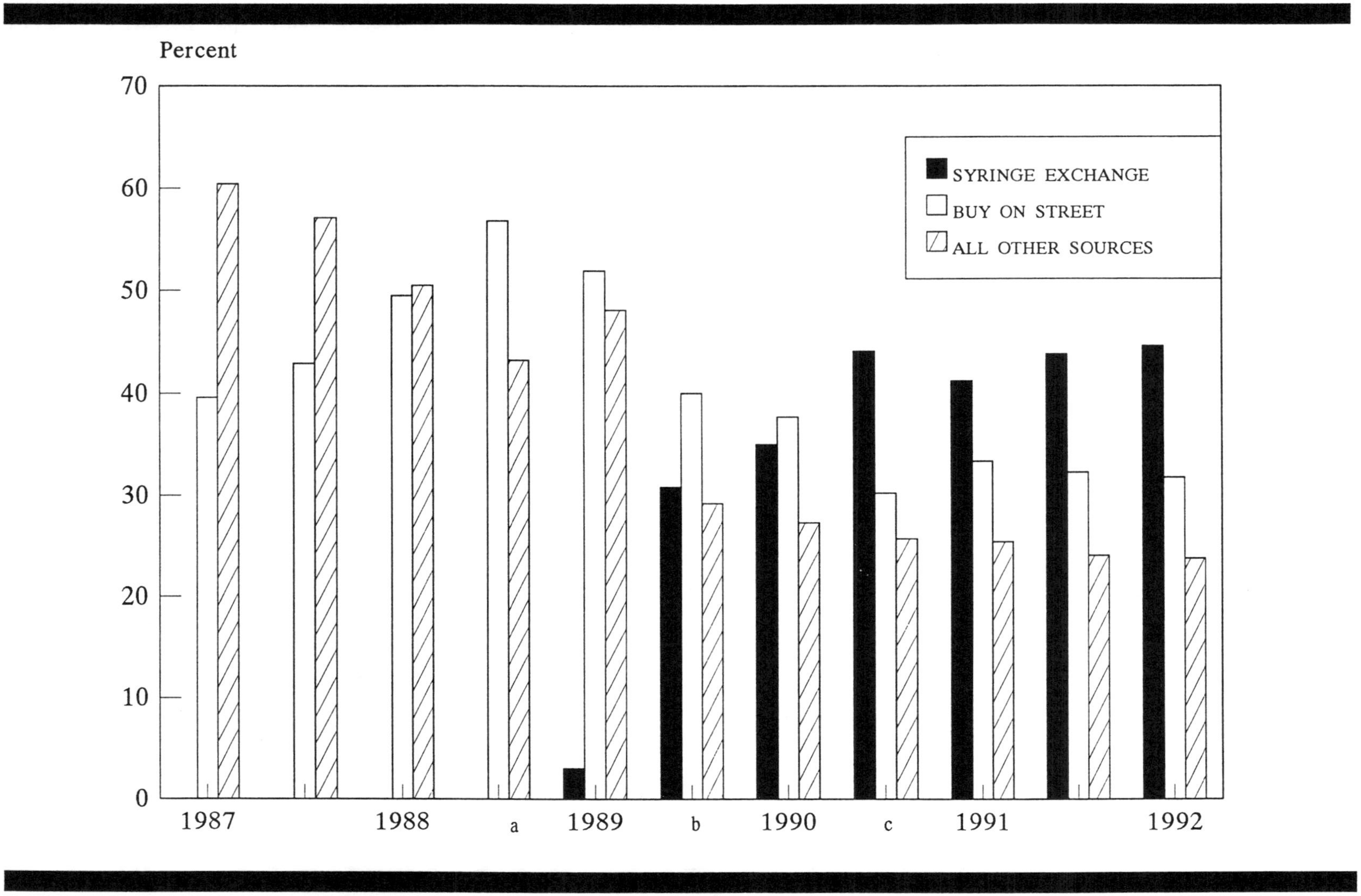

Figure 1: "How do you usually obtain syringes?" San Francisco drug injectors, 1987-1992.
a - Syringe exchange begins Nov. 1988/10 syringe limit. b - May 1989/20 syringe limit.
c - August 1990/syringe limit is abandoned.

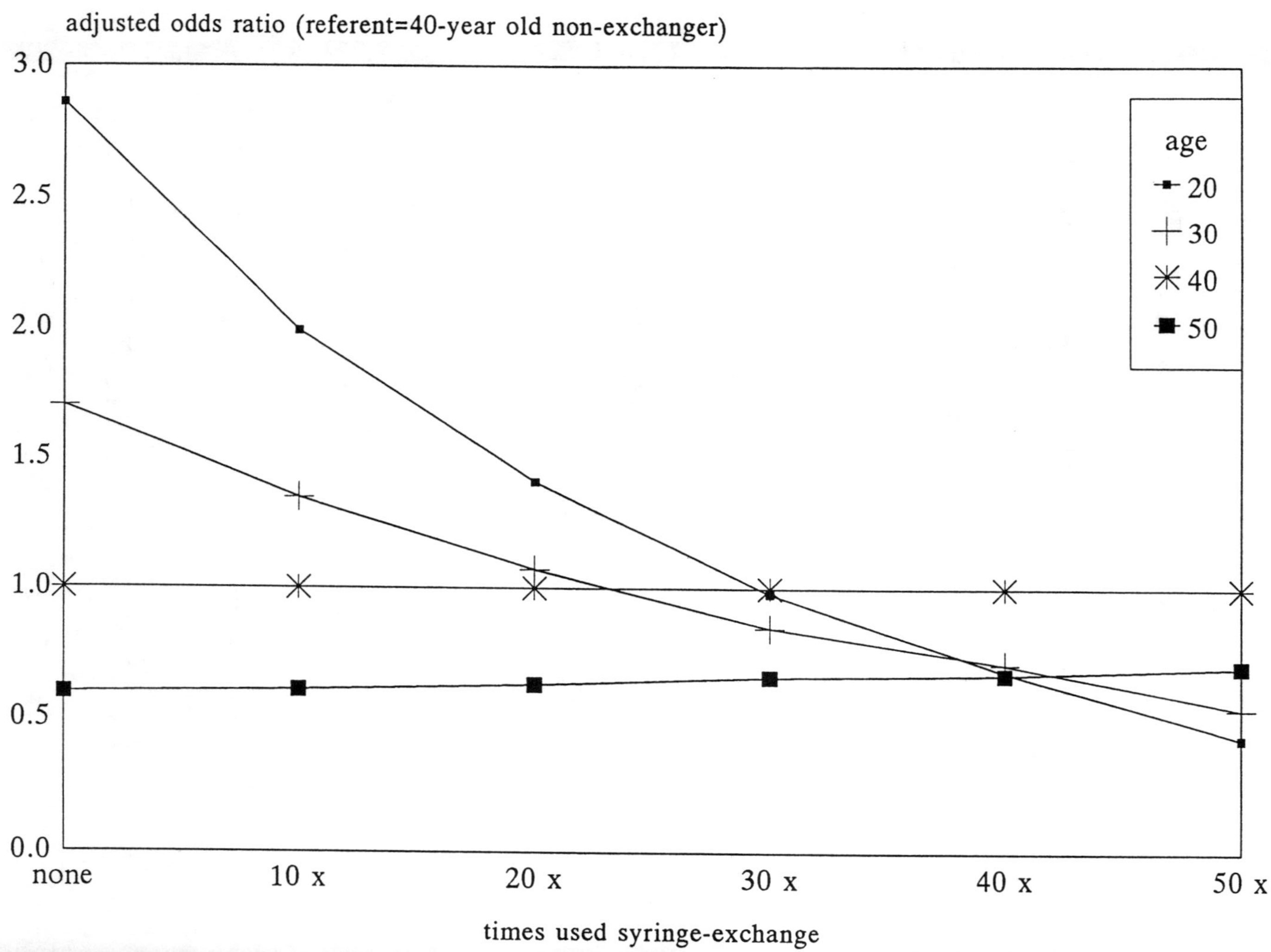

Figure 2: Adjusted odds of needle sharing (30 days) by age and frequency of syringe exchange use in previous year

USING QUALITATIVE METHODS TO EVALUATE NEEDLE EXCHANGE

SHEIGLA MURPHY, Community Health Works,
Institute for Scientific Analysis, San Francisco, California

INTRODUCTION

Injection drug use (IDU) continues to be the second most common risk behavior associated with AIDS in this country and serves as a potential bridge of infectivity to other groups including their non-drug-using sexual partners and children (Centers for Disease Control, 1991a; 1991b; Des Jarlais and Friedman, 1988). IDUs are at increased risk for infection with the AIDS virus through the sharing of needles/syringes, as well as other drug injection paraphernalia (Black, et al., 1986; Chaisson et al., 1987b; Chitwood et al., 1990; Friedland et al., 1985; Hart et al., 1989b; Hopkins, 1988; Inciardi, 1990; Inciardi and Page, 1991; Magura et al., 1989; Marmor et al., 1984; 1987; Page et al., 1991; Schoenbaum et al., 1989).

In the absence of an effective treatment or vaccine, efforts to control the spread of the human immunodeficiency virus (HIV) depend on reduction of risk behaviors (Des Jarlais and Friedman, 1987). Public health interventions have taken the form of prevention campaigns employing the media, educational groups or seminars, and street outreach workers. Decreases in needle sharing have been documented (Chaisson, et al., 1987a; Guydish et al., 1990; Rhodes et al., 1990; Selwyn et al., 1987; Sorensen et al., 1989; Stephens et al., 1991). However, it has also been amply demonstrated that an individual's knowledge of high risk behaviors alone is insufficient to ensure discontinuance of risky activities (Davis-Berman and Brown, 1990; Friedman et al., 1992; Inciardi, 1990; Ottomanelli, et al., 1990; Page et al., 1991).

Thus, despite widespread implementation of legal prevention strategies, the epidemic of HIV infection among injection drug users (IDUs) persists unabated. Consequently, illegal and highly controversial needle/syringe exchanges (NSEs) continue operations in cities across the United States. Currently, there is growing interest among policy makers in information concerning these clandestine AIDS interventions. In this paper, I will describe our ethnographic evaluation of San Francisco's NSE, Prevention Point, focusing the discussion on qualitative methods. I will begin with a brief history of Prevention Point and a description of the study design.

PREVENTION POINT

This full-service exchange has been in operation since 1988. As of May, 1993 services are provided on four evenings a week for two hours at ten stationary locations in the Hunter's Point, Mission, Tenderloin, Western Addition, Polk Gulch and Civic Center districts of San Francisco. These are multi-ethnic neighborhoods with sizable needle using populations.

Like most other NSEs, Prevention Point participants exchange on a one-for-one basis (used-for-sterile) in order to reduce the number of contaminated syringes in circulation. Staff also provide information on safer sex and drug use, referrals to drug treatment programs and health care agencies, and tangible items such as bleach, alcohol wipes, cottons and condoms. Program providers act as conduits to other social services, such as drug counseling and referrals to drug treatment programs, health care services, and HIV-related services.

Prevention Point is staffed by extremely dedicated volunteers. For example, on the night of the 1989 Loma Prieta earthquake, while most San Francisco residents huddled together eating strange culinary combinations from melting freezers, volunteer needle exchangers braved darkened streets to provide services (Personal Communication, 1992). Prevention Point provides services in stationary locations to multi-cultural participants by dedicated providers.

STUDY DESIGN AND RESEARCH OBJECTIVES

Data collection will consist of both ethnographic field observations, depth interviews and closed-ended questions. Field observations will be conducted at five[1] Prevention Point sites. Depth interviews will be conducted with four subsamples: 50 primary exchangers (IDUs who exchange at program sites); 50 secondary exchangers (IDUs who exchange needles/syringes through primary exchangers); 50 non-exchangers (IDUs who do not exchange) and 25 Prevention Point staff. As of September 1993, we have completed field observations at two sites and depth interviews with 14 providers, 11 primary exchangers, 12 secondary exchangers and 14 non-exchangers.

We are conducting this research in order to elicit the following kinds of information: first and foremost, the affect of NSE on the continuation/reduction of needle sharing, as well as sex-related risk behaviors. We are investigating IDUs' perceptions of the factors which influence NSE participation and the barriers to participation. We are gathering information about secondary users of NSE - IDUs who exchange needles through other people and the nature of their relationship (e.g., drug dealer, partner, customer). We are looking at the role of the NSE protocols (e.g., limitations on exchanges, hours of operation, geographic locations) in increasing or decreasing particular types of IDUs' participation and the ways in which various clients/providers experience the intervention. We are examining the role of provision of other services (e.g., referral to drug treatment) in NSE utilization, as well as IDU's involvement with other public health and social services.

---

[1] When we submitted the proposal to NIDA to conduct this evaluation, Prevention Point only had five sites. We are currently preparing a competing supplemental application so that we can do participant observations and depth interviews at all ten sites.

Prevention Point, vis-a-vis other American NSEs, is in a unique position. Shortly after our National Institute on Drug Abuse funded project began in May of 1993, San Francisco's Mayor Jordan declared the city to be in a state of medical emergency. This allowed the Mayor and Board of supervisors to circumvent relevant prescription and paraphernalia laws and allocate public health funds to finance Prevention Point. Thus, our research team is in the very fortunate position of being able to study Prevention Point's transformation from a quasi-legal community-based organization into a publicly-funded social service agency.

In sum, our research objectives are to produce a thorough understanding of the ways in which Prevention Point is currently implemented, utilized and experienced. We will focus on how the program is perceived by participants, non-participants and staff. We will explore the factors which serve as barriers to, or facilitate participation in, NSE. We plan to study not only formal activities and anticipated outcomes, but also informal activities and unanticipated outcomes. Finally, we will provide a detailed description of the impact of this intervention on HIV drug and sex-related risk behaviors. In the following, I will describe the theoretical and methodological perspectives which guide this ethnographic evaluation.

THEORETICAL AND METHODOLOGICAL PERSPECTIVE

In order to achieve our research objectives, we are employing qualitative methods. The philosophical and theoretical perspectives which provide the framework for qualitative methods include phenomenology (Bussis, Chittenden and Amarel, 1973; Carini, 1975), symbolic interactionism and naturalistic behaviorism (Denzin, 1978a; 1978b), and ethnomethodology (Garfinkel, 1967).

A unifying theme running through these varied perspectives is an emphasis on the importance of understanding the meanings of human behavior and the socio-cultural context of interactions. In order to understand any social phenomenon, one must understand the dynamic definitions and patterns of interaction of the social actors. The consequences for methodology of this emphasis is "...the qualitative study of people <u>in situ</u> is a process of discovery. One must find out what the subjects themselves believe they are doing in their own terms rather than impose a preconceived or outsider's scheme of what they are doing" (Lofland, 1971:4).

In order to understand Prevention Point's program operations as they are experienced by staff, clients and non-clients, we are conducting a qualitative process evaluation (Rossi and Freeman, 1989). Traditionally, evaluation research has been criticized by social scientists because of its lack of theoretical sensitivity. This qualitative evaluation research employs a inductive grounded theory approach in order to generate program theory from holistic data gathered through naturalistic inquiry (Glaser and Strauss, 1967; Strauss and Corbin, 1990).

This discovery of program theory will help prevention experts and decision makers understand how Prevention Point functions, why it functions the way it does, and the ways in which outcomes flow from program activities. Prevention experts can use grounded theory to test their own theories of programmatic action, program effects and the relationship between action and effects. Grounded theory evaluation, through its rich and detailed description, takes decision makers into the empirical world as it is experienced by the actors in the setting. Grounded theory evaluation is particularly efficacious in considerations of whether or not to replicate similar programs in other settings (Patton, 1987). It can also be helpful in discovering feasible alternatives to, or modifications of, existing services.

> Process evaluations look not only at formal activities and anticipated outcomes, but they also investigate informal patterns and unanticipated consequences in the full context of program implementation and development. Finally, process evaluations usually include the perspectives of people close to the program about how things are going. A variety of perspectives may be sought from people in dissimilar relationships to the program - inside and outside sources.
> (Patton, 1987:24)

We are studying program implementation by gathering detailed, descriptive information from both clients and staff about what the program is doing in order to answer the following kinds of questions: Who participates in needle exchange? What do Prevention Point clients experience? What services are provided to clients? What other services do they need? What does the staff do? What is it like to exchange needles? What are the differences between the service sites? How does participation affect their drug/sex HIV risk behaviors?

From IDUs who do not participate in NSE (either not at all or indirectly), we are seeking detailed information about the following areas: What do they know about NSE? Why don't they participate in NSE? What are their perceptions of NSE's services, staff and participants? What services do they need? What is their knowledge of and participation in drug/sex related HIV risk behaviors?

Data Collection

As noted previously, data collection consists of ethnographic field observations, depth interviews and closed-ended questions. Field observations will be conducted at 5 Prevention Point sites. At each of the 5 sites, we are conducting field observations for 4 weeks (one evening a week) before respondent recruitment begins and are continuing observations throughout the data collection period. The purpose of field observations is to describe the process of NSE thoroughly and carefully. Information from these observations informs instrument preparation and sample selection. At each site, two or more project staff observes interactions and conducts informal interviews with program participants. Field workers tape record their field notes immediately following each observational period.

By directly experiencing needle exchange, field observers have intimate knowledge of the context of service provision. Trained ethnographic field workers have the opportunity to see things program participants (staff and exchangers) are unaware of due to the routine nature of the experience for them. Field observers form their own understandings of NSE without having to rely totally on the selective understandings/perceptions participants recount during interviews. In sum, the results of our analysis of descriptive data from field notes will allow this study's information users to enter the social world of needle exchange (Patton, 1987; Rossi and Freeman, 1989).

Field workers also conduct observations in the places IDUs congregate (copping areas, bars, etc.) in the neighborhoods surrounding Prevention Point sites. Information from these observations also informs instrument preparation and sample selection. Field notes from these observations are tape recorded and analyzed to develop a more thorough understanding of the social worlds of IDUs who do not exchange.

Depth interviews are being conducted with the four subsamples (providers, primary and secondary exchangers and non-exchangers). We have developed interview guides or lists of topics to be explored. Depth interviewing from an interview guide ensures consistent inquiries with each interview, without precluding the possibility of discovery of other relevant issues. The interview guide serves as a basic checklist. The interviewer is then free to ask questions in a conversational style in a sequence that flows from the respondent's perspective of the situation. Interview guides help focus the interaction while allowing unanticipated topic areas to emerge during the interview.

We also utilize closed-ended questionnaires to enable us to collect relevant demographic data, as well as drug/needle use and NSE utilization history. We include measures of current NSE utilization, needle-sharing and high-risk sexual practices. In addition, questions have been designed to gather information regarding: family of origin; current family and marital relations; work and education; drug and alcohol use histories; arrests and criminal activities; and utilization of social services.

Triangulation

Denzin (1978a) identified four forms of triangulation, or ways of strengthening research designs by building checks and balances into data collection and analysis strategies. We have included three forms of triangulation in the design of this study. The combination of field observations and depth interviews is methodological triangulation, or the multiple use of methods to study a single problem. The process of interviewing staff, participants and non-participants is data triangulation, since we are analyzing program perceptions from diverse perspectives. Finally, each Prevention Point site will be observed by at least two project staff allowing for investigator triangulation. We will then be able to compare field notes from different field workers, further strengthening the resulting information (Denzin, 1978a).

We have chosen a purposeful sampling method employing a maximum variation strategy:

> The logic of purposeful sampling in qualitative methods is quite different from the logic of probabilistic sampling in statistics. The power of statistical sampling depends on selecting a truly random and representative sample which will permit confident generalization from the sample to a larger population. The power of purposeful sampling lies in selecting information rich cases for study in depth (Patton, 1987:53).

Maximum variation sampling aims at capturing the central themes that cut across a great deal of participant variation. The logic of maximum variation sampling presumes any common patterns emerging from great variation are of value in understanding the core experiences of program participants. We will be including in the sample individuals who have had quite different experiences informed by our field work observations and informal interviews with clients and staff. "By including in the sample individuals the evaluator determines have had quite different experiences, it is possible to describe more thoroughly the variation in the group and to understand variations in experiences." (Patton, 1987:54)

Providers

Interviews will be conducted with twenty-five Prevention Point staff. Field observations will inform provider interviewee selection procedures with the intention of capturing the core provider perceptions that cut across variation among providers.

Primary Exchangers

We will recruit fifty adult primary exchangers, ten from each of five sites. The ten interviewees selected will represent the range of variation of NSE participants. Selected exchangers will be asked to participate in this voluntary evaluation of NSE. Ethnographers will record basic observable information (e.g., gender, race) on all those who refuse to participate, as well as recruitees, in order to gather some systematic information about individuals who refuse to participate or who do not show up for appointments.

Secondary Exchangers

We will locate fifty adult secondary users of needle exchange by asking the primary exchangers we interview to refer to the project the individuals for whom they have exchanged. It is difficult to estimate the refusal/no show rate for this sampling procedure. However, if our primary exchangers do not refer enough secondary exchangers, we will recruit other primary exchangers we have not interviewed and ask them to refer respondents until we have 10 interviews from each site or 50 secondary exchangers.

Non-Exchangers

A non-exchanger is an adult IDU who has not been a participant in needle exchange (primarily or secondarily) for three months. They must also have injected at least five times during the past three months. We are including those IDUs who may have stopped exchanging in order to discover the barriers for IDUs who have actually experienced NSE, as well as those who have not. We are going to interview infrequent/new injectors, as well as, frequent/experienced injectors.

Non-exchangers are located via chain referral and field work. Field observations in neighborhoods surrounding Prevention Point sites is being conducted in order to locate non-exchangers for our study. Interviewees are also located by using the snowball sampling or chain referral method (Biernacki and Waldorf, 1981; Watters and Biernacki, 1989). The chain referral method works as follows: one respondent refers us to his/her friends who meet study criteria for the non-exchanger subsample. The referred respondent then refers us to others thus forming chains of respondents. We have initiated chains with interviewees from our current and past drug projects. We select among the non-exchangers located utilizing the maximum variation sampling strategy.

Members of both genders and members of ethnic groups represented at site will be included in each of the four subsamples interviewed from each site.

THE INTERVIEW

The interview process begins with the initial contact with project staff or interviewee/locators. They are briefly informed of confidentiality procedures and an interview appointment will be scheduled as soon as possible. The optimal situation is to interview them on the spot. The time of day, length of interview and interview topics explored often makes scheduling appointments to conduct interviews at a later time, either in their homes or at our field offices, more practical.

At the time of interview, the interviewer begins by acquainting the respondent with the nature of the study and the human subjects protection. After the interviewee has read and signed the consent form, the interview proceeds with the tape-recorded depth interview portion, followed by the closed-ended questions. The process takes approximately two to three hours, therefore, we provide a forty dollar honorarium. Likewise, locators require an adequate remuneration (twenty dollars) for their time spent doing the important work of recruiting respondents. Additionally, the interviewee is asked (with the right of refusal) to provide follow-up tracking information so that s/he can be re-contacted for follow-up.

Immediately following field observations, field observers will tape record key descriptive and narrative material. The depth interviews will be recorded on cassette tapes and then coded and archived by project staff. Also following the interview, the interviewer writes up his/her impressions in a one page summary statement.

QUALITATIVE DATA ANALYSIS

We use the grounded theory method in the analysis of the qualitative data (Charmaz, 1983; Glaser and Strauss, 1967; Strauss and Corbin, 1990). This method's premise is data should be collected and analyzed simultaneously to allow the basic social, social psychological and structural processes inherent in a phenomenon to emerge naturally. We employ this method in an effort to both discover new theory or reconstruct existing theory where it is applicable (Burawoy, et al., 1991). The flexibility of this methodology is perhaps most useful because it allows the researcher to correct mistaken hunches or hypotheses prior to completion of the study. As Borman, et al. (1986:34) note:

> reports of competently done qualitative studies focus upon the flexible, evolutionary and recursive nature of the investigation; the emphasis of the paradigm is upon remaining sensitive to the data and to input from the field. When initial questions of procedures appear to clash with incoming information, the paradigm permits researchers to abandon unworkable lines of inquiry and reformulate new ones that have a better fit. The resulting nested working hypotheses help guide a course of inquiry that leads toward results that closely adhere to the phenomena and have great authenticity. Rather than simply being an ill-thought-through ad hoc operation, the looseness that characterizes qualitative research is one of its defining features and greatest strengths. It permits the researcher to correct mistakes.

While collecting data, the researcher continually makes theoretical, methodological and observational notes which guide him/her through the data-gathering stage naturally into analysis (Schatzman and Strauss, 1973; Strauss and Corbin, 1990). The investigator begins by coding the data immediately after collection. It is imperative as little time as possible elapses between collection and initial analysis. In the coding, the analyst notes patterns which seem salient due to their recurring nature. Either the interviewee has mentioned a given problem/circumstance over and over again during the session, or the researcher has noticed this problem/circumstance is referred to by many interviewees. Through coding the data for salient dimensions, constellations of basic social, social-psychological and structural processes are discovered.

While completing open coding, and throughout the data collection process, we write theoretical and methodological memos. Through memoing the data, we then begin to conceptually connect the diverse codes. In addition, this process helps to clarify holes in the analysis, which provides new directions for data collection. Saturation is reached when continuing redundancy is found in basic social processes and their properties among a number of interviewees.

This will be done in an attempt to deal with what Guba (1978) calls the problems of "convergence and divergence." That is, the discovery of how various pieces of information fit together, or what Strauss and Corbin (1990) called the paradigmatic model. The analyst seeks recurring regularities, between observational and interview data, or patterns that can then be sorted into categories.

> Categories should then be judged by two criteria: "internal homogeneity" and "external heterogeneity." The first criterion concerns the extent to which the data that belong in a certain category hold together or dovetail in a meaningful way....The second criterion concerns the extent to which differences among categories are bold and clear. The existence of a large number of unassignable or overlapping data items is good evidence of some basic fault in the category system (Guba, 1978:53).

The process evaluator then goes back and forth between the data and the emerging paradigm to verify the meaningfulness of the categories and modify the paradigmatic model as necessary.

Along with the tools of the grounded theory method -- coding, memoing, and paradigm building (Glaser and Strauss, 1967; Strauss and Corbin, 1990) -- we utilize other analytic procedures, in particular domain analysis (Spradley, 1979).

Domain Analysis

Since the focus of this study is the investigation of a new culture, with its own specialized and technical jargon, the analytic tool of domain analysis is extremely useful (Olesen and Whitaker, 1968; Spradley, 1979). Briefly, domain analysis attempts to discover most of a culture's principles for organizing symbols into domains. Spradley (1979:107) describes the importance of the semantic relationship to this discovery process:

> A more efficient procedure in identifying domains makes use of the semantic relationship as a starting point. From a growing body of research, it appears that the number of semantic relationships in any culture is quite small, perhaps less than two dozen. In addition, certain semantic relationships appear to be universal. These remarkable facts make semantic relationships an extremely useful tool in ethnographic analysis. Using these relational concepts, the ethnographer can discover most of a culture's principles for organizing symbols into domains.

Conducting domain analyses on the interview/field note data enriches the resulting findings and acts as a sort of validation process for the other analytic procedures. For example, conducting a domain analyses of the semantic term "needle sharing" from the provider, exchanger and non-exchanger interview/observational data should prove very revealing and significant in increasing our knowledge of the cultural meaning of this high risk behavior.

Coding

The first code list will be derived directly from the interviews and will consist of subject areas which, by virtue of the time the respondent spent discussing them and/or their recurrent nature, seem important. We will also begin with an initial set of codes taken roughly from the interview guide, since we generated the topic areas from our research questions about issues relevant to NSE. For example, from our previous research, we anticipate that interviewees will recall their first needle use experiences as turning points in their drug using careers. Thus, as indicated in the qualitative interview guide, we include specific questions about this subject. In this case, we might title a code "initial injection" and designate the appropriate lines of text. The codes will be revised as the data are analyzed. Codes can be modified, collapsed, expanded or dropped as new codes are added to the code list. If "initial injection" does not turn out to be a salient issue after initial coding procedures, the text can be re-coded. On the other hand, if we encounter new subject areas which interviewees discuss (despite their absence from the formal interview guide), we will code them and then incorporate them into the interview guide.

Memoing

The interview will be memoed after coding, at which time the analyst makes theoretical and methodological notes about the data. Basically, the question "What is going on here?" is addressed in a memo. The memos vary in length and often contain direct quotes from the interview that might ultimately be used as data in published material. The memoing is also done on the computer, and the memos are filed according to the code to which they correspond. For example, a passage in the interview in which a provider was discussing her opinions regarding a particular program protocol might be coded "Protocol". We might then make a memo about this activity, possibly including a direct quote from the provider. The memo would then be entered in the "Program Protocol" file, and other such memos would be entered into the same file. Memo-making is the hallmark of the method to be used in this study. While coding the data for prominent dimensions and certainly afterward, the analyst makes theoretical memos to be used in the analysis (Glaser, 1978).

Field Notes

Field notes are incorporated into the analysis of the data in much the same manner as interview data. The field notes are coded and then entered into Folio Views. They are then entered in the appropriate file and are ready for memo-making. These memos are considered data and are treated as such, since interview and field data are complementary. A field worker, in fact, may inadvertently collect interview data while doing field observations, or when interviewing, the interviewer may observe occurrences which might more technically be defined as field observations. In sum, interview and field data, though separate, operate together in the analysis of data.

Data Organization

The data (field notes and memos) is organized according to the code list. Next, coded materials from the interview transcript, the memos and the field notes are entered into code files. A possible category of data, for example, might be "Barriers to NSE." Based on other studies using a similar methodology, we might start with thirty codes and perhaps ultimately collapse them to fifteen.

After approximately five interviews have been transcribed, coded and memoed, the research team will read all the memos and, based upon what they contain, scrutinize the interview guide, possibly emphasizing new areas of investigation. In this way, we probe in areas that are emerging as important and put less emphasis on areas which did not elicit much response and, therefore, did not seem important to the phenomena.

VALIDITY AND RELIABILITY

In exploratory research that is primarily descriptive in nature, validity problems center around these questions: 1) Did the respondent tell the truth? 2) Did the investigators represent the social world, situations and perspectives of the subjects as they see it?

It has been our experience with over seven hundred interviews that, given the assurance of confidentiality, illicit drug users can be relied on to give valid information. Numerous other studies have shown that illicit drug users are usually truthful when interviewed (Ball, 1967; Bonito et al., 1976; Maddux and Desmond, 1975; Nurco, 1975; Stephens, 1972). Nonetheless, we have built into our research some strategies for insuring truthfulness. Many of the respondents are known either directly or indirectly by the interviewers and other respondents. Thus, shared knowledge and mutual experiences make successful deception more difficult. Additionally, asking the same question, worded slightly differently at another point during the interview, helps to expose any inconsistencies in respondents' answers. This is a long and detailed interview, and even a dedicated liar would have difficulty keeping a false story straight.

Strategies for ensuring the validity and adequacy of the data include data source triangulation, researcher and respondent validation and the search for negative cases. Since we conduct field observations and depth interviews, this allows us to employ data triangulation. Another method qualitative researchers use is to seek respondent validation. In previous studies, we have used this method by organizing group sessions with three or more participants as a validating tool. Interviewees become more sociological and abstract in these group sessions and often see themselves as responsible for making sociological sense out of the data in question.

After we develop an analytic framework we are at least provisionally satisfied with, we will informally (while doing fieldwork) interview respondents to ascertain whether our analysis rings true for them. We will conduct these informal interviews with members of each study group with representatives from each site. This validation process will be ongoing from the beginning of data collection and analysis.

Working with a mixed gender multi-ethnic research team will provide the opportunity for researcher triangulation. If the same themes and categories appear in each of our interviews, it will serve as a researcher reactivity check (Hammersley and Atkinson, 1983). Additionally, all the field workers/interviewers will read both memos and drafts of various chapters to verify conceptual relations (Strauss and Corbin, 1990).

In all project publications, we will provide detailed descriptions and in-depth quotations in order to allow readers to understand the program fully and the perspectives of the people represented in this study. This description will be balanced by analysis and interpretation. Verification and validation information will be added wherever relevant. We will include throughout the text explanations concerning the extent of triangulation, validity checks, and supporting evidence for our theoretical framework. This will permit readers to critically evaluate the fit between the data and the analysis.

BIBLIOGRAPHY

Ball, J. (1967) "The Reliability and Validity of Interview Data Obtained from 59 Narcotics Addicts," *American Journal of Sociology* 72:650-654.

Biernacki, P. and Waldorf, D. (1981) "Snowball Sampling: Problems, Techniques and Chain-Referral Sampling," *Sociological Methods and Research*. 10(2):141-163.

Black, J., Dolan, M., DeFord, H., et al. (1986) "Sharing of Needles among Users of Intravenous Drugs," *The New England Journal of Medicine*, 314:446-447.

Bonito, A., Nurco, D. and Shaffer, J. (1976) "The Verdicality of Addicts' Self Reports in Social Research," *The International Journal of the Addictions* 11(5):719-724.

Borman, K., LeCompte, M., Goetz, J. (1986) "Ethnographic and Qualitative Research Design and Why it Doesn't Work," *American Behavioral Scientist*. 30(1):42-57, September/October.

Burawoy, M., Burton, A., Ferguson, A., Fox, K., Gamson, J., Gartrell, N., Hurst, L., Kurzman, C., Salziner, L., Schiffman, J. and Ui, S. (1991) *Ethnography Unbound: Power and Resistance in the Modern Metropolis*. Berkeley and Los Angeles, CA: University of California Press.

Bussis, A., Chittendon, E., and Amarel, M. (1973) *Methodology in Educational Evaluation and Research*. Princeton, N.J.: Educational Testing Service.

Carini, P. (1975) *Observation and Description: An Alternative Methodology for the Investigation of Human Phenomena*. Grand Forks: University of North Dakota Press.

Centers for Disease Control. (1991a) AIDS/HIV Surveillance, National Commission on AIDS Report, July.

Centers for Disease Control. (1991b) The HIV/AIDS Epidemic: The First 10 Years, *Morbidity and Mortality Weekly Report*, 40:357-363, 369, June 7.

Chaisson, R., Osmond, D., Moss, A., et al. (1987a) "HIV, Bleach, and Needle Sharing," *Lancet I*, 8547:1430.

Chaisson, R., Moss, A., Onishi, R., Osmond, D. and Carlson, J. (1987b) "Human Immunodeficiency Virus Infection in Heterosexual Intravenous Drug Users in San Francisco," *American Journal of Public Health*, 77(2):169-172, February.

Charmaz, K. (1983) "The Grounded Theory Method: An Explication and Interpretation." In *Contemporary Field Research* (Ed.) R. Emerson, 109-126. Boston: Little-Brown.

Chitwood, D., McCoy, C. and Comerford, M. (1990) "Risk Behavior of Intravenous Cocaine Users: Implications of Intervention." In National Institute on Drug Abuse Research Monograph 93 (*AIDS and Intravenous Drug Use: Future Directions for Community-Based Prevention Research*), C. Leukefeld, R. Battjes and Z. Amsel (Eds.), National Institute on Drug Abuse Office of Science, Rockville, Maryland.

Davis-Berman, J. and Brown D. (1990) "AIDS Knowledge and Risky Behavior by Incarcerated Females: IV and Non-IV Drug Users," *Social Science Review*, 75(1):8-16, October.

Denzin, N. (1978a) "The Logic of Naturalistic Inquiry." In N. Denzin (Ed.) *Sociological Methods: A Sourcebook*, New York: McGraw-Hill.

Denzin, N. (1978b) *The Research Act*. New York: McGraw-Hill.

Des Jarlais, D. and Friedman, S. (1988) "The Psychology of Preventing AIDS among Intravenous Drug Users: A Social Learning Conceptualization," *American Psychology*, 48:865-870.

Des Jarlais, D. and Friedman, S. (1987) "Target Groups for Preventing AIDS Among Intravenous Drug Users," *Journal of Applied Social Psychology*, 17(3):251-268.

Friedland, G., Harris, C., Butkus-Small, C., et al. (1985) "Intravenous Drug Abusers and the Acquired Immunodeficiency Syndrome (AIDS)," *Archives of Internal Medicine*, 145:1413-1417.

Friedman, S., Neaigus, A., Des Jarlais, D., Sotheran, J., Woods, J., Sufian, M., Stepherson, B. and Sterk, C. (1992) "Social Intervention Against AIDS among Injecting Drug Users," *British Journal of Addiction*, 87:393-404.

Garfinkel, H. (1967) *Studies in Ethnomethodology*. Englewood Cliffs, N.J.: Prentice-Hall.

Glaser, B. (1978) *Theoretical Sensitivity*. Mill Valley, CA: The Sociology Press.

Glaser, B. and Strauss, A. (1967) *The Discovery of Grounded Theory*. Chicago: Aldine.

Guba, E. (1978) *Toward a Methodology of Naturalistic Inquiry in Educational Evaluation.* CSE Monograph Series in Evaluation No. 8. Los Angeles: Center for the Study of Evaluation.

Guydish, J., Abramowitz, A., Woods, W., Black, D. and Sorensen, J. (1990) "Changes in Needle Sharing Behavior Among Intravenous Drug Users: San Francisco, 1986-88," *American Journal of Public Health*, 80(8):995-996.

Hammersley M. and Atkinson, P. (1983) *Ethnography Principles and Practice.* London: Tavistock Publications.

Hart, G., Sonnex, C., Petherick, A., et al. (1989b) "Risk Behaviors for HIV Infection among Injecting Drug Users Attending a Drug Dependency Clinic," *The British Medical Journal*, 298:1081-1083.

Hopkins, W. (1988) "Needle Sharing and Street Behavior in Response to AIDS In New York City." In National Institute on Drug Abuse Research Monograph 80 (*Needle Sharing among Intravenous Drug Abusers: National and International Perspectives*), R. Battjes and R. Pickens (Eds.), National Institute on Drug Abuse Office of Science, Rockville, Maryland.

Inciardi, J. (1990) "HIV, AIDS and Intravenous Drug Use: Some Considerations," *Journal of Drug Issues*, Spring, 20(2):181-194.

Inciardi, J. and Page, J. (1991) "Drug Sharing among Intravenous Drug Users," *AIDS*, 5(6):772-773.

Lofland, J. (1971) *Analyzing Social Settings*. Belmont, California: Wadsworth.

Maddux, J. and Desmond, D. (1975) "Reliability and Validity of Information from Chronic Heroin Users." *Journal of Psychiatric Research* 12: 87-95.

Magura, S., Grossman, J., Lipton, D., et al. (1989) "Determinants of Needle Sharing among Intravenous Drug Users," *American Journal of Public Health*, 79:459-462.

Marmor, M., Des Jarlais, D., Cohen, H., et al. (1987) "Risk Factors for Infection with Human Immunodeficiency Virus among Intravenous Drug Abusers in New York City," *AIDS*, 1:39-44.

Marmor, M., Des Jarlais, D., Friedman, S., Lyden, M. and El-Sadr, W. (1984) "The Epidemic of Acquired Immunodeficiency Syndrome (AIDS) and Suggestions for its Control in Drug Abusers," *Journal of Substance Abuse Treatment*. 1:237-247.

Nurco, D. (1975) "Studying Addicts Over Time: Methodology and Preliminary Findings," *American Journal of Drug and Alcohol Abuse* 2: 183-196.

Olesen, V. and E. Whittaker, E. (1968) "Conditions Under Which College Students Borrow, Use and Alter Slang," *American Speech*, Vol. XLIII, 3, October.

Ottomanelli, G., Kramer, T., Bihari, B., Fine, J., Heller, S. and Mosely, J. (1990) "AIDS-Related Risk Behaviors among Substance Abusers," *The International Journal of Addictions*, 25(3):291-299.

Page, J., Smith, P. and Kane, N. (1991) "Shooting Galleries, Their Proprietors, and Implications for Prevention of AIDS," *Drugs and Society*, 5(1-2):69-85.

Patton, M. (1987) *How To Use Qualitative Methods in Evaluation.* Beverly Hills: Sage Publications.

Personal Communication, 1992. Prevention Point Volunteers.

Rhodes, F., Corby, N., Wolitski, R., Tashima, N., Cathleen, C., Yankovich, D. and Smith, P. (1990) "Risk Behaviors and Perceptions of AIDS among Street Injection Drug Users," *Journal of Drug Education*, 20(4):271-288.

Rossi, P. and Freeman, H. (1989) *Evaluation: A Systemic Approach*. Beverly Hills: Sage Publications.

Schatzman, L. and Strauss, A. (1973) *Field Research: Strategies for a Natural Sociology*. Englewood Cliffs, NJ: Prentice Hall.

Schoenbaum, E., Hartel, D., Selwyn, P., et al. (1989) "Risk Factors for Human Immunodeficiency Virus Infection in Intravenous Drug Users," *The New England Journal of Medicine*, 321:874-879.

Selwyn, P., Feiner, C., Cox, C., et al. (1987) "Knowledge about AIDS and High-Risk Behavior among Intravenous Drug Users in New York City," *AIDS*, 1:247-254.

Sorensen, J., Guydish, J., Costantini, M. and Batki, S. (1989) "Changes in Needle Sharing and Syringe Cleaning among San Francisco Drug Abusers," *New England Journal of Medicine*, 320:807.

Spradley, J. (1979) *The Ethnographic Interview*. New York: Holt, Rhinehart and Winston.

Stephens, R. (1972) "The Truthfulness of Addict Respondents in Research Projects," *The International Journal of the Addictions* 7(3):549-558.

Stephens, R., Feucht, T. and Roman, S. (1991) "Effects of an Intervention Program on AIDS-Related Drug and Needle Behavior Among Intravenous Drug Users," *American Journal of Public Health*, 81(5):568-571, May.

Strauss, A. and Corbin, J. (1990) *Basics of Qualitative Research*. Newbury Park: Sage Publications.

Watters, J. and Biernacki, P. (1989) "Targeted Sampling: Options for the Study of Hidden Populations," *Social Problems*. 36(4):416-430.

OPERATIONAL MODELING OF NEEDLE EXCHANGE PROGRAMS

Edward H. Kaplan

1. Introduction and Motivation

Needle exchange is advocated by many as an intervention to slow the spread of HIV transmission among drug injectors via needle sharing (Des Jarlais and Friedman, 1992; Stimson, 1989). Whether needle exchange achieves this end is difficult to determine via direct observation. Repeated HIV testing of injecting drug users (IDUs) participating in outreach programs is rare relative to the number of outreach programs that exist (for an exception see Ljungberg *et al.*, 1991), while anything approaching a controlled trial pitting the HIV incidence rate among IDUs participating in a needle exchange against incidence in a provably equivalent group of IDUs not exchanging needles is unheard of. Pragmatically speaking, this is not a situation that is likely to change (Des Jarlais and Friedman, 1992).

Given the above difficulties, many researchers have turned to behavioral studies of needle exchange participants. Such studies rely on the presence (or absence) of self-reported changes in risky behaviors (such as sharing frequencies and injection rates) as evidence of the impact of needle exchange (Donoghoe *et al.*, 1989; GAO, 1993; Hagan *et al.*, 1991; Hartgers *et al.*, 1989; Joseph and Des Jarlais, 1989; Watters and Cheng, 1991). Social desirability effects might play a role in skewing self-reported behavioral data. For example, in a program environment where participants are clearly instructed not to share needles, what should one expect in response to a question like "How often do you share needles?" This in itself does not prove that self-reported data are inaccurate. It does mean, however, that it is hard to *know* the degree to which self-reported changes in behavior reflect the truth.

This paper offers a rather different set of ideas for evaluating needle exchange programs. These methods have been described elsewhere as they were developed (Kaplan 1994; Kaplan and Heimer, 1993, 1994), but it seems useful to bring their details together in one place. The common thread in the techniques to be described is the utilization of mathematical models of needle exchange operations in conjunction with objectively observable data such as the volume of needles distributed, the dates of program visitation, the circulation time of needles, and the fraction of returned needles that test positive for HIV. The models lead to testable conjectures that *a priori* could lead to either positive or negative conclusions regarding the effectiveness of needle exchange, while the data enable the statistical testing of these conjectures.

Two different modeling approaches will be described below. The first of these attempts to estimate the incidence of HIV infection among participating drug injectors using nothing other than data describing client visits and the measured level of infection in needles (Kaplan and Heimer, 1994). The second approach develops an operational theory of needle exchange that not only provides an estimate for the relative impact of the program on HIV incidence among participating IDUs, but also provides a compelling explanation for how the physics of needle exchange might conspire to reduce HIV transmission in the absence of major changes in behavior (Kaplan, 1994; Kaplan and Heimer, 1993). Both of these models have been implemented using data collected in conjunction with the evaluation of the legal program operated by the AIDS Division of the New Haven, Connecticut Department of Health, and the results of these studies will be discussed. Technical details involved in both the derivation and interpretation of these models will be stressed, while suggestions for how one might implement these ideas in other settings will be made where appropriate.

While the focus of this paper is on methodology, it is worth stating the results of the New Haven studies up front. The models strongly suggest that needle exchange has reduced needle borne HIV infections among program participants from the beginning of the program in November 1990 through June 1992. One model suggests a relative reduction in transmission on the order of 33%, while the other does not allow rejection of the hypothesis that *no* new infections have occurred among needle exchange participants since the program started.

In July 1992, the purchase of syringes without prescription at Connecticut pharmacies became legal (Valleroy *et al.*, 1993; Weinstein and Hadler, 1993). Coincident with the decriminalization of syringe purchase and sale in Connecticut was a large drop in the number of IDUs participating in the New Haven program. As decriminalization changed the environment in which the New Haven needle exchange was operating in a major fashion, most of the data discussed in this paper will be limited to the first 20 months of the New Haven needle exchange.

2. Estimating HIV Incidence Among Needle Exchange Participants (Kaplan and Heimer, 1994)

2.1 An Idealized Research Environment

To begin, imagine an idealized research environment where one can repeatedly test a cohort of *m* IDUs for HIV infection over time. If the prevalence of HIV infection in the IDUs is denoted by ϕ and the incidence rate of new infections is given by ρ infections per *uninfected* IDU per unit time, then the probability that a randomly selected IDU would become infected within a duration of length δ is given by

$$\Pr\{\text{Infection}\} = (1-\phi)\,(1-e^{-\rho\delta}) \approx (1-\phi)\,\rho\,\delta \equiv \theta\,\delta \tag{1}$$

for sufficiently small values of the product $\rho\delta$ (if $\rho\delta < 0.10$ then the error in the approximation above is no worse than about 5%). Note that this is a short run perspective, in that it is assumed that both the prevalence ϕ and the incidence ρ remain constant over the duration of the study. Let $y_i = 1$ if the ith IDU in the sample *becomes* infected during δ (this assumes that the specific date of infection is unknown, which is reasonable if people are tested only at the beginning and end of the study period, for example), and $y_i=0$ otherwise. First, from data one would discover that approximately $m\phi$ IDUs in the cohort were infected at the start of the study (for the prevalence of HIV infection was assumed to equal ϕ). Second, one would reason that $\Sigma_{i=1}^{m} y_i \approx m(1-\phi)\rho\delta$ based on equation (1) above. The raw incidence rate ρ would thus be estimated by dividing $\Sigma_{i=1}^{m} y_i$ by $m(1-\phi)\delta$ (actually, one would divide $\Sigma_{i=1}^{m} y_i$ by the product of δ and the *observed* number of initially uninfected IDUs, but this latter number is roughly

$m(1-\phi)$). At the end of duration δ, one would have two ways of expressing the incidence rate: the number of new infections per ***uninfected*** drug injector per unit time, given by ρ, or the unconditional number of new infections per IDU per unit time, given by θ. It is easy to show that the expression $\Sigma_{i=1}^{m} y_i/m\delta$ is also the maximum likelihood estimator of θ (again assuming $\rho\delta$ is sufficiently small).

2.2 A Needle Exchange Environment Where Only Needles Are Tested

With the above set of computations in mind for future reference, consider now the more difficult research environment of a needle exchange program. Suppose that no data are available regarding the HIV status of any individual IDU participating in the program, for program officials have decreed that HIV testing might dissuade IDUs from joining the needle exchange. However, data are available regarding the HIV status of samples of ***needles*** returned to the program (this is in fact the situation in the needle exchange operated by the AIDS Division of New Haven's Health Department). Specifically, suppose that for a given IDU the following data are available: the earliest and latest dates of needle exchange (and hence the duration δ that the IDU was exposed to the program), and a series of indicator variables x_1, x_2, ..., x_n corresponding to n returned needles ordered by date of return. The indicator x_i equals one if the ith needle in sequence tests positive, and zero otherwise. What can one infer from such data?

Note that if needles were never shared and all laboratory testing of needles was error-free, the above data record would yield information equivalent to the idealized incidence trial described above. Unfortunately, one expects both laboratory errors and needle sharing to occur. Even in the presence of such distractions, it is possible to estimate ***statistically*** whether a given IDU has become infected. This is because of the following observation: ***whatever*** the laboratory error rates and sharing patterns are, the likelihood that a returned needle will test positive for HIV ***after*** an IDU has become infected ***should be higher*** than the likelihood that a needle returned by the same IDU would test positive ***before*** the IDU becomes infected. One should therefore be able to detect a new infection by observing an upward shift in the fraction of returned needles that test positive.

2.3 A Maximum Likelihood Change Point Model

This intuition can be formalized. Let $\pi(+)$ ($\pi(-)$) denote the probability that needles test positive conditional on their return by an IDU who is in truth infected (uninfected). As this procedure is being applied on an IDU by IDU basis, there is no need for the values of $\pi(+)$ and $\pi(-)$ to be common across IDUs. Indeed, these probabilities allow for differences in needle sharing and needle cleaning patterns across IDUs, in addition to pure laboratory testing errors. Suppose that the IDU in question became infected between the sth and $s+1^{st}$ needles tested. The probability of observing the data record $x_1, x_2, \ldots x_s, x_{s+1}, \ldots, x_n$ is then given by the likelihood function

$$\mathcal{L} = \prod_{i=1}^{s} \pi(-)^{x_i} \left(1-\pi(-)\right)^{1-x_i} \prod_{i=s+1}^{n} \pi(+)^{x_i} \left(1-\pi(+)\right)^{1-x_i}. \quad (2)$$

The model formulated above is a *change point model* (Cox, 1970; Page, 1955), and the unknown parameters $\pi(-)$, $\pi(+)$, and s can be estimated from the data record $x_1, x_2, \ldots, x_n$ via the method of maximum likelihood. Conditional on s, it is clear that the maximum likelihood estimators for $\pi(-)$ and $\pi(+)$ are given by $\Sigma_{i=1}^{s} x_i/s$ and $\Sigma_{i=s+1}^{n} x_i/(n-s)$ unless the former is larger than the latter, in which case the maximum likelihood estimators for *both* probabilities are given by $\Sigma_{i=1}^{n} x_i/n$ (for logic insists that $\pi(+) \geq \pi(-)$). Substituting the above formulas into (2) enables one to conduct a search over $s \in (1,2,3,\ldots,n-1)$ to find that value of s that maximizes the value of $\mathcal{L}$ in (2) above (actually, one only needs to consider those values of s such that $x_s=0$ and $x_{s+1}=1$ in the search process, as is easily shown); call the maximized value of the likelihood function $\mathcal{L}_1$.

Armed with the maximum likelihood estimates for the three change point parameters, it is possible to test the null hypothesis that $\pi(-) = \pi(+) = \pi$, that is, *no* new infection occurred (either because the IDU was already infected, or because the IDU was uninfected and remained so over the study period). Under the null hypothesis, the maximum likelihood estimator for π is given by $\Sigma_{i=1}^{n} x_i/n$. Substituting this value for both $\pi(-)$ and $\pi(+)$ in (2) yields the maximized likelihood under the null hypothesis; call this $\mathcal{L}_0$.

A ***threshold test*** can be established as follows: reject the null hypothesis (and conclude that the IDU became infected) if the ratio $\mathcal{L}_1/\mathcal{L}_0$ exceeds some threshold. Specifically, the null hypothesis will be rejected if the quantity $2\ \ell og\ (\mathcal{L}_1/\mathcal{L}_0)$ exceeds some cutoff denoted by c (this is equivalent to requiring $\mathcal{L}_1/\mathcal{L}_0$ to exceed $e^{c/2}$).

2.4 Statistical Errors and the Change Point Test

Note that even with a testing procedure to determine whether an IDU became infected solely on the basis of needle testing, it is possible that the procedure suggested will lead to erroneous decisions. However, it is also possible to compute the probabilities that such ***statistical*** errors will occur. Specifically, let α denote the probability of concluding that an IDU has become infected ***given no infection actually occurred*** (a Type I error), and β denote the probability of concluding that an IDU has not become infected ***given that infection actually occurred*** (a Type II error). How large might these error probabilities be?

To answer this question requires considering all possible needle testing sequences of size n that ***could*** occur given true underlying values for the parameters $\pi(-)$, $\pi(+)$, and s. There are 2^n possible binary sequences, each one representing a different ordered pattern of positive and negative needle tests. These sequences can be indexed by their binary representation so that in a particular sequence $\mathcal{S}$, the ith element $x_{i\mathcal{S}} = 1$ if and only if

$$\sum_{i=1}^{n} 2^{i-1} x_{i\mathcal{S}} = \mathcal{S} \tag{3}$$

for $\mathcal{S}=0,1,\ldots,2^n-1$; otherwise $x_{i\mathcal{S}} = 0$ (note that for a fixed value of $\mathcal{S}$, equation (3) has a unique solution). In sequence $\mathcal{S}$, the ith needle tests positive if $x_{i\mathcal{S}}=1$, otherwise the ith needle tests negative.

Now, suppose that the data from sequence $\mathcal{S}$ were subjected to the change point test of Section 2.3. The null hypothesis of no new infection would be rejected if $2\ \ell og\ (\mathcal{L}_1/\mathcal{L}_0)$ exceeds the cutoff c. Let $z_{\mathcal{S}}(c)$ be the indicator variable that equals 1 if the cutoff is exceeded (and thus the change point test leads to rejection of the null hypothesis), and 0 otherwise. The overall probability of rejecting the null hypothesis for the change point test is then given by

$$\Pr\left\{ \text{Reject Null Hypothesis} \right\} = \sum_{\mathcal{S}=0}^{2^n-1} z_{\mathcal{S}}(c)\ \Pr\left\{ \text{Sequence } \mathcal{S} \right\}. \tag{4}$$

Equation (4) enables the calculation of the exact probability of rejecting the null hypothesis conditional on the true values of the underlying parameters in the model. For example, suppose that in truth no new infection has occurred, and the probability of any needle testing positive is given by π. The probability of obtaining a particular sequence $\mathcal{S}$ in this circumstance would then equal

$$\Pr\left\{ \text{Sequence } \mathcal{S} \right\} = \pi^{\Sigma_{i=1}^{n} x_{i\mathcal{S}}} (1-\pi)^{n-\Sigma_{i=1}^{n} x_{i\mathcal{S}}} \quad \mathcal{S}=0,1,2,\ldots,2^n-1. \tag{5}$$

Substitution of equation (5) into (4) above then enables the calculation of α for any given sample size n, underlying needle prevalence π, and cutoff criterion c.

Of interest is the following robustness result obtained numerically. Given employment of the threshold criterion $2\ \ell og\ (\mathcal{L}_1/\mathcal{L}_0) > c$, asymptotic maximum likelihood theory might tempt one to relate c to the $1-\alpha$ percentage point of the χ^2 probability distribution with 2 degrees of freedom (Cox and Hinkley, 1974), for the difference in the number of parameters in the change point model (3: $\pi(+)$, $\pi(-)$, and s) and the null hypothesis model (1: π) equals 2. This would not be correct, for the likelihood function of equation (2) is not differentiable with respect to s. However, equations (4) and (5) enable exact computation of the significance level α for comparison with the χ^2 result. The reason for seeking such an approximation is that while the exact computations for α (and β) are possible, they are tedious (for example, a sample of $n = 15$ needles gives rise to $2^{15} = 32{,}768$ different sequences, each one of which must be passed through the change point procedure to determine the value of $z_{\mathcal{S}}(c)$). The 95th percentile of the χ^2 distribution with 2 degrees of freedom is given by 5.991, so setting $c = 5.991$ should yield values of α close to 0.05 if the χ^2 provides reasonable guidance. As reported in Kaplan and Heimer (1994), for sample sizes (n) of 8, 10, 12, and 15, and assumed values of π running from 0.10 through 0.90 in increments of 0.10, the exact significance levels computed ranged from 0.0496 through 0.0663. Thus, even though the use of the χ^2 to select cutoff values is not justified on the theoretical grounds of asymptotic likelihood theory, its use does appear reasonable from the (limited) numerical results obtained. This is of course important, for in any true application of the change point test, one does not know the underlying true value of π (assuming the null hypothesis is correct), while one will also be faced with needle testing sequences of different lengths.

The power of the change point test can also be explored using equation (4) above. Details are provided in the appendix of Kaplan and Heimer (1994). In the numerical computations reported there, the power of a change point test using a cutoff of $c = 5.991$ for samples of size 8, 10, 12 and 15 assuming $\pi(-) = 0.15$ and $\pi(+) = 0.85$ was explored as a function of s, the true change point parameter. With the exceptions of s values equal to 1 or $n-1$, the power obtained was close to or exceeded 50%. For values of s in the middle of the sample ($s \approx n/2$), the power was close to or exceeded 70%.

It therefore seems safe to conclude that for most applications, applying a cutoff of $c = 5.991$ to the change point test described in Section 2.3 results in a Type I error probability of $\alpha \approx 0.05$, and a Type II error probability of $\beta \leq 0.50$. These quantities enable the construction of a procedure for estimating HIV incidence among needle exchange participants based solely on the testing of returned needles.

2.5 Estimating HIV Incidence from Change Point Test Results

To summarize the discussion thus far, a statistical model has been proposed for determining whether or not an individual IDU has become infected based solely on the results of HIV tests on returned needles. The modeling also allows the computation of the statistical significance (α) and power ($1-\beta$) of the test, so the likely size of statistical errors can be known in advance. Now, recall from equation (1) that the probability that an IDU becomes infected over some duration δ approximately equals $\theta\delta$, where θ is the *unconditional* incidence rate, that is, the number of new infections per IDU per unit time. Instead of observing individual tests on IDUs, however, imagine observing the results of change point tests conducted on the sequences of needles returned by program participants. What is the probability that one would conclude an IDU became infected on the basis of a change point test?

Clearly there are two possibilities. First, the IDU in question really became infected (with probability $\theta\delta$), and the change point test had the *power* to detect this new infection (with probability $1-\beta$). Alternatively, the IDU did not become infected (with probability $1-\theta\delta$), but the change point test committed a Type I statistical error, and falsely concluded that the IDU became infected (with probability α). Therefore, the probability $r(\theta)$ that one would conclude an IDU became infected on the basis of a change point test is given by

$$r(\theta) = \theta\delta(1-\beta) + (1-\theta\delta)\alpha = \alpha + (1-\alpha-\beta)\theta\delta. \qquad (6)$$

By analogy with Section 2.1, let $y_i = 1$ if the change point test performed on the sequence of needles returned by the ith IDU suggests that infection has occurred (i.e. $2 \log (\mathcal{L}_1/\mathcal{L}_0) > c = 5.991$ for the ith sequence of needles), and $y_i = 0$ otherwise, $i=1,2,\ldots,m$. A very simple test of the hypothesis that *no* new infections have occurred among the IDUs returning the needles can be constructed by setting $\theta=0$ (as required by the hypothesis of no new infections). In this case, $r(\theta) = \alpha$, thus the total number of rejected change point tests $\Sigma_{i=1}^{m} y_i$ follows the binomial probability distribution with parameters m and α. It is then an elementary task to compute the probability that at least as many rejected change point tests as actually observed would occur solely due to chance.

It is also possible to estimate θ via maximum likelihood. Given δ_i, the duration of exposure of the ith IDU to the needle exchange as discerned from the dates of first and last program visits (or perhaps more appropriately, from the dates of first and last visits from which returned needles were tested for HIV), the probability of observing a rejected change point test follows equation (6) after substituting δ_i for δ; call this probability $r_i(\theta)$. As a consequence, the probability of observing the particular set of change point results for all m IDUs is given by

$$\mathcal{L}(\theta) = \prod_{i=1}^{m} r_i(\theta)^{y_i} \big(1-r_i(\theta)\big)^{1-y_i}. \tag{7}$$

Maximizing $\mathcal{L}(\theta)$ over θ subject to the constraint that $\theta \geq 0$ can be achieved directly. The maximum likelihood estimator $\hat{\theta}$ will equal zero for any change point significance level $\alpha \geq \Sigma_{i=1}^{m} y_i\delta_i \,/\, \Sigma_{i=1}^{m} \delta_i$; otherwise, $\hat{\theta}$ is the unique root of the equation

$$\sum_{i=1}^{m} y_i\delta_i \,/\, r_i(\theta) = \sum_{i=1}^{m} (1-y_i)\delta_i/\big(1-r_i(\theta)\big). \tag{8}$$

Note that if $\delta_i=\delta$ for $i=1,2,\ldots,m$, then equation (8) yields a simple formula for $\hat{\theta}$, given by

$$\hat{\theta} = \frac{\Sigma_{i=1}^{m} y_i - m\alpha}{(1-\alpha-\beta)\; m\delta}. \tag{9}$$

In the idealized world of perfect statistical testing, both α and β would equal zero, yielding $\hat{\theta} = \Sigma_{i=1}^{m} y_i/m\delta$, the same result cited in Section 2.1.

2.6 Application to the New Haven Needle Exchange: The Syringe Tracking and Testing System and Statistical Results

The data structures alluded to above have been realized as part of the evaluation of New Haven's needle exchange program. The unique ***syringe tracking and testing system*** (or STT) implemented in New Haven works as follows (Kaplan and O'Keefe, 1993): all participants in the program receive a code name of their own choosing. In addition, all needles distributed by the program are endowed with a unique tracking code. When the program started, these codes were placed by hand with a paint pen directly on outbound syringes, and covered with transparent tape for protection (non-detachable needle/syringe pairs are distributed by the program, so the terms needle and syringe are used interchangably). Since the fall of 1992 syringes have been tracked by bar code. At the time exchange transactions occur, outreach workers record the date, location, and code name of the person receiving the needles. When needles are returned to the program, the date, location, and code name of the person returning the needles are also recorded. Consequently, a complete record of syringe transactions and client participation is compiled.

In addition to syringe tracking, samples of returned needles are tested for the presence of HIV-1 proviral DNA using polymerase chain reaction (PCR) techniques developed by Robert Heimer (see Heimer ***et al.*** (1992a)). Recognizing that a simple random sample of returned needles would be weighted heavily to reflect those who exchange most often, a two-stage sampling procedure has been implemented to achieve greater client coverage. Needles are exchanged in batches of at most five. In the first sampling stage, all syringes are retrieved from returned batches of at most two, while two syringes are taken from batches of size three through five. The second stage systematically samples every 10th needle selected in the first stage. From November 1990 through June 1992, this procedure selected 2,813 of the 49,405 needles distributed for testing.

The change point models were implemented on a subset of the needle testing data reported above. First, testing results were available only for needles returned by the end of May 1992 at the time this study was undertaken. Second, only those clients who had returned at least five tested needles were considered for analysis, recognizing the inability of the change point test to provide meaningful results for smaller values of n. The STT provided a total of 1,920 needles representing 132 different clients with at least five tested needles (averaging 14.5 tested needles per client). Just over 42% of these needles tested HIV positive via PCR. Exposure times were taken as the time between the first and last dates tested needles were returned inclusive. The total derived exposure time was 34,903 person days in the needle exchange, averaging 264 days per client.

Of the 132 change point tests conducted, six rejected the null hypothesis of no infection using the cutoff $c = 5.991$. If one was to simply divide this number by the total exposure time, one would estimate an unconditional HIV incidence rate of 6.3 new infections per 100 needle exchange clients per year. However, this ignores the chance errors one can expect from applying the change point test.

Having observed that $\Sigma_{i=1}^{132} y_i = 6$, a Type I error probability of $\alpha = 0.05$ associated with the change point test (as suggested by numerical studies) easily accounts for the data. Under the null hypothesis that no new infections occurred (that is, that $\theta = 0$), the probability of observing six or more rejected change point tests is given by the binomial tail probability

$$\Pr\left\{ \text{Number of Rejections} \geq 6 \right\} = \sum_{i=6}^{132} \binom{132}{i} 0.05^{i}\, 0.95^{132-i} = 0.6512. \qquad (10)$$

Given that one has more than a 65% chance of observing the change point results assuming that $\theta = 0$, ***it is not possible to reject the hypothesis that in the New Haven needle exchange, no new infections have occurred among those IDUs studied.***

The maximum likelihood approach supports this point as well. The value of $\Sigma_{i=1}^{132} y_i\delta_i \,/\, \Sigma_{i=1}^{132} \delta_i = 0.0398$. For any $\alpha \geq 0.0398$, $\hat{\theta} = 0$, and as numerical studies of the change point test suggest that α is in the neighborhood of 0.05, it is indeed the case that $\hat{\theta}=0$.

It is worth mentioning at this point that these results were not in any way preordained. It could have been the case that the change point test rejected the null hypothesis for a large percentage of those clients studied. It is important to note that at the conventional significance level of 5%, one would not be able to reject the null hypothesis of no new infections unless 12 or more change point tests suggested that infections had occurred. Given that only half that number was actually observed suggests that in the New Haven needle exchange program, the incidence rate of new infections is not high. Furthermore, since more than 42% of the needles tested HIV positive, it is clear that this population had a positive HIV incidence rate in the past.

While the change point model provides an approach to estimating HIV incidence among needle exchange participants, it does not explain *how* needle exchange operations might be expected to effect HIV transmission rates. Doing so requires deeper understanding of the *physics* of needle exchange. Models describing the physical workings of needle exchange and implications for disease transmission are described next.

3. The Physics of Needle Exchange (Kaplan, 1994)

3.1 A Qualitative Overview

This section of the paper formalizes a *circulation theory* of needle exchange developed over the past two years. Before presenting the mathematical and statistical details of this theory, however, it is useful to summarize the intuition underlying the key ideas. The mathematical arguments that follow provide a rigorous mechanism for expressing and testing this intuition.

To begin, try to imagine the HIV status of a needle from the moment it is introduced into a population of drug injectors. Many different experiences are possible, but at any moment in time a needle may be viewed as either contaminated or not. Needles can only become infected following use by an HIV infected IDU, though not all needles necessarily become contaminated following such use (also, effective post-injection bleaching may render some needles non-infectious in spite of having been used by infected IDUs). Infected needles can become decontaminated for a variety of reasons, including effective pre-injection bleaching (though not all bleaching is effective), dilution of infectious blood with the blood of uninfected IDUs following several shared injections, or natural inactivation of the virus. Whatever the relative contamination and decontamination rates are per needle, clearly the longer a needle remains in circulation, the higher the likelihood that the needle in question becomes infected.

Aggregating the stochastic infection processes for individual needles across all needles in the population leads to an average level of infection among all needles at any point in time. This average level may be interpreted as the probability that a needle selected at random is contaminated with HIV. In addition to the relative contamination and decontamination rates, the average level of infection depends on the distribution of needle circulation times, with stochastically longer circulation times associated with higher average levels of infection in the needles.

Needle exchange may be thought of as a mechanism that operates directly on the distribution of needle circulation times (Kaplan and Heimer, 1993). First, note that by *exchanging* needles, the total number of needles in circulation does not change in theory for a law of conservation of needles applies: the rate with which needles are distributed is balanced by the rate with which needles are returned. To the extent that one believes that HIV transmission among IDUs is a function solely of the *number* of needles in circulation, then, one should not expect needle exchange to change matters much. Instead, what one achieves by exchanging needles is the *interruption* of the needle circulation process. This stochastically reduces the length of time for which needles remain in the population. ***The greater the rate with which needles are exchanged, the greater the reduction in needle circulation times.*** This is the key operational link between needle exchange programs and HIV transmission, for reducing needle circulation times acts via the stochastic infection process to lower the average level of infection in the population of needles. The intuition is simple: if needles are available for shorter periods of time *per needle*, then the likelihood that different IDUs will use the same needle declines. In effect, needle exchange causes needles to share fewer people.

Reducing the mean level of infection in circulating needles is important, for those who persist in sharing needles are in effect sampling from the population of needles in circulation. If the mean level of infection in needles declines, then the chance that a person who persists in sharing needles will encounter a contaminated needle also declines. Since one can only become infected via needle sharing from contaminated needles, it follows that the incidence rate of HIV infection by needle sharing will be proportional to the average level of infection in circulating needles. The ***relative*** success of a needle exchange in reducing HIV transmission can therefore be measured by the ***relative*** drop in the level of infection in circulating needles.

The theory summarized above does not imply that needle exchange is an instant success. To be effective in reducing HIV incidence, the theory suggests that exchange programs must exchange needles with sufficient rapidity to reduce circulation times by a large amount. Another important point is that this theory offers *no* support for the contention that needle exchange reduces HIV transmission among anyone not participating in the program. Needle exchange ***might*** cause a reduction in such transmission (perhaps via averting sexually transmitted infections to non-injecting sex partners of client IDUs, or via the placement of non-client IDUs in drug treatment programs), but the analysis developed here does not consider such possibilities. The fair interpretation of what follows is that the physics of needle exchange alone can conspire to confer protective benefits to those who regularly exchange needles.

The validity of the theory can be tested providing the requisite data are available to do so. Such data have been assembled via New Haven's syringe tracking and testing system. Less exhaustive approaches to data collection could also yield sufficient information for applying the ideas presented below, as will be discussed briefly later on.

With the above intuition firmly in mind, it is time to explore the physics of needle exchange.

3.2 The Needle Infection Process

As described above, circulating needles are always in one of two states, HIV-contaminated or uncontaminated. Aiming for simplicity, a two-state continuous time Markov process is proposed as a model for the dynamics of needle infection. Uncontaminated needles are assumed to become infected with rate λ per uncontaminated needle per unit time, while HIV-contaminated needles become uncontaminated with rate μ per contaminated needle per unit time. The perspective is again short term in that the epidemiological and biological processes that contribute to λ and μ as described in Section 3.1 are assumed to remain stable. Thus, the prevalence of infection (ϕ), needle injection, sharing and cleaning rates, and viral inactivation rates are all assumed constant over the period of study, leading to stable values of λ and μ. Let $\pi(t)$ denote the probability that a needle that has been circulating for t time units is HIV-contaminated. Following standard Markov process theory (Bhat, 1984), $\pi(t)$ can be found from the recursion

$$\pi(t+\Delta t) = (1-\pi(t))\ \lambda\ \Delta t + \pi(t)\ (1-\mu\ \Delta t) + o(\Delta t). \tag{11}$$

Letting $\Delta t \to 0$ in equation (11) leads to the first order linear differential equation

$$\frac{d\pi(t)}{dt} + (\lambda+\mu)\ \pi(t) = \lambda \tag{12}$$

which solves to yield

$$\pi(t) = \frac{\lambda}{\lambda+\mu} + \left(\pi_0 - \frac{\lambda}{\lambda+\mu} \right) e^{-(\lambda+\mu)t} \tag{13}$$

where π_0 is the probability that the needle is already HIV-contaminated when introduced to the population (and should equal zero if the needle in question was provided via a needle exchange program). Equation (13) quantifies the intuition described earlier, in that the probability that a needle is HIV-contaminated increases from π_0 to the equilibrium value of $\lambda/(\lambda+\mu)$ with increasing circulation time.

3.3 The Needle Circulation Process

Equation (13) describes the probability that a needle is HIV-contaminated following a fixed circulation time of duration t. However, there are many needles circulating at any moment in time. Of interest is the mean level of infection in those needles circulating at any moment in time, that is, the probability that a randomly selected circulating needle is infected.

To compute this probability requires a model of the needle circulation process. Let random variable **T** denote the complete length of time for which a needle remains in the population, and random variable $\mathbf{T_R}$ denote the complete length of time for which a ***circulating needle selected at random*** remains in the population. The random variable $\mathbf{T_R}$ is thus obtained by ***length biased sampling*** or ***random incidence*** (Cox, 1962; Drake, 1967), for the likelihood of finding a complete circulation interval of a given duration is proportional to both the frequency with which such intervals occur and the duration of the interval itself. The probability density of random variable $\mathbf{T_R}$ is related to the density of random variable **T** by the equation

$$f_{T_R}(t) = \frac{t f_T(t)}{E(T)} \qquad (14)$$

where E(T) denotes the expected circulation time, and probability densities are denoted by f.

It is now necessary to obtain the probability density function for the ***elapsed*** circulation time of a needle selected at random from the population. Note that conditional upon selecting a needle with a ***complete*** circulation interval equal to, say, u, the elapsed circulation time will simply be distributed uniformly between 0 and u. Therefore, the probability density function for the ***elapsed*** circulation time of a needle selected at random (elapsed circulation time is denoted by random variable T_E) is given by

$$f_{T_E}(t) = \int_{u=t}^{\infty} (1/u)\, f_{T_R}(u)\, du = \frac{1-F_T(t)}{E(T)} \qquad (15)$$

where $F_T(t)$ is the *cumulative distribution function* associated with the original circulation time distribution.

The probability that a circulating needle selected at random is HIV-contaminated, $E[\pi(T_E)]$, is therefore equal to

$$E[\pi(T_E)] = \int_0^{\infty} \pi(t)\, f_{T_E}(t)\, dt. \tag{16}$$

Equation (16) is a general result, in that it shows how to obtain the average level of infection in circulating needles for *any* needle infection process (not just the Markov process considered earlier) and for *any* needle circulation process. However, in studies conducted thus far, only the Markov infection process has been considered in concert with an ***exponential*** circulation time probability density function given by

$$f_T(t) = \frac{1}{\tau} e^{-t/\tau} \tag{17}$$

where τ is the mean circulation time. The exponential possesses the special property that the distribution of ***elapsed*** circulation times equals the original distribution of circulation times (the so-called ***memoryless*** property). The average level of infection in circulating needles for the Markov-exponential model, denoted by $\bar{\pi}(\tau)$, is thus given by

$$\bar{\pi}(\tau) = \int_0^{\infty} \left\{ \frac{\lambda}{\lambda+\mu} + \left(\pi_0 - \frac{\lambda}{\lambda+\mu} \right) e^{-(\lambda+\mu)t} \right\} \frac{1}{\tau} e^{-t/\tau}\, dt$$

$$= \frac{\pi_0 + \lambda\tau}{1 + (\lambda+\mu)\tau}. \tag{18}$$

Equation (18) again has the correct intuitive properties. Note that as τ approaches 0, $\bar{\pi}(\tau)$ approaches π_0 as it should, while as τ becomes very large, $\bar{\pi}(\tau)$ approaches the equilibrium value $\lambda/(\lambda+\mu)$.

Having established a model describing the average level of infection in circulating needles at a random moment in time, it is possible to consider how needle exchange effects this mean level of infection. This is the subject of the next section.

3.4 Needle Exchange Reduces Circulation Times

Needle exchange physically interrupts the needle circulation process by replacing circulating syringes with new ones every time an exchange transaction occurs. Thus, the physical result of needle exchange is to shorten the circulation times of needles. A specific hypothesis is offered for the nature of the relationship between needle exchange and circulation times. Let ν denote the rate with which needles are exchanged per ***IDU*** per unit time, and $\tau(\nu)$ denote the mean circulation time that results when needles are exchanged with rate ν. The mean ***removal rate*** of needles from the population when a program with exchange rate ν is in force will be denoted by $\xi(\nu)$. Clearly $\xi(\nu) = 1/\tau(\nu)$ by definition.

In the absence of needle exchange (ν=0), there will still be some baseline removal rate ($\xi(0)$) and mean circulation time ($\tau(0)$) in the population of needles. However, as ν increases, one expects $\xi(\nu)$ to increase as well. In particular, let

$$\xi(\nu) = a + b\nu \qquad (19)$$

represent the impact of needle exchange on the removal rate of needles (the parameters a and b are both non-negative). The parameter a denotes the baseline removal rate (so $\tau(0)=1/a$), while b may be interpreted as a ***transfer coefficient*** converting needle distribution per client to needle removal per circulating needle. The coefficient b accounts for the difference in the population size of clients and the population size of needles (the greater the ratio of clients to needles, the greater the value of b). In addition, b allows for the possibility of substitution effects, in that the availability of needles from an exchange program may partially substitute for needles previously obtained from other sources (the greater the degree of substitution, the lower the magnitude of b).

The models above present a compact theory of the physical effect of needle exchange. To recap: implementing a needle exchange program with an exchange rate of ν needles per client per unit time is hypothesized to increase per needle removal rates ($\xi(\nu)$) in accordance with equation (19). This reduces the average circulation time among circulating needles, for $\tau(\nu)$ equals $1/\xi(\nu)$. Reducing $\tau(\nu)$ reduces $\bar{\pi}\big(\tau(\nu)\big)$ in accordance with equation (18).

As HIV transmission via needle sharing requires injection with a contaminated needle, it is reasonable to consider the relative reduction in the mean level of HIV infection in circulating needles as a measure of the relative reduction in HIV incidence. The key evaluation performance measure to be considered is therefore equal to

$$\text{Relative Reduction} = 1 - \bar{\pi}\big(\tau(\nu)\big) \;/\; \bar{\pi}\big(\tau(0)\big). \qquad (20)$$

To compute ***absolute*** reductions in incidence requires an estimate of the baseline HIV incidence rate before needle exchange began. Such estimates are not available via the theory advanced here, but can be obtained from other back-of-the-envelope calculations to be demonstrated shortly if actual observations from field studies are not available (which will most often be the case).

3.5 Back-of-the-Envelope Estimates of Baseline HIV Incidence Rates

If one wishes to estimate the actual number of infections prevented via a needle exchange program, one requires estimates of baseline HIV incidence among those IDUs participating in the program. This in itself is a difficult task as noted in Section 1. What follows are some very simple suggestions for producing ballpark estimates of baseline HIV incidence. The idea is not to be precise, but rather to develop a range of values that can be combined with equation (20) to produce upper and lower bounds on the actual number of infections averted by needle exchange.

The first suggestion borrows from an established result in epidemiology: for any disease in equilibrium (i.e. ***steady state***), the ***prevalence*** of the disease equals the product of the ***incidence rate*** and the ***mean duration of infectiousness*** (Mausner and Kramer, 1985). As a note of independent interest, this result is actually of much greater generality. For example, in the theory of stochastic service systems (better known as ***queueing theory***), the mean number of customers in the system equals the product of the customer arrival rate and the average sojourn time in the system for any ***workload conserving*** system in equilibrium, a result known as ***Little's Theorem*** (Gross and Harris, 1985). One sees the analogy immediately: new infections correspond to arriving customers, prevalent infections correspond to customers in the system, and the duration of infectiousness corresponds to the sojourn time in the system.

Queueing theory aside, one can invoke the prevalence/incidence law if one believes that the HIV epidemic has become (locally) endemic among drug injectors. Following our notation of Section 2, an estimate of the unconditional incidence rate θ is given simply by

$$\theta = \phi \gamma \tag{21}$$

where ϕ is the prevalence of HIV infection, and γ is the mean ***progression rate***, and can be thought of as the reciprocal of the duration of infectiousness. In applying this relationship, "duration of infectiousness" means the length of time during which an infectious IDU is behaving in a manner that is capable of spreading disease. The usual assumption among AIDS epidemic modelers is to set γ equal to the reciprocal of the mean time from HIV infection through the development of AIDS symptoms (Anderson and May, 1991; Kaplan, 1989). While it is possible that IDUs with frank AIDS may continue to share needles or engage in unprotected sexual activity, it is also possible that HIV-infected IDUs cease risky behavior before complete progression to AIDS.

There are some caveats that must be applied to equation (21). First, this relation is only sensible if one does believe that the epidemic has achieved an equilibrium level of infection. This may be true for drug injectors in some areas of the United States such as the northeastern seaboard (i.e. New York City and environs). Second, not all drug injectors are infected via needle sharing, and it is only such infections that the physics of needle exchange can prevent. While it is not known precisely what percentage of new infections among IDUs are sexually acquired (Nelson *et al.*, 1992; Schoenbaum *et al.*, 1989), some researchers have produced estimates as high as 40% (Dr. James Kahn, personal communication). Therefore, it is reasonable to discount the result of equation (21) to account for possible sexual transmission. A final caveat is that in employing equation (21), one either has a prevalence estimate among program IDUs at baseline, or one uses prevalence information from other sources. If the prevalence value used is a ***community*** value, then there may be selection effects of unknown form if those participating in the needle exchange are not representative of all IDUs in the relevant population. Some might argue that those likely to be engaged in a needle exchange are those most likely to look after their own health, an argument for reducing the prevalence among program clients relative to a community value. Alternatively, others might note that needle exchanges seem to attract older drug injectors, an argument for raising the prevalence relative to a community value. Rather than systematically attempting to sort these biases out, the suggestion offered here is to use equation (21) to create a range of plausible values for which credible arguments exist. An example of this will be illustrated later.

A second suggestion for estimating baseline incidence involves the application of the well-known ***backcalculation*** technique for reconstructing aggregate HIV incidence data from reported AIDS incidence data corrected for reporting delays (Brookmeyer, 1991; Brookmeyer and Gail, 1988). Backcalculation employs the consensus relationship between HIV infection and AIDS in the form of a convolution integral. Letting $\mathcal{A}(t)$ denote (lag corrected) AIDS incidence at time t (measured in the ***number*** of cases per unit time), $\mathcal{H}(t)$ denote the HIV incidence rate at time t (measured in the ***number*** of infections per unit time), I denote the random variable representing the time needed to progress from HIV infection through AIDS, and $f_I(\cdot)$ denote the probability density function of I (assumed known), the backcalculation model can be represented as

$$\mathcal{A}(t) = \int_0^t \mathcal{H}(u)\, f_I(t-u)\, du. \tag{22}$$

The logic of backcalculation is simple: in order for $\mathcal{A}(t)$ AIDS cases to have been reported at time t, how many HIV infections *must* have occurred at earlier points in time?

Backcalculation can be applied to AIDS incidence data specific to drug injectors to obtain a rough idea of HIV incidence rates in that population. It is well known that backcalculation offers little information about recent HIV incidence (for the nature of the incubation time distribution precludes the development of AIDS cases shortly after HIV infection occurs). However, one can still develop an idea about the magnitude of HIV incidence from backcalculation. For example, one might conjecture an HIV incidence function with a constant incidence rate for the past several years, and use backcalculation to obtain an estimate of this incidence rate.

Of course, assuming one has been able to obtain an incidence estimate among IDUs in a given geographical area via backcalculation, it must be remembered that this estimate pertains to the IDU population as a whole, and also accounts for all possible sources of infection. Thus, one first needs to ask what percentage of the incidence estimated can be assigned to needle exchange clients at baseline. If one believes that clients are representative of all IDUs in the community, for example, then one could multiply the incidence rate obtained by the ratio of the number of program participants to the number of IDUs in the community. This of course assumes that one has available an estimate of the number of drug injectors in the community, a number which itself is very hard to come by. The figure resulting from the above scaling might be adjusted up or down depending upon one's beliefs regarding the likelihood of infection among needle exchange clients relative to IDUs at large as discussed above. Also, one should discount the resulting figure to account for HIV infections acquired via sources other than needle sharing.

Lest the reader begin to think that there are so many uncertainties operating here as to render the above suggestions worthless, recall that the idea is not to produce a precise estimate, but rather to produce a range of plausible values. While one may not know the exact number of IDUs in a city, for example, one can reasonably place bounds on the population size using data sources such as arrest records, drug treatment data, and mortality data (Aldrich *et al.*, 1990; Frischer *et al.*, 1993; Newmeyer, 1988), not to mention common sense (e.g. is it reasonable to believe that more than 5% of a city's population regularly injects drugs?). Again, the idea is to consider a credible range of values that will lead to a range of baseline incidence levels. The approach will be illustrated shortly.

3.6 Application to the New Haven Needle Exchange Program

It is possible to apply the ideas of the past several sections to the evaluation of the New Haven needle exchange program due to the availability of data from the syringe tracking and testing system as described in Section 2.6 above. The sampling procedure for obtaining needles for testing was already described there, and the fraction of tested needles distributed in a given month that subsequently tested HIV positive via PCR is taken as an empirical measure of $\bar{\pi}$, the mean level of infection in circulating needles *among program clients*. As the exchange program will accept *any* needles in exchange for new ones, there is no reason to believe that those needles returned represent a biased selection of all needles in circulation.

Needle distribution rates per client (ν) were defined monthly as the number of needles distributed by the program in a given month divided by the number of clients who visited the program *at least once* during the month in question. Mean needle circulation times were also indexed by month of distribution. As needles are typically exchanged in batches of at most five per visit, mean circulation times are defined as the average elapsed time between needle distribution and return for returned needles normalized by the average number of needles distributed per batch, to obtain an average circulation time *per needle*. Such normalization ensures that the circulation times attributed to needles *individually* exchanged four times per week (i.e. in batches of size one) are equivalent to circulation times for needles exchanged weekly in batches of size four, for example.

To gain a feel for the scale of needle exchange operations in the New Haven program, Figure 1 reports the number of distinct client visits, as well as the number of clients who visited the program each month since program inception through June 1993. That the decriminalization of syringe possession without prescription in Connecticut pharmacies apparently had a major impact on participation in the program is evident from this graph. If one focuses on the 20 months prior to July 1992 however, one notes that visitation frequency increased more rapidly than client participation, suggesting that the same clients were exchanging needles more frequently. This in turn suggests that needle circulation times should have fallen over time due to the increasing frequency of exchange.

Figure 2 documents the inbound and outbound flow of needles in the New Haven program over time. Again the apparent impact of syringe decriminalization in July 1992 is visible. Also visible, however, is the close match between the number of needles distributed and returned over time. The closeness of this match is important, for it shows that for the New Haven program, the "law of conservation of needles" is approximately correct. It is clear that there is some leakage in the system. Some of this can be attributed to program policy whereby newly enrolling IDUs with no needles to exchange can receive a single "starter" needle, following which all exchanges are in theory to occur on a one for one basis. However, the amount of leakage that actually occurred exceeds what can be explained by this policy, indicating that in some transactions clients received more needles than they returned as a result of clerical error or deliberate deception.

A major claim of the theory advanced is that more frequent exchanging should lead to a reduction in mean needle circulation times. Focusing now only on the 20 months from November 1990 through June 1992 inclusive, Figure 3 shows that mean circulation times have been reduced. Thus, needle exchange appears to be interrupting the needle circulation process in the manner intended.

Equation (19) affords another empirical test of the physics of needle exchange. Figure 4 plots $\xi(\nu)$ (defined monthly as the reciprocal of the mean circulation time) versus the distribution rate ν itself. The strength of the linear relationship is clear from the figure. Simple linear regression yields the empirical relation

$$\hat{\xi}(\nu) = \underset{(0.01992)}{0.04255} + \underset{(0.00206)}{0.03492}\,\nu. \qquad (r^2 = 94.1\%) \quad \text{(standard errors in parentheses)} \tag{23}$$

Of great interest is the estimated value of $\hat{a} = 0.04255$, for an estimate of pre-needle exchange circulation times is provided by $\hat{\tau}(0) = 1/\hat{a} = 23.5$ days. As of the end of July 1992, circulation times had been reduced to between two and three days, so the reduction in needle circulation times appears to be substantial.

Equation (18) proposes a specific expression for the mean level of infection in circulating needles as a function of mean circulation times. Using the circulation time and PCR test results for the first 20 months of the program, it is possible to estimate the unknown parameters π_0, λ and μ via maximum likelihood. Specifically, letting $n_{POS}(i)$ denote the number of needles that tested positive for HIV via PCR in month i, $n_{NEG}(i)$ denote the number of needles that tested negative in month i, and $\bar{\pi}(\tau_i)$ equal equation (18) with mean circulation time equal to $\bar{\tau}_i$ (the observed mean circulation time for month i), the likelihood function constructed is given by

$$\mathcal{L} = \prod_{i=1}^{20} \bar{\pi}(\tau_i)^{n_{POS}(i)} \left(1-\bar{\pi}(\tau_i)\right)^{n_{NEG}(i)}. \tag{24}$$

This function was maximized numerically using the GAUSS maximum likelihood routine (GAUSS, 1992). The resulting maximum likelihood estimates are given by $\hat{\pi}_0 = 0.0016$ (standard error = 0.028); $\hat{\lambda} = 0.3675$ (standard error = 0.0676); and $\hat{\mu} = 0.1665$ (standard error = 0.0824).

A number of results are worth mentioning. First, as all tests were performed on needle exchange needles, one would expect that $\pi_0 = 0$. This intuition is confirmed statistically, as the maximum likelihood estimate obtained is not significantly different from 0. Second, the fit of the model can be gauged from Figure 5, which plots both observed and modeled mean infection levels in the needles over time. There are four clear outliers that cannot be explained by the theory, but the general fit of the model appears reasonably good.

Third, it is possible to conduct two "holdout" tests of the model. At the beginning of the needle exchange, 160 "street needles" that were delivered to the program in exchange for new needles were selected for HIV testing via PCR. Of these 160 needles, 108 (or 67.5%) tested HIV positive (Heimer *et al.* 1992b; Heimer *et al.*, 1993). Now, while the true pre-needle exchange circulation times are in truth unknown, equation (23) affords the previously mentioned estimate of 23.5 days. Substituting this into equation (18) with the estimated parameters cited above yields an estimate of $\bar{\pi}(\tau(0))$ equal to 0.6375 (standard error = 0.0529 incorporating fluctuations due to the sample size of 160 street needles). That the prediction obtained is in such close accord with the level of infection in the street needles, ***needles which were not employed in estimating the parameters of equation (18)***, provides a certain degree of confidence in the model.

The second holdout test involves needles retrieved from an illegal underground needle exchange program that existed prior to the establishment of the legal program. It is interesting (and perhaps surprising) to note that the reach of this program was apparently not great, for among 851 clients of the legal exchange responding to surveys over the course of the last two years, only 12 stated that they formerly obtained needles from underground programs in New Haven (contrasted to more than 70% of such respondents who stated that they purchased needles or obtained them "off the street"). While this statistic is not intended as a precise measure of the fraction of IDUs who used the underground program, it does suggest that this fraction could not have been large. Of 180 needles tested from the underground program, 113 (or 62.8%) tested HIV positive via PCR (Heimer *et al.*, 1992b; Heimer *et al.*, 1993), extremely close to the prediction of equation (18). It is again important to point out that the needles from the underground program were *not* used to calibrate the model. A negative implication of this result, however, is that it appears that the underground program in question did not achieve a sufficient turnaround of needles to significantly change HIV transmission patterns. This example should again help to convince the reader that the results of these studies are not preordained. Negative results are possible, and occasionally they are obtained as in the example of the underground program.

Returning to the legal needle exchange program, however, it appears that the impact of needle exchange on interrupting the needle circulation process, and hence the HIV transmission process, has been considerable. As the mean circulation time of needles appears to have been reduced to near 3 days, equation (20) suggests a relative reduction in HIV transmission on the order of 33% (obtained by setting $\tau(0) = 23.5$ days and $\bar{\pi}(23.5) = 0.6375$). While this sounds impressive, recall that this is only a relative reduction in incidence ***via needle borne infections among needle exchange participants***. To translate this relative reduction into an actual number of infections averted requires producing a range of baseline incidence estimates.

Consider first the equilibrium method based on equation (21). Prevalence surveys among New Haven drug injectors are not common, but a range of estimates are available. Data from the CDC national seroprevalence surveys included drug injectors sampled at a sexually transmitted disease clinic in New Haven, of whom 35.6% tested HIV positive (CDC, 1990). On the high end, 67% of African American men entering a drug treatment program tested HIV positive (Dr. Patrick O'Conner, personal communication), while early attempts to estimate HIV prevalence among needle exchange participants using more assumption laden models yielded estimates in the neighborhood of 60% (Kaplan and Heimer, 1992). To be comprehensive, baseline HIV prevalence among needle exchange clients will be assumed to lie somewhere between 30% and 70% inclusive.

A number of studies have documented that the mean (or median) time between HIV infection and AIDS is approximately 10 years in duration (Bacchetti and Moss, 1989; Brookmeyer and Goedert, 1989; Freund and Book, 1990; Muñoz *et al.*, 1989). Therefore, the mean progression rate γ will be set equal to 0.10 per infected IDU per year. Equation (21) then suggests that aggregate HIV incidence at baseline among IDUs resides somewhere between three and seven infections per 100 IDUs per year.

However, not all of these infections would have been transmitted via needle sharing. A number of researchers have documented that drug injectors do become infected sexually (Nelson *et al.*, 1992; Schoenbaum *et al.*, 1989), and some researchers have pegged the fraction of all infections due to sexual transmission among IDUs as high as 40% (Dr. James Kahn, personal communication). For now, it will be assumed that 30% of all infections among drug injectors are acquired sexually, reducing the baseline incidence of needle borne HIV infections to between 2.1 and 4.9 per 100 IDUs per year. The New Haven data suggest a *relative* reduction in incidence on the order of 33%. Thus, the number of infections prevented is estimated to fall between 0.7 and 1.6 per 100 needle exchange participants per year. As roughly 200 IDUs have participated in the needle exchange on a monthly basis over the time period considered, the *absolute* number of infections prevented is estimated to fall between 1.4 and 3.3 annually. If one assumed that 40% of all infections were transmitted sexually instead of the 30% figure used above, the estimated number of infections averted would fall between 1.2 and 2.8. Given all available information, this approach suggests that roughly speaking, the New Haven needle exchange prevented between 1 and 3 infections annually.

The second approach suggested relies on backcalculation combined with estimates of the number of drug injectors in New Haven. The backcalculation model was implemented using the Weibull incubation density estimated by Brookmeyer and Goedert (1989); the median incubation time for this function equals 10 years. Using seven years of AIDS incidence data for New Haven drug injectors yielded a mean HIV incidence rate of approximately 160 infections per year. Again assuming that 30% of all infections are sexually acquired, this leaves a baseline annual incidence rate of 112 needle borne infections among New Haven's drug injectors. Early attempts to estimate the number of drug injectors in New Haven yielded estimates in the vicinity of 2,300 (Kaplan and Soloshatz, 1993), while it is difficult to believe that more than 5% of New Haven's population of 129,000 actively inject drugs, which yields an upper bound of 6,450 for the number of active drug injectors. Considering a range on the population of IDUs from 2,000 through 7,000 suggests that the average needle exchange client population of 200 represents between 2.86% and 10% of the population of all drug injectors. Multiplying these percentages by the estimated 112 infections acquired via needle sharing yields a baseline between 3.2 and 11.2 infections annually. Finally, applying the 33% relative reduction suggests that between 1.07 and 3.73 infections have been averted annually. If it was instead assumed that 40% of all infections derived from sexual exposure, the estimated number of infections averted would fall between 0.92 and 3.2 per year, a range very close to that obtained from the equilibrium model.

3.7 A Note on the Consequences of Laboratory Testing Errors

It seems prudent at this point to discuss briefly the consequences of laboratory testing error on the analysis above, for in effect it has been assumed that all tests on needles yield correct responses regarding HIV status. The somewhat surprising result is that were one to take laboratory testing errors into account in the analysis, one would discover that the modeled impact of needle exchange would increase.

To see why this is the case, let $\bar{\pi}_0$ and $\bar{\pi}_1$ denote the true average levels of infection in circulating needles before and after a needle exchange has been implemented (and assume $\bar{\pi}_0 > \bar{\pi}_1$), and $\tilde{\pi}_0$ and $\tilde{\pi}_1$ denote the ***measured*** level of infection before and after the advent of needle exchange. Finally, let σ denote the ***sensitivity*** of the PCR test (that is, the conditional probability that an HIV-positive needle will test positive), and ψ denote one minus the test ***specificity*** (so ψ is the probability that a needle erroneously tests positive given that it is in truth uncontaminated). The observed quantities $\tilde{\pi}$ are related to the true quantities $\bar{\pi}$ by the simple equation

$$\tilde{\pi} = \bar{\pi}\,\sigma + (1-\bar{\pi})\,\psi = \psi + (\sigma-\psi)\,\bar{\pi}. \qquad (25)$$

First, note that the ***apparent*** difference in the mean level of infection among circulating needles is given by

$$\tilde{\pi}_0 - \tilde{\pi}_1 = (\sigma-\psi)\ (\bar{\pi}_0 - \bar{\pi}_1) \le \bar{\pi}_0 - \bar{\pi}_1 \qquad (26)$$

assuming that the probability a truly infected needle tests positive is at least as large as the probability that a truly uninfected needle tests positive, an assumption that is patently true for any reasonable HIV testing procedure. For example, in pilot trials of the PCR approach reported by Heimer *et al.* (1992a), 28 of 30 known HIV infected needles tested positive, while 0 of 64 known HIV negative needles tested positive. What this means is that the ***true*** reduction in the mean level of infection in circulating needles ***is at least as large*** as the measured reduction in the mean level of infection.

However, the main result of the last section relies not on the absolute reduction in the mean level of infection in circulating needles, but rather upon the ***relative*** reduction in this quantity. Here too, however, ignoring laboratory error proves to be conservative, for taking equations (25) and (26) together shows that

$$\frac{\tilde{\pi}_0 - \tilde{\pi}_1}{\tilde{\pi}_0} = \frac{(\sigma-\psi)\ (\bar{\pi}_0-\bar{\pi}_1)}{\psi + (\sigma-\psi)\bar{\pi}_0} = \frac{\bar{\pi}_0 - \bar{\pi}_1}{\bar{\pi}_0 + \psi/(\sigma-\psi)} \le \frac{\bar{\pi}_0 - \bar{\pi}_1}{\bar{\pi}_0} \qquad (27)$$

again providing that $\sigma \ge \psi$, a perfectly reasonable assmption. Equation (27) shows that the ***actual*** relative reduction will be ***at least as large*** as the ***measured*** relative reduction in the mean level of infection in circulating needles. Thus, failing to account for laboratory testing errors actually lends the analysis a degree of conservatism not discussed until now.

3.8 A Note on Data Collection for Model Implementation Elsewhere

The syringe tracking and testing system provides an exhaustive approach to collecting the data needed for studying the physics of needle exchange. This approach proved feasible in New Haven where the volume of needles exchanged is limited due to both the number of IDUs and program policy capping the number of needles exchanged per visit. However, in other programs serving greater numbers of clients or operating without a cap on needles exchanged per visit, it is not practical to track all distributed syringes.

What are needed are sufficient data for computing the following quantities at different points in time: the number of needles distributed per client per unit time (ν); the mean needle circulation time (τ), and the mean level of infection in circulating needles ($\bar{\pi}(\tau)$). If one wishes to conduct "holdout" tests as discussed in Section 3.6, then one also needs an estimate of $\bar{\pi}(\tau(0))$, that is, the mean level of infection in needles in the absence of needle exchange. Such data enable empirical tests of equations (18) and (19) which are at the heart of the theory developed.

To estimate the needle distribution rate requires knowing two things for a given time period: the total number of needles distributed, and the total number of clients served (as distinct from the total number of client *visits*). The first of these numbers should be easily determined from program records. If individual counting of outbound needles proves difficult because of the pressures associated with actually exchanging needles, one should still be able to determine the volume of needles distributed by subtracting the inventory of needles on hand at the end of the time period in question from the inventory of needles available at the start of the period (adjusting for the arrival of fresh inventory if necessary). The number of clients served in a given time period can be counted in a variety of ways. One approach is simply to ask clients "Is this your first visit to the program in (MONTH OF ACCOUNTING PERIOD)?" and keep track of the number of people who say yes. The required quantity ν is then given by division.

Needle circulation times can be estimated via banding studies similar to that reported by Guydish *et al.* (1991) in San Francisco. All needles distributed on a given day can be banded with a given color or other identifying mark. When needles are returned on subsequent days, one records the number of banded needles returned each day. Doing so over time will lead to a frequency distribution of circulation time for returned needles, from which a mean can be computed. It is also important to gain a feel for the average *number* of needles distributed per exchange transaction, so that the mean circulation time can be normalized to a *per needle* measure. Short of counting all needles distributed with each transaction, it is possible to obtain an estimate of mean batch size by sampling transactions. For example, outreach workers could record the number of needles exchanged for every fifth, or every tenth transaction, and divide the total number of needles distributed in *sampled* transactions by the number of *sampled* transactions to obtain an estimate of the mean batch size.

Finally, samples of returned needles must be tested for HIV. A simple sampling mechanism would be to maintain two sharps containers for needle return. The first one (or two) needles returned with any transaction could be deposited into the first container (the *sampling* container), while the remainder would be deposited into the second container. Needles selected for testing would then be selected randomly from the first container. While PCR was used to test needles in the New Haven studies, EIA tests have been used to test needles in other settings (Chitwood *et al.*, 1990; Wodak *et al.*, 1987), and recent modifications of EIA protocols have produced results that surpass PCR in terms of test quality (Myers *et al.*, 1993).

4. A Roll Call of Results from the New Haven Studies: What Was Learned versus What Might Have Been

Sections 2 and 3 of this paper have presented the details of two distinct modeling approaches for use in evaluating needle exchange programs. Both of these approaches were applied to data collected in conjunction with the New Haven needle exchange, and both suggest that needle exchange has had considerable impact on HIV transmission among program participants.

What cannot be overstated, however, is the fact that ***had the data been different, the models could have led to different results***. To be very clear about this, a roll call of the results of the New Haven studies will now be presented, along with a listing of what *might* have resulted from different data.

First, the change point/incidence model of Section 2 did not allow rejection of the null hypothesis that no new infections occurred among needle exchange clients. Given that more than 40% of tested needles were HIV positive, it is clear that the HIV incidence was non-zero in the past in this population. It could have been the case that the change point test led to rejecting the hypothesis of no new infection in 12 or more of the 132 instances considered. In fact, it could have been the case that *many* change point tests led to rejection. This would have resulted in rejection of the hypothesis of zero incidence, and led to a high estimated incidence rate. That this did not occur suggests that needle exchange is helping rather than hurting matters.

The analysis of Section 3 affords several opportunities for contemplating what might have been. It was shown that the "law of conservation of needles" held approximately. This did not have to be the case. The number of needles distributed could have exceeded the number of needles returned by 20%, or even 50%, ruining the claim that the program is a needle *exchange*. However, the total number of needles distributed between November 1990 and June 1993 (80,292) exceeds the total number returned to the program over the same time period (78,067) by only 2.9%.

To be effective, it was argued that needle exchange must reduce needle circulation times. That mean circulation times fell over time is clear from Figure 3. This did not have to occur. Had participating needle exchange clients failed to visit the program with increasing frequency over time, circulation times would not have fallen. It could have been the case that observed circulation times remained the same or even increased.

Equation (19) provided a direct test of the notion that increasing needle exchange frequency reduces circulation time. The data strongly supported the postulated relation. This did not have to be the case. It could have been that the relationship postulated was not borne out by the data. Equation (19) also suggests that in the absence of needle exchange, needle circulation times were in the neighborhood of three weeks! Again, it could have been the case that the estimated pre-needle exchange circulation times were no different from the circulation times observed in the study, a result that would have constituted a strike against the efficacy of needle exchange.

The mean level of infection in needles observed generally conforms to the mathmatical expression derived from theory, though there are four outliers to be sure. However, it could have been the case that there was no conformance whatsoever between the theory and the data. The level of infection in needles could have remained constant over time, or could even have displayed a statistically significant *upward* trend, something which would have constituted a very serious strike against the needle exchange.

This did not happen. That the model was able to reasonably predict the level of infection in needles from two holdout samples, street needles and underground exchange needles, provides additional confidence in the results.

Of the two modeling approaches advanced, the methods of Section 2 yield a maximum likelihood incidence estimate of zero, while the methods of Section 3 produce a range of post-needle exchange incidence estimates from one through four per hundred IDUs per year. These two results are not inconsistent, for while the best incidence point estimate from Section 2 is zero, rates as high as four per hundred per year are well within the noise level associated with the estimation technique.

In sum, the models advocated could have led to conclusions suggesting that needle exchange is ineffective. That they have led to the opposite conclusion, namely, that needle exchange has prevented infections among program clients, is a result of the ***data***, not a result of the ***models***. The modeling approaches advocated thus meet what is perhaps the most basic premise of all scientific research, namely, that of ***falsifiability***. Things could have gone the other way. They did not.

5. A Note on Validating Mathematical Models with Special Reference to AIDS

How should one think about the validation of mathematical models in general? While being able to fit a model to observed data is clearly an important criterion, it is not the only one. Norman Bailey (1994) identifies other criteria to consider when attempting to validate public health models of HIV and AIDS, including cross-checking with other research results and preliminary prediction of future events (or backcasting of prior events). That the majority of needle exchange research published to date claims to support the efficacy of needle exchange cannot be disputed. Earlier modeling studies relying on behavioral data and assumptions in addition to only limited syringe tracking and testing data also led to similar conclusions (Kaplan and O'Keefe, 1993). In the case of the "holdout" samples described earlier, it was possible to successfully backcast the level of infection in needles for data that had not been employed in calibrating the model.

That models are routinely employed in studies of the AIDS epidemic is perhaps a theme worth pursuing momentarily. Consider the simple problem of estimating the number of HIV infections that have occurred in the United States. Many readers will be familiar with estimates in the neighborhood of 1 million infected persons, but how does one know? *No one has ever counted!* The most credible estimates are those that derive from a mathematical model, specifically, the backcalculation method as exemplified by the work of Brookmeyer (1991) and Brookmeyer and Gail (1988). Why should one believe the resulting estimates from backcalculation? It is possible to match predicted *AIDS* incidence with what is observed, but HIV incidence remains invisible! The faith in backcalculation follows to a great extent from one's belief in the *process* represented by the model.

A similar example involves studies that have attempted to estimate the probability of HIV transmission during individual acts of sexual intercourse between discordant pairs (i.e. one infected, one uninfected). These studies have *not* been conducted in a manner where the uninfected partner is tested following each act of unprotected sex for obvious reasons. The most commonly cited estimates of the per sex act *infectivity* follow from very simple *models* of risk compounding and population heterogeneity (Kaplan, 1990; Shiboski and Jewell, 1992; Wiley *et al.*, 1989). Again, it is the process embodied in the modeling which leads one to gain some confidence in the nature of the results obtained.

What modeling offers is a language for making these processes explicit. In fact, modeling offers something that a controlled experiment cannot. Even if one discovered via a controlled experiment that the HIV transmission rate among needle exchange participants was less than among an otherwise equivalent group of IDUs without access to needle exchange, one would not know *why* needle exchange had the effect it had. One would not be able to formulate suggestions for what to expect from needle exchanges operating under a different set of circumstances from those in the experiment. To be sure, a controlled experiment would offer the best evidence possible for the effect of the *specific* needle exchange program tested. Precise measurements for one such program, however, may not be worth as much as a set of general principles that can be explored in a variety of settings (such as the relationships between needle exchange rates, needle circulation times, and the mean level of infection in circulating needles, for example). The generation of such principles is one of the major benefits of modeling.

6. Concluding Thoughts

Operational modeling is not the method of choice most needle exchange researchers have settled upon, and it is not the intent of this paper to suggest that the techniques developed here are the only ones worth pursuing. It is, however, important to stress the unique features of this approach to program evaluation. The operational modeling of needle exchange leads to a number of falsifiable conjectures regarding program function and HIV transmission risks that can be tested empirically. Operational modeling relies on objectively observed program data and other available public health information as opposed to behavioral information estimated from surveys of needle exchange clients. The modeling philosophy espoused throughout this paper is but an instance of the application of the methods of *operations research* which have been applied successfully to business (Cook and Russell, 1989), industry (Nahmias, 1989), public service systems (Drake *et al.*, 1972; Larson and Odoni, 1981) and health care (Eddy, 1980; Willemain and Larson, 1977). When viewed as a methodology for evaluating an AIDS prevention program such as needle exchange, operational modeling may appear both suspicious and arcane. However, when viewed within the historical context of the field of operations research, the approach espoused is well-grounded methodologically.

The purpose of evaluating programs in general and needle exchange in particular is to provide information useful for decision making (Larson and Kaplan, 1981). Public health decision makers seriously interested in needle exchange do *not* need information regarding program efficacy with the same precision required to land a spacecraft on the moon. Rather, the task at hand is to decide if *sufficient* evidence exists to break the state of equipoise regarding the usefulness of needle exchange. The results of the New Haven studies add weight to the arguments of those who advocate needle exchange programs on the grounds of HIV incidence reduction. Whether this additional weight is sufficient to break the state of equipoise, however, is for public health policy officials to decide.

To recap, this paper has presented the details of a new set of techniques developed explicitly for the purpose of evaluating needle exchange programs. These methods have been applied to the evaluation of the legal needle exchange program operated by the New Haven Health Department. Field data filtered through the lens of operational modeling suggest strongly that the operations of needle exchange have reduced needle-borne HIV transmission risks among participating drug injectors. The weight of the evidence greatly favors the contention that, at least in New Haven, HIV transmission has slowed as a result of needle exchange.

Acknowledgments

The PCR approach to testing needles for the presence of HIV proviral DNA was developed by Dr. Robert Heimer, Assistant Professor of Medicine at Yale University. He has supervised all laboratory operations from the start of our evaluation studies with the able assistance of Ms. Bini Jariwala. The syringe tracking and testing database has grown considerably, and managing this database is the responsibility of Ms. Coleen Klansky at the Yale University School of Management. It is frightening to imagine how this project would fare without her skills in information management. Mr. Kaveh Khoshnood, a doctoral candidate in Epidemiology and Public Health, continues to provide research assistance in the evaluation of the New Haven needle exchange. This research does not take place in a vacuum, and I feel it appropriate to acknowledge the stimulating environment provided by other Yale colleagues dedicated to AIDS research of all stripes, including Drs. Phil Alcabes, Rick Altice, Gerald Friedland, Jeanette Ickovics, Alvin Novick, Peter Selwyn, Ann Williams, and David Paltiel (now at Harvard's School of Public Health). I thank Dr. Edwin Cadman, Chair of the Department of Internal Medicine at Yale, for having sufficient interest in this research to pay for it when no external funding was available. That situation has thankfully changed, and it is a pleasure to acknowledge the National Institute on Drug Abuse for support under grant R01-DA07676-02 (Dr.

Peter Hartsock, Project Officer) and the Robert Wood Johnson Foundation for support under grant 20049 (Dr. Paul Jellinek, Project Officer). Finally, none of this work would have been possible without the cooperation of the New Haven Health Department. Regardless of one's feelings about needle exchange, no one can deny that Ms. Elaine O'Keefe, former AIDS Division Director; Mr. William Quinn, Director of Health Services; and the entire outreach staff of the needle exchange program care deeply for the clients they serve. Their concern and dedication cannot be overstated.

References

Aldrich MR, Mandel J and Newmeyer JA (1990). A spreadsheet for AIDS: Estimating heterosexual injection drug user population size from AIDS statistics in San Francisco. *Journal of Psychoactive Drugs* 22(3):343-349.

Anderson RM and May RM (1991). *Infectious diseases of humans: Dynamics and control*. Oxford University Press, Oxford, England.

Bacchetti P and Moss AR (1989). Incubation period of AIDS in San Francisco. *Nature* 338:251-253.

Bailey NJT (1994). Prediction and validation in the public health modelling of HIV/AIDS. *Statistics in Medicine* (in press).

Bhat UN (1984). *Elements of applied stochastic processes*. John Wiley and Sons, New York.

Brookmeyer R (1991). Reconstruction and future trends of the AIDS epidemic in the United States. *Science* 253:37-42.

Brookmeyer R and Gail M (1988). A method for obtaining short-term projections and lower bounds on the size of the AIDS epidemic. *Journal of the American Statistical Association* 83:301-308.

Brookmeyer R and Goedert JJ (1989). Censoring in an epidemic with application to hemophilia associated AIDS. *Biometrics* 45:325-335.

CDC (1990). *National HIV seroprevalence surveys*. Centers for Disease Control and Prevention, Atlanta (HIV/CID/9-90/006, Table 1).

Chitwood D, McCoy C, Inciardi J, *et al*. (1990). HIV seropositivity of needles from shooting galleries in south Florida. *American Journal of Public Health* 80:150-152.

Cook TM and Russell RA (1989). *Introduction to management science*. Prentice Hall, Englewood Cliffs, New Jersey.

Cox DR (1962). *Renewal theory*. Methuen and Company, London, England.

Cox DR (1970). *The analysis of binary data*. Chapman and Hall, London, England.

Cox DR and Hinkley DV (1974). *Theoretical statistics*. Chapman and Hall, London, England.

Des Jarlais DC and Friedman SR (1992). AIDS and legal access to sterile drug injection equipment. *Annals of the American Academy of Political and Social Science* 521:42-65.

Donoghoe M, Stimson G, Dolan K and Alldritt L. (1989). Changes in HIV risk behaviour in clients of syringe-exchange schemes in England and Scotland. *AIDS* 3:267-272.

Drake AW (1967). *Fundamentals of applied probability theory*. McGraw Hill, New York.

Drake AW, Keeney RL and Morse PM (eds.) (1972). *Analysis of public systems*. MIT Press, Cambridge, Massachusetts.

Eddy DM (1980). Screening for cancer: Theory, analysis, and design. Prentice-Hall, Englewood Cliffs, New Jersey.

Freund HP and Book DL (1990). Determination of the spread of HIV from the AIDS incidence history. *Mathematical Biosciences* 98:227-241.

Frischer M, Leyland A, Cormack R *et al*. (1993). Estimating the population prevalence of injection drug use and infection with human immunodeficiency virus among injection drug users in Glasgow, Scotland. *American Journal of Epidemiology* 138:170-181.

GAO (1993). *Needle exchange programs: Research suggests promise as an AIDS prevention strategy*. United States General Accounting Office Report Number GAO/HRD-93-60, Washington, DC.

GAUSS (1992). *Maximum likelihood*. GAUSS 3.0 Applications, The GAUSS System Version 3.0, Aptech Systems Incorporated, Maple Valley, Washington.

Gross D and Harris CM (1985). *Fundamentals of queueing theory*. John Wiley and Sons, New York.

Guydish J, Clark G, Garcia D *et al*. (1991). Evaluating needle exchange: Do distributed needles come back? *American Journal of Public Health* 81:617-619.

Hagan H, Des Jarlais DC, Purchase D *et al*. (1991). The Tacoma syringe exchange. *Journal of Addictive Diseases* 10:81-88.

Hartgers C, Buning E, van Santen G *et al*. (1989). The impact of the needle and syringe-exchange programme in Amsterdam on injecting risk behaviour. *AIDS* 3:571-576.

Heimer R, Myers S, Cadman E *et al.* (1992a). Detection by polymerase chain reaction of human immunodeficiency virus Type I proviral DNA sequences in needles of injecting drug users. *Journal of Infectious Diseases* 165:781-782.

Heimer R, Kaplan EH and Cadman C (1992b). Prevalence of HIV-infected syringes during a syringe-exchange program. *New England Journal of Medicine* 327:1883-1884.

Heimer R, Kaplan EH, Khoshnood K *et al.* (1993). Needle exchange decreases the prevalence of HIV-1 proviral DNA in returned syringes in New Haven, Connecticut. *American Journal of Medicine* 95:214-220.

Joseph SC and Des Jarlais DC (1989). Needle and syringe exchange as a method of AIDS epidemic control. *AIDS Updates* 2:1-8.

Kaplan EH (1989). What are the risks of risky sex? Modeling the AIDS epidemic. *Operations Research* 37:198-209.

Kaplan EH (1990). Modeling HIV infectivity: Must sex acts be counted? *Journal of Acquired Immune Deficiency Syndromes* 3:55-61.

Kaplan EH (1994). A method for evaluating needle exchange programs. *Statistics in Medicine* (in press).

Kaplan EH and Heimer R (1992). HIV prevalence among intravenous drug users: Model-based estimates from New Haven's legal needle exchange. *Journal of Acquired Immune Deficiency Syndromes* 5:163-169.

Kaplan EH and Heimer R (1993). What happened to HIV transmission among drug injectors in New Haven? *Chance* 6(2):9-14.

Kaplan EH and Heimer R (1994). HIV incidence among needle exchange participants: Estimates from syringe tracking and testing data. *Journal of Acquired Immune Deficiency Syndromes* 7:182-189.

Kaplan EH and O'Keefe E. (1993). Let the needles do the talking! Evaluating the New Haven needle exchange. *Interfaces* 23(1):7-26.

Kaplan EH and Soloshatz D (1993). How many drug injectors are there in New Haven? Answers from AIDS data. *Mathematical and Computer Modelling* 17:109-115.

Larson RC and Kaplan EH (1981). Decision-oriented approaches to program evaluation. *New Directions for Program Evaluation* 10:49-68.

Larson RC and Odoni AR (1981). *Urban Operations Research.* Prentice-Hall, Englewood Cliffs, New Jersey.

Ljungberg B, Christensson B, Tunving K *et al.* (1991). HIV prevention among injecting drug users: Three years of experience from a syringe exchange program in Sweden. *Journal of Acquired Immune Deficiency Syndromes* 4:890-895.

Mausner JS and Kramer S (1985). *Epidemiology: An introductory text*. W.B. Saunders Company, Philadelphia, Pennsylvania.

Muñoz A, Wang M-C, Bass S *et al*. (1989). Acquired immunodeficiency syndrome (AIDS)-free time after human immunodeficiency virus type 1 (HIV-1) seroconversion in homosexual men. *American Journal of Epidemiology* 130:530-539.

Myers SS, Heimer R, Liu D and Henrard D (1993). HIV DNA and antibodies in syringes from injecting drug users: A comparison of detection techniques. *AIDS* 7:925-931.

Nahmias S (1989). *Production and operations analysis*. Richard D. Irwin Incorporated, Boston, Massachusetts.

Nelson KE, Vlahov D, Muñoz A *et al*. (1992). Incident HIV-1 infections in a cohort of intravenous drug users (IVDUs). Presented at the VIII International Conference on AIDS, Amsterdam, The Netherlands (Abstract PoC 4698).

Newmeyer JA (1988). The prevalence of drug use in San Francisco in 1987. *Journal of Psychoactive Drugs* 20:185-189.

Page ES (1955). A test for a change in a parameter occurring at an unknown point. *Biometrika* 42:523-527.

Schoenbaum EE, Hartel D, Selwyn PA *et al*. (1989). Risk factors for human immunodeficiency virus infection in intravenous drug users. *New England Journal of Medicine* 321:874-879.

Shiboski SC and Jewell NP (1992). Statistical analysis of the time dependence of HIV infectivity based on partner study data. *Journal of the American Statistical Association* 87:360-372.

Stimson G (1989). Syringe-exchange programmes for injecting drug users. *AIDS* 3:253-260.

Valleroy L, Weinstein B, Groseclose S *et al*. (1993). Evaluating the impact of a new needle/syringe law: Surveillance of needle/syringe sales at Connecticut pharmacies. Presented at the IXth International Conference on AIDS, Berlin, Germany (Abstract PO-C24-3189).

Watters J, Cheng Y-T and the Prevention Point Research Group (1991). Syringe exchange (SE) in San Francisco: Preliminary findings. Presented at the VII International Conference on AIDS, Florence, Italy (Abstract ThC 99).

Weinstein B and Hadler JL (1993). Impact of new legislation on needle and syringe purchase and possession - Connecticut, 1992. *Morbidity and Mortality Weekly Report* 42:145-148.

Wiley JA, Herschkorn SJ and Padian NS (1989). Heterogeneity in the probability of HIV transmission per sexual contact: The case of male-to-female transmission in penile-vaginal intercourse. *Statistics in Medicine* 8:93-102.

Willemain TR and Larson RC (1977). *Emergency medical systems analysis: Papers on the planning and evaluation of services*. Lexington Books, D.C. Heath and Company, Lexington, Massachusetts.

Wodak A, Dolan K, Imrie A *et al*. (1987). Antibodies to human immunodeficiency virus in needles and syringes used by intravenous drug abusers. *Medical Journal of Australia* 147:275-276.

Figure 1
Client Participation and Visitation

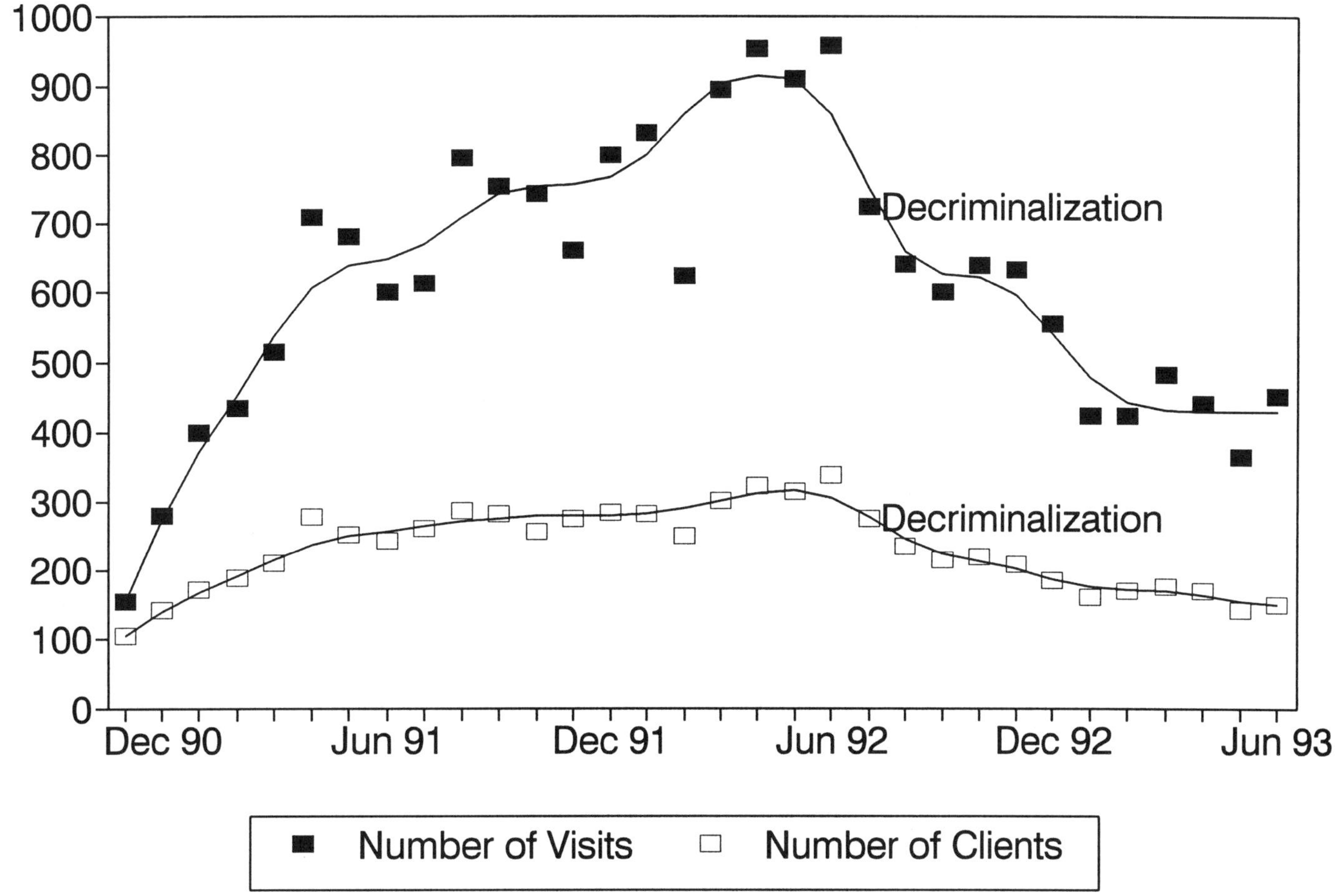

Figure 2
Volume of Needle Exchange

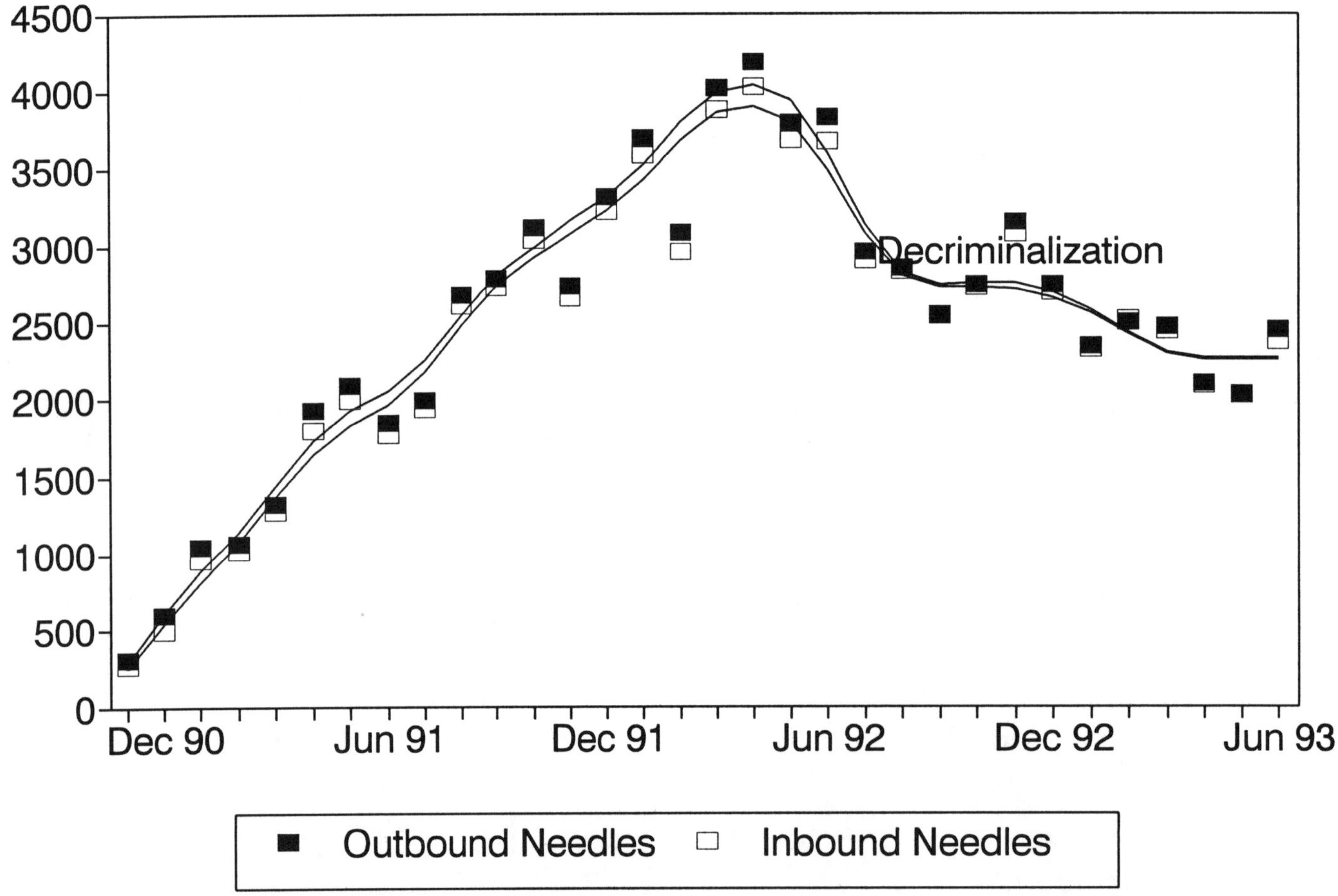

Figure 3
Mean Needle Circulation Time

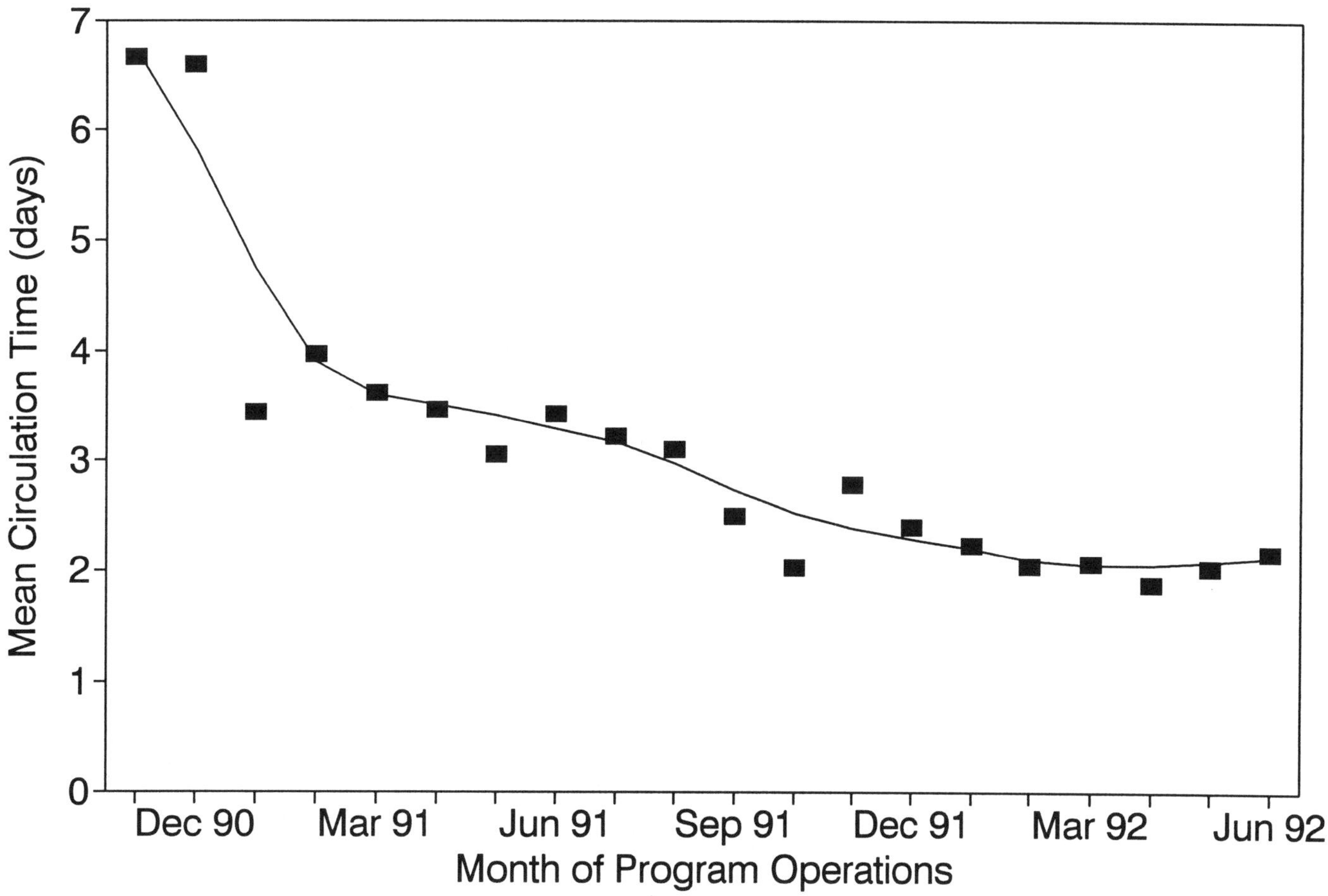

Figure 4
Needle Exchange and Removal Rates

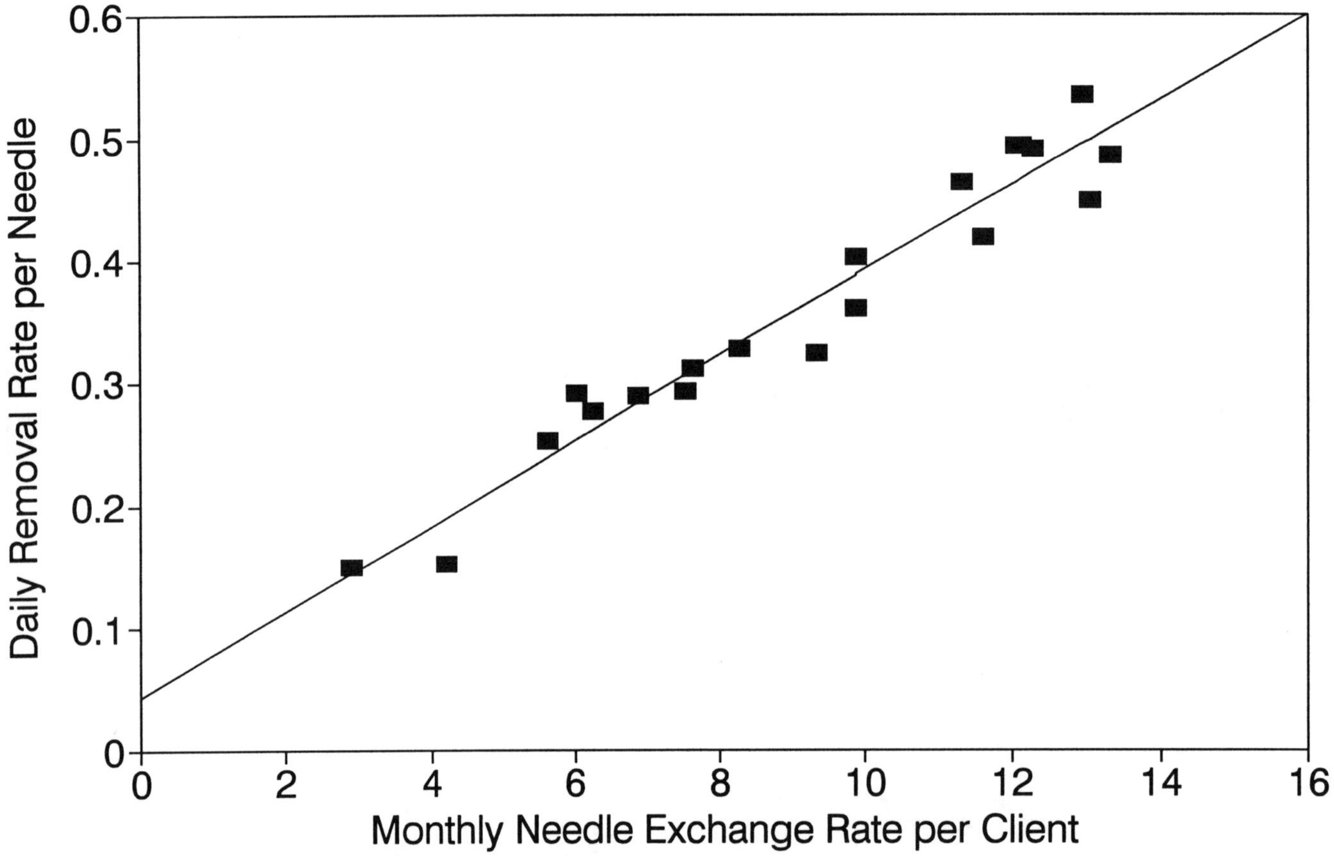

Figure 5

HIV Infection in Needles over Time

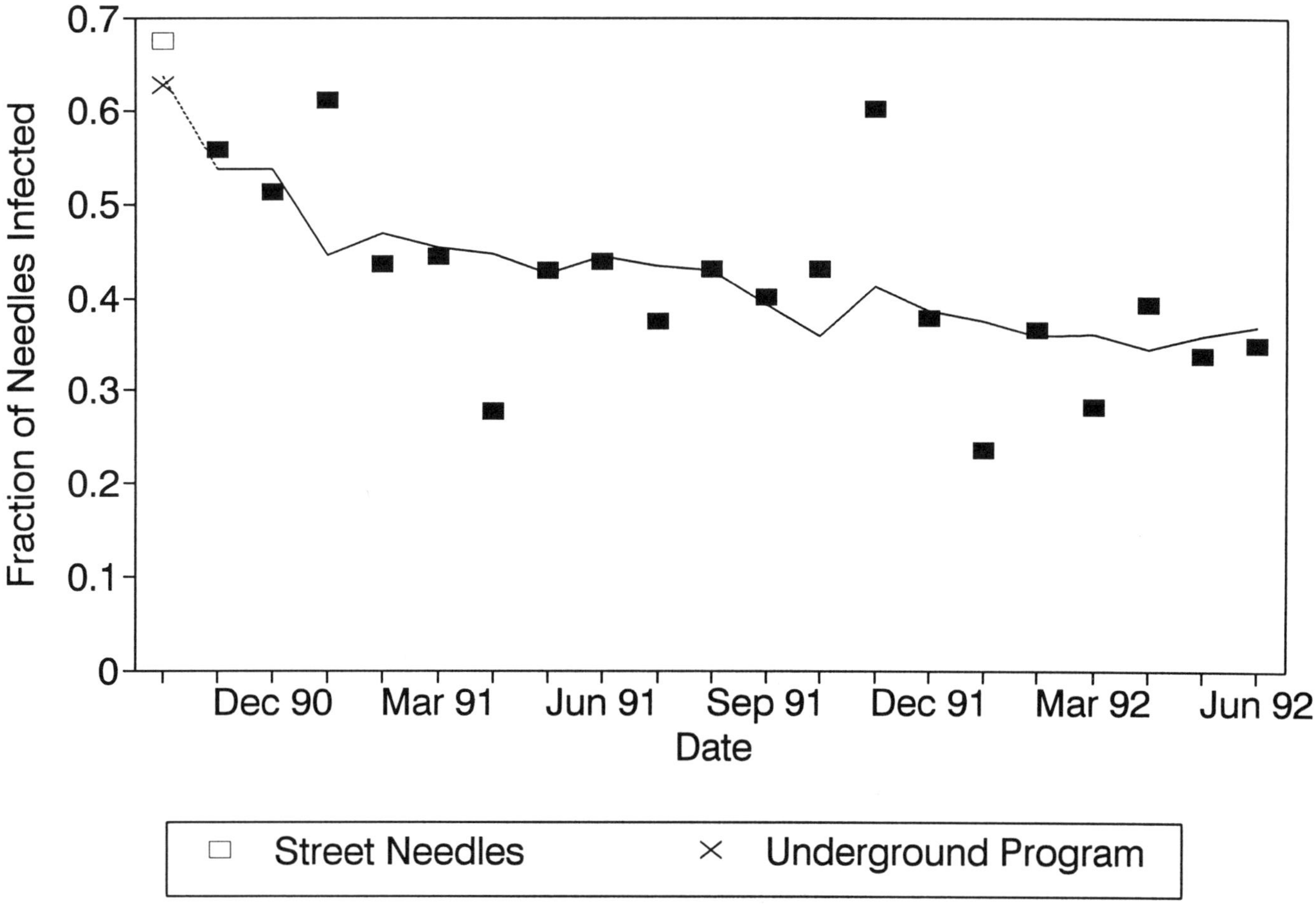

DISCUSSION: EVALUATION METHODS

ROBERT BOOTH

Robert Booth observed that, on one hand, quantitative evaluation methods are especially appealing because of the typically large sample sizes they employ, their use of statistical inference, and their generalizability. On the other hand, they are subject to biases and problems of recall and social desirability. Such methods are also subject to threats to internal validity, particularly one-shot case studies and studies using cross-sectional designs, in which it is difficult to parcel out the influence of historical trends on observed differences. Some statistical procedures have been developed to attend to these difficulties, but the use of experimental designs that strengthen the grounds for inference is preferable.

He commented that qualitative methods are also appealing, in that the yield from qualitative methods has a richness and detail often lacking in quantitative approaches. In addition, qualitative methods can uncover information that survey research often misses. However, qualitative research is often threatened by issues of sampling bias and sample size.

Booth described mathematical modeling as a particularly strong methodology, especially as operationalized by Edward Kaplan. Kaplan's approach is intuitively appealing; it yields a conservative estimate of effectiveness; its limitations, Booth noted, are its exclusive focus on needles and their exchange and the attribution of HIV reduction solely to needle exchange. Other interventions and other factors may also play a role in how injectors obtain and use needles. In addition, although exposure time can be calculated in the model, because the focus is on needles and not on people, one does not know how many people use a needle; one knows only the length of time the needle was in circulation.

Looking at the context of program evaluation, particularly quantitative methods, which have dominated the literature to date, Booth stated that the evidence clearly suggests that HIV risk behaviors, particularly needle risk behaviors, have declined over time. The decline is possibly due to the interventions that have been implemented, the media, word of mouth, or other factors. Evidence of the decline, however, has been found in cross-sectional research designs, one-shot case studies, pre-post-quasi-experimental designs, true experimental designs, time series designs, and other designs.

He said that evidence also suggests that risk has not been totally eliminated; addicts sometimes find themselves in situations in which it is difficult to follow risk reduction protocols. These findings are supported in evaluations of drug treatment programs, community-based outreach interventions, educational office-based interventions, pre- and post-HIV testing and counseling, and needle exchanges. Indeed, risk reduction in the absence of intervention has also been reported.

This is not to say, he went on, that any and all interventions work or that behaviors will change without interventions, although they may. Nor does it mean that needle exchanges are no better or worse than other interventions. Indeed, data have shown that participants in needle exchange programs differ demographically from participants in drug treatment and other interventions and that participants in drug treatment differ from those involved in street-based outreach programs. As was said a number of times during the workshop, different programs attract different types of people and people at different stages of their addiction, and *all* the intervention programs may be necessary.

What are lacking in the evaluations discussed over the past two days, other than in a few studies, are rigorous tests of program effectiveness, Booth concluded. Nearly 10 years ago, Mark Lipsey wrote an article entitled "Evaluation: The State of the Art and the Sorry State of the Science" (Lipsey, Crosse, Dunkle, et al., 1985). He noted that most studies conducted under the label of program evaluation embody at least the rudiments of experimental methods. The telltale signs of quantitative measurement are there, some attempts have usually been made at control comparison or use of baseline groups, and cause-and-effect thinking is evident, even when there is little resemblance to classical randomized experiments. However, he said, program evaluation is often poorly done within the experimental paradigms, and he cited two reasons for this. First, there are numerous practical difficulties in matching good research designs to practical program circumstances. Second, social scientists, for the most part, are not very well trained to do methodologically exacting research under field conditions. To this Booth added a third reason: outcome evaluation is more exciting than process evaluation. Hence, in his view, program evaluation has not only neglected theory, but attention to the treatments or interventions provided--that is, the intervention dose--has been neglected. The result is that treatments or interventions have been represented as black boxes. Moreover, the vast majority of studies of risk reduction programs that involve some sort of experimental design represent the treatment or intervention level as a dichotomy. That is, they assume that each member of the treatment or intervention group receives the same treatment and each member of the control group receives nothing. When outcomes show success, they are due to the treatment, and when outcomes show failure, they are due to failure of the treatment. However, the lack of outcome success may be due to the failure of the research, not of the treatment or intervention.

Needle exchange programs are particularly difficult to evaluate, he observed, in part because the standards for good research are more stringent than for other interventions, notably community-based outreach interventions, and in part because the research itself may be a deterrent to program participation. Consequently, Booth recommended the use of multiple methods to evaluate needle exchange programs, including quantitative and qualitative studies, mathematical modeling, and use of what have been referred to as *focal-local indicators*, such as those used in the Tacoma and Portland studies reported on earlier, in which the researchers looked at hepatitis-B prevalence and incidence over time. In addition to hepatitis data, other indicators would include HIV and AIDS cases, drug-related crimes and arrests, and sexually transmitted diseases. Such investigations would require an extended period of time. In addition, he asked for recognition that any single indicator, as well as any single method, has its limitations.

He summarized by saying that most effectiveness studies have not taken into account the influence of other interventions or temporal trends in subject populations. Participants in needle exchanges or community outreach programs are considered as existing in a vacuum. Sterile needles can be obtained from sources other than needle exchanges, and behavior modifications can occur, in the absence or in the presence of needle exchange, unrelated to needle exchange. Noting that a number of presenters at the workshop have argued for looking at multiple interventions rather than attribute change to single interventions, he concluded that there is a need to focus on single interventions while measuring the landscape of other possible influential factors.

Booth ended by mentioning the important issue of retention, which has been stressed repeatedly in evaluations of drug treatment programs. In the context of needle exchange programs, the issue becomes: What are the criteria for success regarding retention in a program?

REFERENCE

Lipsey, M. W., S. Crosse, J. Dunkle, J. Pollard, and G. Stobart
1985 Evaluation: The state of the art and the sorry state of the science. *New Directions for Testing and Measurement* 27:7-28.

BLEACH DISTRIBUTION PROGRAMS

HIV-1 PREVENTION: INTERDISCIPLINARY STUDIES AND REVIEWS ON EFFICACY OF BLEACH AND COMPLIANCE TO BLEACH PREVENTION PROTOCOLS

Clyde B. McCoy, Comprehensive Drug Research Center and Department of Epidemiology, University of Miami, Florida; Paul Shapshak, Comprehensive Drug Research Center and Departments of Psychiatry, Neurology, and Pathology, University of Miami, Florida; Syed M. Shah, Comprehensive Drug Research Center, University of Miami, Florida; H. V. McCoy, Comprehensive Drug Research Center, University of Miami, Florida, and Department of Public Health, Florida International University, Miami, Florida; James E. Rivers and J. Bryan Page, Comprehensive Drug Research Center and Departments of Psychiatry and Epidemiology, University of Miami, Florida; Dale D. Chitwood, Comprehensive Drug Research Center and Department of Sociology, University of Miami, Florida; Norman L. Weatherby, Comprehensive Drug Research Center and Department of Epidemiology, University of Miami, Florida; James A. Inciardi, Comprehensive Drug Research Center, University of Miami, Florida, and Center for Drug and Alcohol Studies, University of Delaware, Newark; Duane C. McBride, Department of Behavioral Sciences, Andrews University, Berrien Springs, Michigan; Deborah C. Mash, Comprehensive Drug Research Center and Department of Neurology, University of Miami, Florida; and John K. Watters, Institute for Health Policy Studies, University of California, San Francisco

SUMMARY

A major federally-funded approach to human immunodeficiency virus (HIV-1) prevention for injecting drug users (IDUs) includes teaching them to always rinse their needles/syringes with household bleach and water before use. This report describes interdisciplinary studies and reviews of the extent to which HIV-1 can be found in injection equipment and the efficacy of bleach as a disinfectant, and the compliance of IDUs to bleach cleansing protocols, under simulated field conditions.

Bloody needle/syringe units collected from Miami, Florida, shooting galleries or from community outreach prevention participants were selected for these studies. Groups of needle/syringe units were cleansed with bleach using a standard technique taught to IDUs in community outreach programs. Cleansed and uncleansed groups of needles/syringe units were then tested for the presence of HIV-1.

Participants (450) in a NIDA federally funded intervention project were tested on the ability to recall and perform bleach cleansing protocols taught six months earlier. IDUs demonstrated high compliance on basic elements, but somewhat less so with each detailed steps of the protocol.

The data demonstrate the efficacy of bleach rinses in reducing the risks of HIV-1 infection from needle/syringe units and indicate that the teaching and self-demonstrations of a bleach cleansing method to IDUs should be part of a total AIDS prevention effort to increase efficacy and compliance.

INTRODUCTION

In their attempt to understand the transmission of HIV-1, and therefore the potential for reducing and preventing its spread, researchers have viewed the transmission in several ways, characterizing the spread of HIV-1 among high risk groups such as the gay population and injecting drug users (IDUs), prostitutes and sexual partners of IDUs. This characterization of high risk groups sometimes clouded the issue that transmission occurred because of high risk behaviors occurring between individuals, one of whom had already been infected with HIV-1 regardless of whether the individual was a member of such the risk group or not. These high risk behaviors therefore can be characterized as often being carried out in high risk environments such as bath houses, crack dens, shooting galleries, and places of prostitution. These high risk environments provide useful access points for the study of the transmission of HIV-1.

Since it was first described in 1981, acquired immune deficiency syndrome (AIDS) has been concentrated in the United States among people who engage in certain high-risk behaviors. Intravenous and other injecting drug users represent the second highest risk group after homosexual and bisexual men and comprise an increasing percentage of all new cases of AIDS.

RISKY PRACTICES

HIV-1 is transmitted among IDUs by the sharing and/or pooling of contaminated injecting apparatus and associated paraphernalia, as well as by the sharing of injection drugs themselves from contaminated equipment/paraphernalia. The intravenous administration of heroin, cocaine, and other drugs typically includes a practice known within injecting drug subcultures as "booting." The practice involves the aspiration of venous blood back into a syringe for the purpose of mixing the drug with blood, while the needle remains inserted in the vein. The mixed blood/drug solution is then injected back into the vein. Injecting drug users value the mixing of blood for several reasons: some repeated pumping and drawing back of the blood-drug mix allows the user to titrate the dose and avoid overdose or the full effects of potential contamination often present in drug preparations; the drawing of blood into the syringe also indicates that the needle has hit a usable vein; some believe that this "pre-mixing" enhances a drug's effects. Since injecting drug users often inject with needles and syringes previously used by others, particularly if they are administering the drugs in "shooting galleries" (places where injecting drug users gather to take drugs), booting increases the probability that HIV-1 will remain in a syringe to be transmitted to the next user.

"Frontloading" and "backloading" are IDU drug sharing practices conducted in group settings, possibly but not necessarily in the injecting equipment rented and shared in shooting galleries. These practices were recently reported in the professional literature by investigators of community outreach and intervention projects sponsored by the National Institute on Drug Abuse.[8,9] In groups using these practices, all of the chosen or available drug(s) are pooled for mixing and distribution among the present agreed-upon participants. One participant will measure the prepared drug(s) solution by drawing it into his/her syringe and checking the number of cc units. After calculating each person's equal share by dividing the amount by the number of participants, each user receives his/her allocation by either "backloading" (ejecting it from the syringe of the mixer directly into the other users' open syringes) or "frontloading" (ejecting all but the mixer's own share back into the "cooker" [or mixing container], with each user then drawing up their own share). In either method, if the mixer/distributor has HIV-contaminated injection equipment (which may even be his/her personal apparatus), each of the other users can be HIV-infected, even though they have not shared needle/syringes or even if they have used their own personal "works," sterile used or even new equipment.

RISKY ENVIRONMENTS

It is common knowledge that the likelihood of performing many behaviors is increased in certain physical environments that are identifiable by characteristic behavior of the group(s) who habituate that setting or locale; this is sometimes called a *contextual effect*. Therefore, the likelihood that individuals will engage in behavior representing, in general, high risk for HIV infection is increased when they are among many others engaging in such behavior and their risk is elevated even further when the rate of HIV seropositivity is high among the group being emulated. Environments such as bath houses, houses or areas of prostitution, and shooting galleries represent this scenario.[10]

Frequent injection in "shooting galleries" long has been considered to be particularly associated with HIV infection among IDUs.[11,12,13] In these environments, individuals rent used needle and syringe units which typically are reconditioned to extend their usable life far beyond nine uses, which is the average number reported by injection drug users who reuse their own or share their personal injecting equipment with others.[14] The risk-laden practices of "frontloading" and "backloading" are also more likely to occur in these group environments.[8,9]

Research and clinical observation suggest that "booting", the use of shooting galleries, and the sharing of needles combine to explain the increasing proportion of injecting drug users infected with HIV-1[26,27]. The sharing of needle/syringe units has been well documented as a primary vector for the spread of the AIDS virus among IDUs.[1,2,3] In particular, frequency of injection in shooting galleries has been associated with HIV-1 seropositivity among IDUs.[4,5,6] Recent studies have identified the presence of HIV-1 antibody in a large sample of needle/syringe units collected from shooting galleries in Miami, Florida.[7,8] In an effort to reduce exposure to HIV-1 among out-of-treatment IDUs, a number of behavioral risk reduction programs has been initiated in communities with high rates of injecting drug use and AIDS.[9,10] Instruction in the cleansing of needle/syringe units with full-strength household bleach is one of the practical skills taught to participants in these programs who choose to continue injecting drugs.[11] This cleansing technique was first implemented on a large scale in 1986 in a San Francisco AIDS prevention program for out-of-treatment IDUs.[12,13,14] Given the general lack of needle exchange programs in the United States, and internationally,[15,16,31,32,33] such risk reduction efforts remain as one of the more significant *modus operandi* for reducing the spread of HIV-1 among IDUs.

Two important separate, but complementary, issues surround the utilization of bleach as a preventive measure to reduce the risk of transmitting the HIV-1 from contaminated needle/syringe units: 1) the efficacy or actual effectiveness of bleach in the decontamination of the needle/syringe units, and 2) the compliance to the cleansing protocol taught in these prevention programs - how reliably do IDU's actually carry out the procedures that are taught?

More recently, information presented at a public health workshop at Johns Hopkins in Baltimore prompted the release of two important and unique federal bulletins which resulted in additional questions about what the specific decontamination protocol should be.[17,18] This series of events has inspired an attempt to accelerate related research and its dissemination, further examining both the effectiveness of bleach and the implications of these new findings for compliance to protocols.

A multi-disciplinary research team has been carrying out a series of collaborative studies on these issues for the past several years. This article presents the research procedures and findings of these interdisciplinary studies that attempt to establish empirical bases underlying revised guidelines and protocols that will increase the effectiveness of risk reduction strategies utilized in community prevention programs.

While household bleach has been shown to inactivate HIV-1 in clinical and laboratory settings,[19] there have been few studies which have directly examined the efficacy of bleach disinfection of injection equipment under conditions which realistically approximate the field conditions faced by IDUs.[20,21].

Six separate, but interdependent, sets of experiments combining field, laboratory and clinical techniques and methodologies are presented in this paper as outlined below.

I. Prevalence of HIV-1 in field-collected needles and syringes.

II. Testing the efficacy of bleach in needles and syringes collected from field conditions and randomized for bleach cleansing.

III. Inactivation of HIV-1 with bleach: Results under laboratory conditions.

IV. Inactivation of HIV-1 with bleach: Results under approximated field conditions

V. Results of tests utilizing diluted bleach

VI. Bleach utilization and compliance among participants in a community prevention program.

PREVALENCE OF HIV-1 IN FIELD COLLECTED NEEDLES AND SYRINGES

When the University of Miami researchers began their first series of studies, they reviewed studies of HIV-1 in needles and syringes and discovered that there were no reports that assessed the extent to which injection equipment owned by shooting galleries is positive for HIV-1 antibodies. A study of needle exchange programs in Sydney, Australia, had determined that antibodies for HIV-1 were present in 3.1 percent of 1,544 needle/syringe units exchanged at two exchange centers.[22] More recently, studies of needle exchange programs in the U.S. also tested a large sample of needle/syringe units.[31-33] The University of Miami researchers suspected that risk of exposure to HIV-1 probably is higher in shooting galleries. There, each individual rents works that may have been used by others and passed on to others later. Needle/syringe units are routinely reconditioned to extend their useful life far beyond the average nine uses reported by injecting drug users in Miami who reuse or share personal works.[7]

In order to examine the potential for HIV-1 transmission through the use of injection equipment available in these high-risk settings, needle/syringe units were collected from these shooting galleries frequented by parenteral drug users in Miami and were tested for antibodies to HIV-1 (see Table 1). "Fifteen of 148 needles (10.1 percent) tested positive for HIV-1 antibody. Seropositivity rates did not vary by the day of the week of collection, nor by shooting gallery from which they were collected. When the needle appeared to contain blood residue, 20.0 percent were positive versus 5.1 percent with no visible blood residue. These findings suggest that needles/syringes used in shooting galleries are likely to serve as reservoirs and/or vectors of transmission of the HIV-1 virus, and that although visual inspection of the needle/syringe may be useful in lessening the chance for transmission, even the visually "clean" needles may result in transmission of infection.[7]

Based upon this study, a probability matrix was constructed to determine the likelihood of infection in number of days given the two conditions of blood visibility and non-visibility in the syringes[8] (see Table 2). The data indicate that given the assumptions of randomness and a 10.1% likelihood of needle/syringe contamination with seropositive blood, a user shooting up just once a day in a gallery would have a 90% chance of encountering an HIV-1 contaminated needle/syringe (or 10% likelihood of not encountering one) within 22 days. Shooting up 3 times a day in a gallery (and using a different needle/syringe each time) reduces the number of days to 7, and shooting up 5 times a day further reduces the time for a seropositive encounter to within 4 days. We should point out that, depending on the drug used, the personal schedule of the user, and the number of pooled needles versus clients, those who shoot more than once a day could be using the same needle/syringe more than once a day (which may or may not have been used by other individuals). A cocaine shooter, for example, may come in for three quick hits on a single occasion, using the same house-issued needle/syringe consecutively all three times.

RANDOMIZED STUDY OF FIELD COLLECTED NEEDLES/SYRINGES

The second set of studies also focused upon the environment of shooting galleries, and in addition to estimating the extent of HIV-1 in needle/syringe units, addressed the effects of bleach cleansing. While household bleach has been shown to inactivate HIV-1 in clinical and laboratory settings, there have been few studies which have directly examined the efficacy of bleach disinfection of injection equipment under conditions which realistically approximate the field conditions faced by IDUs. Assessing the extent of HIV-1 in needle/syringe units and the efficacy of bleach in decontamination of any HIV-1 present followed the overall study design presented in Figure 1. The research design called for (a) the controlled collection of needle/syringe units from representative shooting galleries in Miami, (b) testing these in the laboratory for presence of HIV-1, and (c) testing the efficacy of bleach in the decontamination process.

In order to provide a more definitive validation of bleach cleansing methods, used needle/syringe units were collected from shooting galleries in Miami and randomized into two groups. One group was cleansed using the standard technique taught to National AIDS Demonstration Research (NADR) project participants in the Miami community outreach prevention program, while the other remained uncleansed. Both the cleansed and the uncleansed groups were then tested for antibodies to HIV-1.

Used needle/syringe units were collected from four separate shooting galleries in Miami. These were among the most frequently mentioned galleries patronized by IDUs enrolled in the Miami National AIDS Demonstration Research project. Shooting galleries again were chosen as the source of the needle/syringe units, based upon the extent of HIV-1 presence found in the study discussed above[7,8]. In addition, collecting the needle/syringe units in a systematic manner from similar sources (the shooting galleries) provided a more controlled study approach that also permitted randomization.

Each gallery was located in a different inner-city area known for its high rates of drug use. Field observations at additional Miami shooting galleries indicated that the four sites from which the needle/syringe units were gathered were typical of area shooting galleries and were similar and from the same parts of the city as galleries reported in earlier studies.[7] Access to each of the four galleries was gained through the efforts of a staff outreach worker who had established a network of contacts with the IDU population in Miami. All shooting gallery operators rented used injection equipment to their clients for $2. Each operator was paid a flat fee of $24 per specimen collection visit by the outreach worker and did not participate in the selection of the needle/syringe units.

During a three-month period in late 1991, needle/syringe units that recently had been used in the shooting galleries (up to 24 hours earlier) were collected each morning by the outreach worker and brought to the Comprehensive Drug Research Center at the

University of Miami. Approximately 15 to 20 needles/syringes were brought in each week.

Laboratory Control Study

Prior to conducting the study of the field-collected needle/syringe units, it was necessary to validate the laboratory measures which would be used. Blood from three seropositive IDUs (confirmed by p24 antigen capture assay and Western Blot) was drawn into 24 needle/syringe units. These seropositive subjects were in an early asymptomatic stage of HIV-1 infection based on interviews and physical examination. Eight needle/syringe units were filled with blood from each subject, emptied, and left undisturbed overnight.

Twelve needle/syringe units (four from each of the three subjects) were then cleansed with bleach using the standard National AIDS Demonstration Research (NADR) projects technique.[11,34] Full-strength household bleach (5.25% sodium hypochlorite, volume/volume), was drawn up through the needle to completely fill the syringe. After emptying, the needle/syringe unit was again filled with bleach and emptied a second time. It was then flushed twice with water. Time intervals for experiments with needles were measured by observing a precision laboratory clock.

Laboratory procedures were done as previously described[23,24]. After the cleansing, 0.5 ml volumes of phosphate-buffered saline (PBS) solution was then used to rinse each of the 12 bleach-cleansed and the 12 uncleansed needle/syringe units. Thin wires were used as catheter plungers to dislodge debris and promote the rinses when necessary. The PBS solutions were then tested for antibodies to HIV-1 using the Western Blot procedure. Western Blot detection of antibodies to HIV-1 was performed using licensed kits from Biorad Laboratories according to the manufacturer's instructions (Biorad Inc., Hercules, CA). The Western Blot procedure was sensitive down to 30 nanoliters of serum from HIV-1 positive individuals (data not shown).

The results of the laboratory control study revealed that the PBS rinses from all (100%) of the 12 HIV-1-contaminated needle/syringe units that were rinsed with bleach and water tested negative for HIV-1 antibodies. All (100%) of the PBS rinses from 12 needle/syringe units that were not rinsed with bleach and water tested positive (Table 3). These results validated the methodology for the simulated field cleansing of the needle/syringe units collected from the Miami shooting galleries.

Simulated Field Cleansing of Used Needles/Syringes

Using a method previously described,[7] the needle/syringe units were graded as to appearance and only those showing visible blood were selected and numbered. These were then randomized into two groups using a table of random numbers and sent directly to the Retroviral Immunodiagnostic and Research Laboratory at the University of Miami where they were identified only by number.

A laboratory staff member cleansed the 121 needle/syringe units in the first group with household bleach using the method described above. The other group of 116 needle/syringe units remained uncleansed. All needle/syringe units were then rinsed with phosphate-buffered saline (PBS) solution and tested using the Western Blot procedure.

A total of 11 needle/syringe units (3 from the bleach cleansed group and 8 from the uncleansed group) tested indeterminate on Western Blot according to the specifications of the manufacturer. In an attempt to resolve the indeterminate classification, the volume of rinse solution tested in the Western Blot was increased three-fold. New test results remained indeterminate, nevertheless, and these needle/syringe units were excluded from the analysis.

The results of testing the needle/syringe units, collected from four Miami shooting galleries, are provided in Table 4. Of the 108 needle/syringe units not rinsed with bleach and water, more than half of these tested positive for HIV-1 antibodies and 44 percent tested negative. Of the 120 needle/syringe units, rinsed with bleach and water, none (0%) of these tested positive with Western Blot for HIV-1 antibodies.

These findings suggest that needle-syringe units used in shooting galleries are likely to serve as reservoirs and/or vectors of transmission of HIV-1. Further, they suggest that simple visual inspection of needle-syringe units might lessen individual risk of infection if the IDU were to react to observed residue by properly cleansing the dirty equipment with bleach and water. At the same time, the fact that even visually "clean" needle-syringe units tested HIV-1 antibody positive suggests that appearance is not a reliable indicator of the potential for contracting the virus.

Given that the seropositivity rates of these visibly bloody needle/syringe units were much higher than in our earlier studies, we thought it would be instructive to update the probability matrix, including the 5%-10% seropositivity of the earlier studies with the 52% of the most recent study. The relative probability of exposure in number of days to a contaminated needle representing varying rates of seropositivity found in the shooting galleries is provided in Figure 3.

The Miami researchers constructed probability graphs, similar to the matrix discussed earlier, based upon rates observed from both studies, to determine the likelihood of exposure to HIV via a contaminated needle-syringe unit in shooting galleries (see Figure 2). Given the assumptions of randomness and a 10 percent likelihood of needle-syringe unit contamination, they estimate that a user "shooting up" just once per day in one of these galleries would have a 90 percent chance of encountering an HIV-contaminated unit within 22 days. More frequent injection events decreased the days-to-exposure: injecting three times per day (assuming a different unit were used each time) reduced the number of days to 7; shooting five times per day raises the risk to 4 days. When the assumption is changed to the 52 percent rate observed in the second study, the once-per-day shooting gallery user might have a 90 percent chance of exposure to HIV-contaminated equipment in just 3 days.

There are, of course, other variables which can effect these probabilities, such as the personal schedule of the user and the drug used. For example, a cocaine user may come in for three quick "hits" on a single occasion, using the same house injecting unit each time. The investigators note that the more important points from their analysis are: the risk of infection stemming from injecting equipment reuse and rental practices in shooting galleries is extremely high, and explaining these 'odds' in understandable and persuasive terms should be an educational priority in any HIV risk-reduction strategy.

As can be determined by viewing our overall research design (Figure 1), the initial intent was to culture any virus contained in the rinses from the needle/syringe units after processing in the laboratory. However, virus could not be consistently cultured from the rinses of the needle/syringe units collected from the field, as would be required in order to gain the precision and conclusive evidence needed by these types of experiments. When viruses were filtered using 0.2 micron pore-size filters, it was difficult to isolate the virus consistently from the subsequent cultures. Filtration was performed in order to eliminate microbial contamination in rinses of needle/syringe units from the field. In addition, filtration of rinses from needle/syringe units exposed to HIV-1 infected blood in the laboratory also resulted in a significant reduction in the ability to isolate viruses from the rinses (data not shown).

Therefore, in our attempt to determine bleach efficacy, our studies had to take a different direction and rely more strongly upon other laboratory experiments, as discussed below.

INACTIVATION OF HIV-1 PELLETS WITH BLEACH

Due to the difficulties of consistently culturing the rinses directly from the needle/syringe units as described above to obtain the necessary precision, different laboratory techniques were utilized. We undertook another series of tests to derive a more precise estimate of the optimal dilution of bleach (*e.g.*, 100% or 10% strength) and exposure time (15 seconds, 30 seconds, etc.) required to inactivate HIV-1[23].

HIV-1 was pelleted from infected cell culture supernatants at 13,000 relative centrifugal force in micro-centrifuge tubes. These HIV-1 pellets were exposed to bleach for various periods of time, ranging from 15 seconds to 5 minutes. After gently removing the bleach from the tubes, the pellets were suspended immediately in cell culture medium and used to infect normal donor peripheral blood mononuclear cells (PBMNCs) using standard techniques[23,24]. The PBMNC cultures were maintained for up to 28 days and were assayed for virus production at weekly intervals by determination of HIV-1 p24 in the culture medium (using kits purchased from Abbott Laboratories, Inc., Chicago, IL., and according to manufacturer instructions).

The viability of normal PBMNCs was determined after treatment with bleach. After exposure to bleach for 15, 30, 45, 60 seconds, the suspensions of cells were immediately diluted to 50 ml (100-fold) using RPMI medium containing 500 units/ml each of penicillin and streptomycin, and 1% of fetal calf serum. Time intervals were measured with the use of a precision reverse count down laboratory timer. Cells were killed by exposure to 30 seconds or longer of undiluted bleach.

HIV-1 was completely and consistently inactivated by undiluted household bleach at all tested exposures of 30 seconds or longer. As summarized in Table 5, HIV-1 was not completely inactivated at shorter intervals of exposure to bleach. The p24 antigen concentrations reported in Tables 5 and 6 are averages for triplicate experiments at the indicated bleach exposure time periods. HIV-1 was not consistently inactivated at exposures to undiluted bleach durations less than 30 seconds such as 15 seconds.

INACTIVATION OF HIV IN BLOOD USING BLEACH APPROXIMATING FIELD CONDITIONS

The latest series of experiments uses three modifications of the above-reported experiments to improve the laboratory simulation of conditions under which IDUs are exposed to HIV-1. First, the most recent experiments used HIV-1 infected blood from human study drug users who were participants in federally funded community outreach projects. Second, blood was left in syringes for various periods of time up to 24 hours, to simulate needles utilized in shooting galleries. Third, the cleansing procedure taught in the Miami community HIV-1 risk reduction program was simulated in the laboratory when treating the needle/syringe units with bleach as described[24]. Specifically, blood from red top and (heparinized) green top tubes was drawn into needles/syringes and expelled leaving 50 ul of visible blood within the needle/syringe. After bleach treatments specified in Table 6 using the procedures described above,[24] cultures were produced from the PBS rinses.

Results of these studies concluded that undiluted bleach treatment of the needle/syringe units inactivated HIV-1 consistently after an exposure of 30 seconds duration. Exposure to bleach for 15 seconds was unreliable for inactivation of HIV-1 in needle/syringe units left at room temperature. Without bleach treatment, virus was isolated from needles/syringes that remained up to 24 hours at room temperature.

TESTS UTILIZING DILUTED BLEACH

Earlier studies had shown some effectiveness using 10% volume/volume dilutions of bleach[19]; however, others have questioned the effectiveness of 10% bleach at short time intervals of exposure[25]. Although our primary results are that undiluted bleach is effective at inactivating HIV-1 in micro-pellets and in needle/syringes (clotted and unclotted blood) at 30 seconds of exposure, we also investigated the lack of effectiveness of 10% diluted bleach.

Ten percent bleach was shown to result in 10% viability of nPBMNCs after 24 hours of exposure whereas undiluted bleach killed cells within 30 seconds. Up to five minutes of exposure of micropellets of HIV-1 to 10% bleach resulted in no inactivation whereas undiluted bleach inactivated HIV-1 within 30 seconds. Exposure of clotted blood (from HIV-1 seropositive drug users) in needle/syringes simulating shooting gallery conditions as described above, to 10% bleach for 30 seconds did not result in virus inactivation whereas the use of undiluted bleach did inactivate HIV-1 under these conditions (Tables 5 and 6).

BLEACH UTILIZATION AND COMPLIANCE

While there are many issues surrounding the efficacy of bleach *per se* in reducing the risks of infection from contaminated needle/syringe units, there are also issues surrounding the compliance by IDUs to any recommended protocols for cleansing of needle/syringe units.

These issues are germane to overall effectiveness and are similar for any prevention/intervention/therapeutic program. Overall effectiveness depends upon the two aspects of the intervention: efficacy of the bleach cleansing process and compliance to protocol. Although both efficacy or compliance have a theoretical range of total completeness to nothing being completed in most protocols, each is only completed with partial success (see Figure 3). Even if a protocol has proven to be highly effective under controlled conditions, whether it will be utilized faithfully and reliably depends upon a number of factors including its acceptability as well as its availability and accessibility. Total adherence in carrying out the specifics of the protocol also depends upon the knowledge, recall, and skills of the client or patient.

Compliance refers to how well IDUs heed the educational messages presented and/or reliably follow the cleansing procedures taught to them. Unfortunately, behavioral intervention programs that teach needle-syringe cleansing with bleach generally report poor or unreliable compliance by IDUs with the "works"-cleansing protocols being taught. Indeed, discussions of techniques to improve compliance are prominent in both the scientific and informal settings when representatives from risk reduction sites and sponsoring agencies gather.

The University of Miami research group availed itself of the opportunity to study compliance factors in its community outreach center wherein a variety of research assessments and prevention/intervention strategies that target drug users at high risk for HIV and related diseases. Our investigations focused on the specific compliance-influencing factors of protocol recall and knowledge, as demonstrated by skills performance.

Shortly following enrollment in an HIV risk reduction study, a cohort of IDUs were taught a bleach cleansing procedure that was "standard" among similar projects in a national program sponsored by the National Institute on Drug Abuse. Briefly, this procedure involves: filling the syringe with 100% bleach, twice; discarding the waste appropriately, i.e., not back into the bleach container; and, similarly following with two water rinses. As all project participants were sought for follow-up assessments for any possible changes in HIV status and/or risk behaviors, the Miami investigators decided also to study two aspects of the compliance issue: 1) whether the IDUs had sufficient recall of the protocol (procedures and materials), and 2) whether they could demonstrate retained knowledge by performing skills taught to them months earlier.

The recall/performance checklist was pretested and revised appropriately. Role play respondents assisted in assessing inter-rater reliability. Two objective examiners and four staff examiners who would conduct the tests took part in the evaluation. There was 100% agreement on all needle cleaning performance items. The consistency of rating of different raters for the same questions revealed 100% agreement of six raters on seven needle cleaning recall items, 67% agreement on one item, and 50% agreement on one item. Agreement was 100% on all seven condom use performance items. The raters were instructed on consistency of observing and marking the items on which there was disagreement prior to implementation of the instrument. Below we report only the results of the bleach cleaning items.

The intervention protocol was based on learning theory, drawing upon concepts similar to those of Edgar Dale (Figure 4). It presented the materials in written and verbal forms, where expectations generally are that only 10-20% of the material will be remembered, but also in visual form and by simulated situations and experiences, training techniques reported to have much greater (up to 90%) potential for yielding knowledge recall and skills retention.

The results of assessments for 450 IDU project participants revealed that more than 90 percent were able to demonstrate the basic elements of skills that had been taught to them six months earlier (Table 7). More than three-fourths of those who used the bleach flushed it twice. However, as one analyzes each step of the protocol as taught, greater variability and complexity of determining and gaining compliance are noted. For each step in the protocol, there is greater potential for non-compliance (Table 8). As the criteria of the protocol become more detailed, less adherence is noted. Although 83% used two or more bleach rinses, as opposed to one rinse, recall and performance of greater details of the protocol were not demonstrated as reliably. For example, only 43 percent of the assessed participants retracted the plunger fully to completely fill the syringe. Almost one-half (47.1%) of the participants only partially fill their works with bleach, and 28.3% of these participants go through this process only once rather than twice, as taught.

Although these data do not inform us of actual adherence in the field situation, they are instructive regarding those bleach cleansing steps which need special emphasis. They also remind us that, regardless of how effective bleach may be in killing the virus, the probability of reliable performance of protocol procedures is contingent upon the number of steps and precision required. These data also should be a reminder to policy makers, program planners, and practitioners to be attentive to all program requirements and components, avoiding those that are likely to complicate the protocol. This is a simple but important lesson from these data, as we all seek ways to improve efficacy, compliance, and utilization of HIV risk reduction efforts.

DISCUSSION

These interdisciplinary field, clinical and laboratory studies used needle/syringe units that were collected from the field or that were prepared simulating field conditions to determine the efficacy of bleach as an HIV-1 disinfectant and compliance to a bleach cleansing protocol. The studies demonstrate the difficulties involved in conducting research to confirm the efficacy of a bleach cleansing technique similar to those currently being taught in many AIDS risk reduction programs.

It is alarming that more than 50% of the cleansed needle/syringe units collected more recently from shooting galleries tested positive for antibody to HIV-1, illustrating the potential of exposing other IDUs to HIV-1. In the study conducted two years previously, the seropositivity of needle/syringe units with visible blood residue collected from three Miami shooting galleries was only 20%.[7,8] These data emphasize the necessity of continuing to provide and expand prevention programs even in high prevalence settings. Existing public health agencies need to employ all possible intervention strategies in order to reduce the risk of transmission of HIV-1 from infected needles and syringes.

These must include new efforts to increase availability and utilization of personal sterile injection equipment and to decrease the amount of needle sharing among users who are not successful in abstention from drugs. While recognizing that these strategies are preferred, it also must be recognized that because of the difficulties of implementing these strategies for all IDUs, a new protocol for needle cleansing needs to be developed which utilizes all the new data available. Additional research is needed to fill in the gaps of information, especially concerning compliance issues.

However, the results of the Miami laboratory studies demonstrate that two bleach cleansing steps, totaling 30 seconds, followed by two water rinses, can be effective in the inactivation of HIV-1 in clotted and unclotted blood.

Our results underscore the appropriateness of ascertaining better whether IDUs who continue to inject are aware of this cleansing method, and whether they can actually perform the procedure correctly. Intervention programs for IDUs should conduct skills evaluation assessments in which participants go through the steps of the bleach cleansing technique in the presence of an interventionist or counselor using actual needle/syringe units. Incorrect practices can be noted to the IDU by the counselor, who then can demonstrate the correct technique and require the IDU to repeat the steps of the procedure. Also, direct observation of field situations should be conducted.

An additional consideration involves expanding the locations where bleach cleansing can be taught, going beyond demonstration projects to existing public health facilities so as to educate as many IDUs as possible in the use of recommended techniques. Alternative HIV-1 testing programs could demonstrate this cleansing method in their pre-test counseling sessions with IDUs. All of these discussions should begin with the importance of drug cessation and preferred use of sterile equipment.

As with other risk reducing behavioral changes, however, bleach cleansing must be practiced consistently, i.e., before every injection with a used needle and syringe. Perceived social norms within IDU networks can be powerful determinants of such behavior.[2] Norms supporting bleach cleansing, promulgated by outreach workers, who are often recovering addicts themselves, can bring about changes in injection practices, making bleach use or use of personal sterile needle/syringe units an intrinsic part of the injection ritual. Since bleach cleansing can take less than one minute to complete, success of the interventions may require very little alteration of existing patterns of needle use.

Based upon the research reported at a conference at Johns Hopkins and upon McCoy's and Shapshak's research reported in the February issue of *Journal of AIDS*, intervention programs have already changed their protocols to include instructions for the necessary exposure of 30 seconds.[23,24] Since the exposure time was not an issue before this recent research, none of the protocols had previously emphasized the exposure time required. Therefore, the standard protocols that were being practiced among intervention programs needed to incorporate this new information into their procedures to give greater assurance that the HIV-1 will be inactivated.

Several examples illustrate differential responses of practical applications to attain the required 30 second exposure time. The Miami intervention site has maintained the standard protocol except to advise the clients to have minimal exposure of no less than 15 seconds with each of the two bleach flushes followed by two water rinses. The San Francisco site has opted for more bleach flushes, recommending five such bleach cleansing steps with the reminder that bleach must be inside the syringe and needle for at least 30 seconds. The additional bleach flushes might mechanically remove more residue and possibly provide greater exposure time of the bleach under the assumption that the clients will respond more to a number of flushes than holding the bleach longer in the syringes on fewer flushes. The Dayton, Ohio, and Denver, Colorado intervention sites recommend one bleach flush of at least 30 seconds, thinking that compliance would be greater with one such flush. Therefore, these three sites represent three different ways of carrying out the latest recommendations of 30 seconds of exposure to the bleach. Further research is required to determine whether any of these three different responses will bring about greater compliance than the others.

CONCLUSION

The exposure of HIV-1 infected blood to undiluted bleach, under varying conditions, including clotted blood, for durations of 30 seconds comprising two bleach rinses and followed by two water rinses, continues to be a laboratory defined standard for the inactivation of HIV-1. If this standard is implemented in a needle/syringe cleansing protocol which is correctly and reliably used by IDUs, the procedure will assist those who cannot abstain from drug use in reducing their risks of exposure to HIV-1 infection.

ACKNOWLEDGMENTS

Dr. T. Stephen Jones (Centers for Disease Control, Atlanta, Georgia) and Dr. Harry Haverkos (National Institute on Drug Abuse) are acknowledged for critical review of the manuscript. This work was supported in part by grants from the National Institute on Drug Abuse: DA04433, DA04787, DA06227, DA06910, DA07909 and from the National Institute of Mental Health: MH 50240.

REFERENCES

1. Des Jarlais DC, Friedman SR, Stoneburner RL. HIV-1 infection and intravenous drug use: critical issues in transmission dynamics, infection outcomes, and prevention. *Rev Infect Dis*. 1988;10:151-157.

2. Turner CF, Miller HG, Moses LE, eds. AIDS and IV drug use. In: *AIDS, Sexual Behavior, and Intravenous Drug Use*. Washington, DC: National Academy Press; 1989:186-255.

3. Schoenbaum EE, Hartel D, Selwyn PA et al. Risk factors for human immunodeficiency virus infection in intravenous drug users. *N Engl J Med*. 1989;321:874-879.

4. Chaisson RE, Bachetti P, Osmond D, Brodie B, Sande MA, Moss AR. Cocaine use and HIV-1 infection in intravenous drug users in San Francisco. *JAMA*. 1989;261:561-565.

5. McCoy CB, Khoury EL. Drug use and the risk of AIDS. *Am Behav Sci*. 1990;33:419-431.

6. Celentano DD, Vlahov D, Cohn S, Anthony JC, Solomon L, Nelson KE. Risk factors for shooting gallery use and cessation among intravenous drug users. *Am J Public Health*. 1991;81:1291-1295.

7. Chitwood DD, McCoy CB, Inciardi JA, McBride DC, Comerford M, Trapido E, McCoy V, Page B, Griffin J, Fletcher MA, Ashman MA. HIV-1 seropositivity of needles from shooting galleries in South Florida. *Am J Public Health*. 1990;80:150-152.

8. Inciardi JA, Page JB, McBride DC, Chitwood DD, McCoy, CB, McCoy HV, Trapido EJ. The risk of exposure to HIV-1-infected needles in shooting galleries. Chapter in: *The American Drug Scene*, Inciardi, JA. and Karen MacElrath (Edition), Roxbury Press, Los Angeles. (In press).

9. Chitwood DD, Inciardi JA, McBride DC, McCoy CB, McCoy HV, Trapido E. A Community Approach to AIDS Intervention: exploring the Miami Outreach Project for Injecting Drug Users and Other High Risk Groups. Westport, CT: Greenwood Press, 1991.

10. McCoy CB, Rivers JE, Khoury EL, et al. An emerging public health model for reducing AIDS related risk behavior among injecting drug users and their sexual partners. *Drugs and Society*. 1993;7(3/4):143-159.

11. McCoy CB, Chitwood DD, Khoury EL, Miles CE. The implementation of an experimental design in the evaluation of an intervention to prevent AIDS among IV drug users. *J Drug Issues*. 1990;20:215-222.

12. Watters JK, Newmeyer JA, Feldman HW, Biernacki P. Street-based AIDS Prevention for Intravenous Drug Users in San Francisco: Prospects, Options, and Obstacles. In: *Community Epidemiology Work Group Proceedings: Volume II*. Washington, DC: U.S. Government Printing Office 1986;I:37-42.

13. Watters JK, Downing M, Case P, Lorvick J, Cheng Y-T, Fergusson B. AIDS prevention for intravenous drug users in the community: Street-based education and risk behaviors. *Am J Community Psychology*. 1990;18:587-596.

14. Newmeyer JA. Why bleach? Fighting AIDS contagion among intravenous drug users: The San Francisco experience. *J Psychoactive Drugs*. 1988;20:159-163.

15. Wodak A, Dolan K, Imrie AA, Gold J, Whyte BM, Cooper DA. Antibodies to the HIV-1 in needles and syringes used by IV drug abusers. *Med J Aust*. 1987;147:275-276.

16. Ljungberg B, Christensson B, Tunving K, Andersson B, Landvall B, Lundberg M, Zall-Friberg AC. HIV-1 prevention among injecting drug users: three years of experience from a syringe exchange program in Sweden. *J Acquir Immune Defic Syndr*. 1991; 4:890-895.

17. Community Alert Bulletin, National Institute on Drug Abuse, March 25, 1993.

18. HIV/AIDS Bulletin CDC, CSAT, NIDA, March 25, 1993

19. Resnick L, Veren K, Salahuddin MS, Tondreau S, Markham P.D. Stability and inactivation of HTLV-III/LAV under clinical and laboratory environments. *JAMA*. 1986;255:1887-1891.

20. Newmeyer J, Drew L, Miner R. HIV-1 transmission in simulated conditions of sharing of hypodermic equipment. *J Acquir Immune Defic Syndr*. 1990;10:1019-1021.

21. Satter SA, Springthorpe VS. Survival and disinfectant inactivation of the Human Immunodeficiency Virus: a critical review. *Rev Infect Dis*. 1991;13:430-437.

22. Wolk J, Wodak A, Morlet A, et al: Syringe HIV-1 seroprevalence and behavioral and demographic characteristics of intravenous drug users in Sydney, Australia, 1987. *AIDS* 1988; 2:373-377.

23. Shapshak P, McCoy CB, Rivers JE, Chitwood DD, Mash DC, Weatherby NL, Inciardi JA, Shah SM, and Brown BS. Inactivation of human immunodeficiency virus-1 at short term intervals using undiluted bleach. *J Acquir Immune Defic Syndr*. 1993;6:218-219.

24. Shapshak P, McCoy CB, Shah SM, Page JB, Rivers JE, Weatherby NL, Chitwood DD, and Mash DC. Preliminary laboratory studies of inactivation of HIV-1 in needles and syringes containing infected blood using undiluted household bleach. *J Acquir Immune Defic Syndr*. 1994;7:754-759.

25. Aranda Anzaldo A, Viza D, and Busnel R.A., Chemical inactivation of HIV in Vitro, *J of Viral Methods*. 1992;37:71-82.

26. Chitwood, Dale D., Clyde B. McCoy, and Mary Comerford. "Risk Behaviors of Intravenous Cocaine Users: Implications for Intervention." National Institute on Drug Abuse. 1989.

27. Curran, J., H. Jaffe, A. Hardy, W. Morgan, R. Selik, and T. Dondero. Epidemiology of HIV infection and AIDS in the United States. *Science.* 1988;239;610-616. 28.

28. Koester S. Copping, running and paraphernalia laws: Contextual variables and needle risk behavior among injection drug users in Denver. *Human Organization.* (in press, 1993).

29. Koester S. and Hoffer L. Indirect Sharing: additional risks of HIV transmission during drug preparation and injection. *Scientific Meeting of NIDA Cooperative Agreement Projects*, Flagstaff, AZ, Fall, 1993.

30. McCoy CB, Inciardi JA. Sex drugs and the secondary spread of HIV. Roxbury Publications, Los Angeles, (in press).

31. *New England Journal of Medicine*, Vol. 327, No. 26, pp.1883-1884, December 24, 1992.

32. *Chance*, Vol. 6, No.2, pp.9-14, July, 1993.

33. *Needle Exchange Programs*, GAO/HRD-93-60, March, 1993.

Table 1

SEROPOSITIVITY OF NEEDLE/SYRINGE UNITS WITHOUT AND WITH VISIBLE BLOOD

Appearance	Total tested (n)	Proportion HIV AB+ (%)
No visible blood	98	5.1
Visible blood	50	20.0
Total	148	10.1

Chitwood DD, McCoy CB, Inciardi JA, McBride DC, Comerford M, Trapido EJ, McCoy HV, Page JB, Griffin J, Fletcher MA and Ashman MA. "HIV Seropositivity of Needles from Shooting Galleries in South Florida": *American Journal of Public Health*. 1990;80(2): 150-152.

Table 2

NUMBER OF DAYS BEFORE THERE IS A 90% PROBABILITY OF A SEROPOSITIVE NEEDLE/SYRINGE ENOUNTER AT VARYING FREQUENCIES OF INJECTION

Visible Blood		No Visible Blood	
1x per day	22 days	1x per day	44 days
2x per day	11 days	2x per day	22 days
3x per day	7 days	3x per day	15 days
4x per day	5 days	4x per day	11 days
5x per day	4 days	5x per day	9 days

Inciardi JA, Page JB, McBride DC, Chitwood DD, McCoy CB, McCoy HV, Trapido EJ. "The Risk of Exposure to HIV-Contaminated Needles in Shooting Galleries." Chapter in: *The American Drug Scene*. Roxbury Press, Los Angeles (In Press).

Table 3

WESTERN BLOT RESULTS FROM BLEACH CLEANSED AND UNCLEANSED NEEDLE/SYRINGE UNITS TO VERIFY LABORATORY METHODOLOGY

Bleach Cleansed	Total Tested	Percent HIV-1 Ab+
	N	%
Yes	12	0
No	12	100

Table 4

PRESENCE OF HIV ANTIBODIES IN NEEDLES IN SOUTH FLORIDA EFFICACY OF BLEACH INTERVENTION

	Number of Needles (%)	
Treatment	Positive	Negative
No bleach rinse n=116	60(52%)	56(48%)
With bleach	0(0%)	120(100%)

Abs detected by Western Blot
Three needles could not be used due to blockage

Table 5

INACTIVATION OF HIV-1 BY UNDILUTED HOUSEHOLD BLEACH

Duration of Exposure	Average concentration of p24 antigen in supernantants of cultures infected with virus treated for indicated time: pg/ml (standard deviation)
0	$\geq$ 100
15 seconds	31 (26)
25 seconds	13 (13)
30 seconds	0
45 seconds	0
60 seconds	0
2.5 minutes	0
5 minutes	0

Shapshak P, McCoy CB, Rivers JE, Chitwood DD, Mash DC, Weatherby NL, Inciardi JA, Shah SM, Brown BS. "Inactivation of Human Immunodeficiency Virus-1 at Short Time Intervals Using Undiluted Bleach" *Journal of Acquired Immune Deficiency Syndromes* 6:218-219, 1993.

Table 6

BLEACH INACTIVATES HIV-1-INFECTED BLOOD IN NEEDLES AT SHORT TIME INTERVALS

Treatment	HIV-1 p24 (pg/ml) Treatments					
	Undiluted Bleach					
Duration of Treatment	15 Seconds	N[a]	30 Seconds	N	No Bleach	N
3 hours	[b]		0	3[c], 3[d]	100	3[c], 3[d]
6 hours	100	3[c]	0	3[c], 3[d]	100	3[c]
18 hours			0	3	100	3[c]
24 hours	0	3[c]	0	3	100	3[c], 3[d]

[a]N: number of cultures at each indicated experimental condition.
[b]: blank; not done.
[c]: blood, clotted in needles, from red top tubes.
[d]: blood from green top tubes.

Shapshak P, McCoy CB, Shah SM, Page JB, Rivers JE, Weatherby NL, Chitwood DD, Mash DC, "Preliminary laboratory studies of inactivation of HIV-1 in needles and syringes containing infected blood using undiluted household bleach," *J Acquir Immune Defic Syndr* 1994;7:754-759.

Table 7

SKILLS/COMPLIANCE EVALUATION
NEEDLE CLEANING SKILLS DEMONSTRATION: BASIC ELEMENTS

	Filled Needle/Syringe with Bleach % of Total (N)	Filled Needle/Syringe with water % of Total (N)	% of Those Using Bleach Disposing Appropriately % of Total (N)	% of Those Using Water Disposing Appropriately % of Total (N)
Yes	90.2 (406)	94.8 (427)	91.9 (373)	92.0 (393)
No	9.8 (44)	5.1 (23)	8.9 (33)	8.0 (34)

Table 8

SKILLS/COMPLIANCE EVALUATION
NEEDLE CLEANING SKILL DEMONSTRATION: DETAILED

Filled Needle/Syringe With Bleach	% of Total (n)	Number of Times Needle/Syringe Filled: One Row % (n)	Two or More Row % (n)	Discarded Waste Appropriately Row % (n)
Completely*	43.1 (194)	17.0 (33)	83.0 (161)	94.3 (183)
Partially	47.1 (212)	28.3 (60)	71.7 (152)	89.6 (190)
Did not fill	9.8 (44)			
Filled Needle/Syringe with Water				
Completely*	50.4 (227)	11.9 (27)	88.1 (200)	92.5 (210)
Partially*	44.4 (200)	25.0 (50)	75.0 (150)	91.5 (183)
Did not fill	5.1 (23)			
TOTAL	100.0 (450)			

*The Plunger in the syringe had to be fully drawn back; otherwise, it was recorded as partially filled.

FIGURE 1

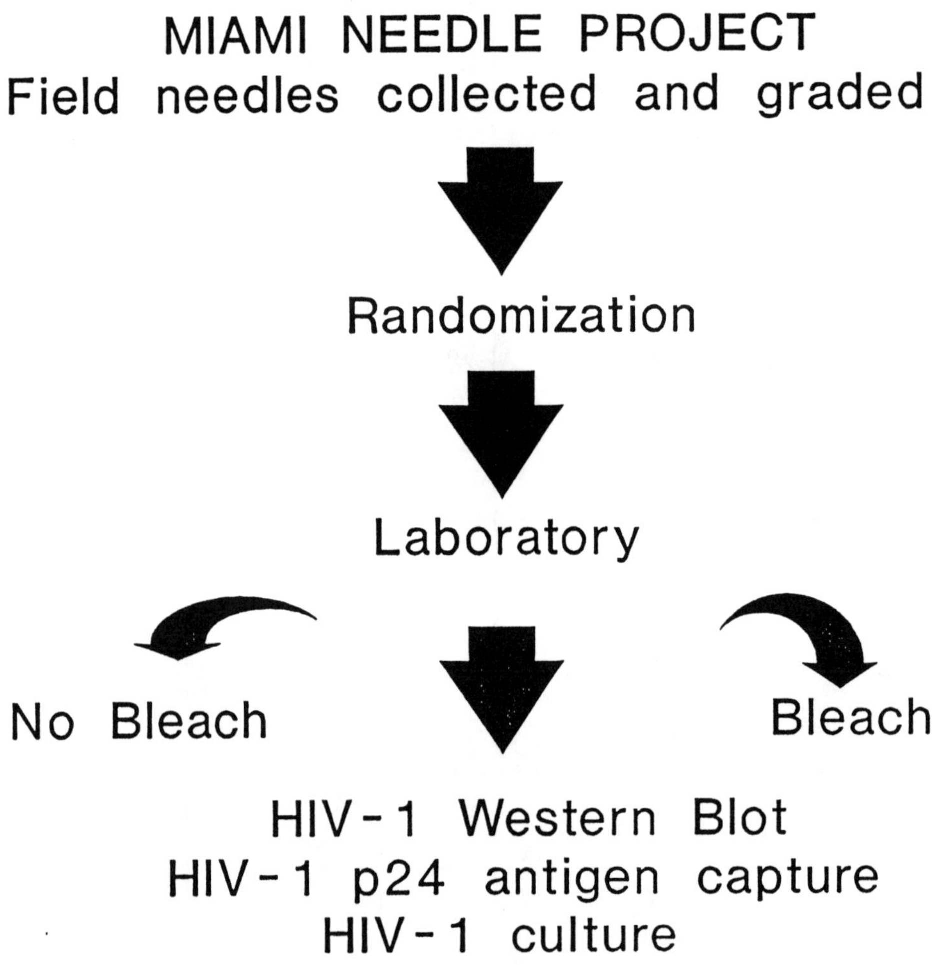
MIAMI NEEDLE PROJECT
Field needles collected and graded
Randomization
Laboratory
No Bleach
Bleach
HIV-1 Western Blot
HIV-1 p24 antigen capture
HIV-1 culture

FIGURE 2

Relative Probability (90%) of exposure within a number of days with different syringe seropositivity rates (5%, 10% & 56%)

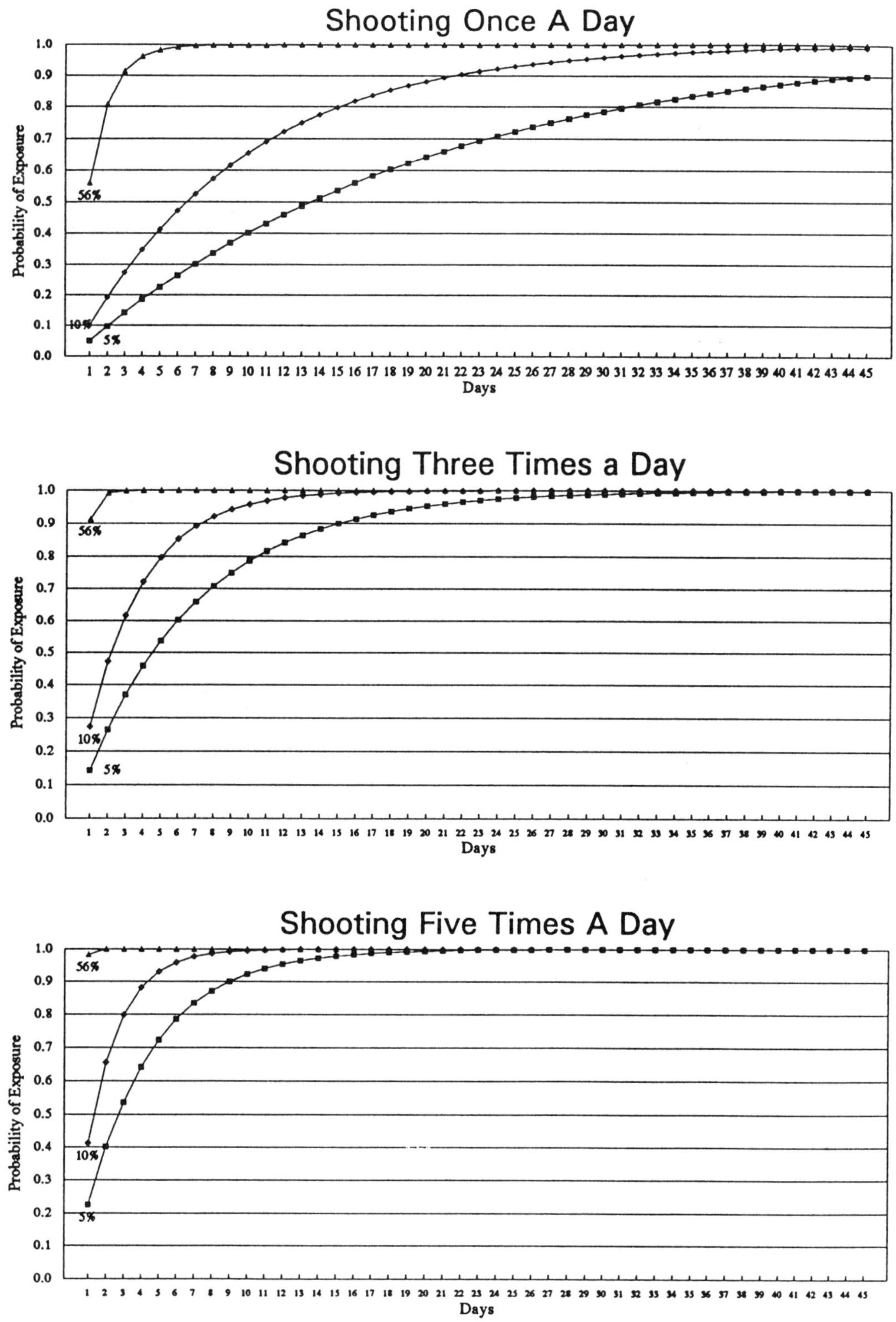

Figure 3

MEASUREMENT AND POLICY ISSUES OF PROTOCOL RECOMMENDATIONS /UTILIZATION

INTERVENTION/THERAPEUTIC PROTOCOL

None -----> Partial -----> Complete

Effectiveness
Compliance

EFFECTIVENESS

None -----> Partial -----> Complete

Risk Reduction (Prevention)
Curative Value
- Increase Survival
- Decrease Mortality
- Increase Satisfaction
  - Quality of Life
- Decrease Pain
- Efficacy
  - (Costs/Benefits)

COMPLIANCE

None -----> Partial -----> Complete

Knowledge
Recall
Skills
Adherence

UTILIZATION

None -----> Partial -----> Complete

Availability
Accessibility
Acceptability

FIGURE 4.

DALE'S LEARNING CONE OF EXPERIENCE *

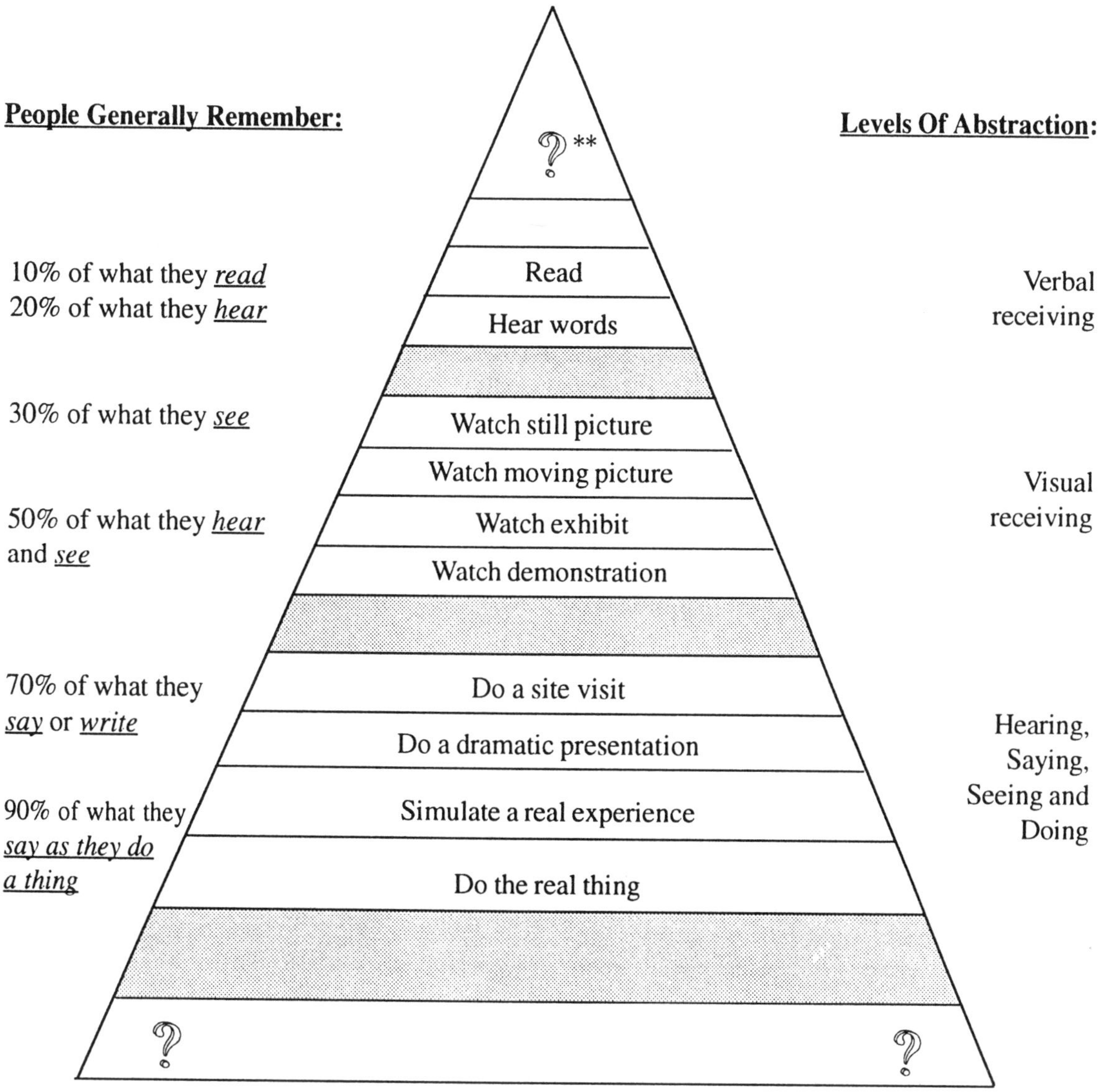

* See Wiman and Mierhenry, Educational Media, Charles Merrill, 1969, for reference to Edgar Dale's "Cone of Experience."
** Question marks refer to the unknown.

INACTIVATION AND DISINFECTION OF HIV: A SUMMARY

LINDA S. MARTIN, National Institute for Occupational Safety and Health, Centers for Disease Control and Prevention, Atlanta, Georgia

In 1983 a retrovirus was isolated and classified as the causative agent of AIDS (1). Laboratories began research with the human immunodeficiency virus (HIV) soon after. Because of the serious consequences of infection with the virus, the susceptibility of the virus to chemicals and disinfectants was investigated (2,3,4).

Before discussing the results of these and other studies, it is necessary to review the principles of viral inactivation and the categories of disinfectants as they relate to microorganisms. The following definitions and tables are adapted from the third and fourth editions of Seymour S. Block's book entitled "Disinfection, sterilization, and preservation" (5). Martin Favero and Walter Bond, Centers for Disease Control and Prevention (CDC) Hospital Infections Program, wrote the chapter on sterilization, disinfection and antisepsis in the hospital (6).

"Sterilization" is the use of physical or chemical procedures to destroy all microbial life, including large numbers of highly resistant bacterial endospores. The major process types include moist heat by steam autoclaving, ethylene oxide gas, and dry heat. A variety of chemical germicides have also been used (5,6).

"Disinfection" eliminates nearly all recognized pathogenic microorganisms, but not necessarily all microbial forms on inanimate objects. The effectiveness of a disinfection procedure is controlled by the nature and number of microorganisms, the amount of organic material, the type and condition of the materials to be disinfected, and the temperature (5,6).

"Decontamination" is a process of treatment that renders a device, instrument, or environmental surface safe to handle but does not necessarily mean that it is safe for patient use (5,6).

"Antisepsis" is the process of inhibiting or destroying microorganisms on skin or living tissue (5,6).

As shown in Table 1, bacterial spores are the most difficult form of microorganisms to inactivate or "kill" (6). The most resistant organisms in the vegetative state are in the class of *Mycobacteria*. The high level of resistance is due to the very waxy coating which confers more resistance to aqueous germicides than found with other vegetative bacteria. Following *Mycobacteria*, in descending order of resistance, are the nonlipid or small viruses, fungi, vegetative bacteria, and lipid or medium sized viruses, the least resistant organisms. HIV and hepatitis B virus (HBV) are both in the last category. Why are lipid viruses more susceptible to chemical germicides than other forms of microorganisms? Klein and Deforest outlined the principles of viral inactivation (7). Viruses and vegetative bacteria are generally similar in their susceptibility to physical agents such as heat, ionizing irradiation, and UV light. All viruses are generally susceptible under appropriate conditions to broad spectrum germicides such as the halogens, some alcohols, and glutaraldehyde. Viruses do differ in their susceptibility to lipophilic germicides. These compounds have an affinity for lipid-containing viruses and some, but not all, nonlipid containing viruses (7).

Susceptibility to chemical disinfectants of most viruses can be predicted on the observation that the presence of lipid in a virus is uniformly associated with a high degree of susceptibility to all germicides. The absence of lipid and small size is associated with resistance to lipophilic germicides, but the absence of lipid and larger size is similar to lipid containing viruses (7,8).

E.H. Spaulding proposed three levels of germicidal action to properly carry out strategies for disinfection in hospitals. These include high, intermediate and low and are based on the fact that microorganisms can be categorized into several groups according to their innate resistance to a spectrum of physical or chemical germicidal agents (9). In Table 2, the Environmental Protection Agency (EPA) product label terminologies are compared with the CDC germicidal process terminology (6,9). Depending on the intended use, chemical germicides are regulated by the EPA, the Food and Drug Administration, or both. Germicides intended for use only on environmental surfaces are regulated only the EPA.

Does HIV react to disinfectants as predicted by Klein and Deforest? This question can be answered based on laboratory studies. First, the experimental laboratory conditions must be defined, then the results must be interpreted based on comparisons with the laboratory conditions and the conditions that may exist in body fluids such as blood. In the human body, cell free HIV enters the CD4+ lymphocyte and can either become latent in the cell or replicate resulting in new virus being released into the surrounding milieu where virus may infect another CD4+ cell. The number of infected cells/ml in an infected individual's blood is estimated to be about 100-1000. The titer of cell free virus is estimated to be about 100 or less. Both cell-free HIV and infected cells may be present in the circulating blood.

In the laboratory, cell free HIV can be grown in CD4+ tissue culture cells. Generally, the virus containing supernatant fluid is harvested and the titer of cell free virus ranges from 10^4 to 10^6 per unit volume, titers higher than generally found in blood. The amounts of protein and other organic materials in laboratory tissue culture fluid are usually less than that found in blood.

Laboratory inactivation studies have been performed by mixing an equal volume of virus containing fluid and disinfectant for varying periods of time. Following the inactivation process, serial dilutions of each test disinfectant and controls were plated into CD4+ cells. After 7 days, the supernatant fluids from each dilution were harvested and tested for presence of virus using an ELISA. Additional incubation time may be needed to detect low levels of virus remaining following the inactivation step. The lack of viral replication indicated inactivation of the virus by the disinfectant. Controls must be done to determine if the test disinfectant killed the indicator CD4+ cells which would also result in no detection of viral replication (3).

Prior to the routine use of the ELISA assay to detect presence of virus, reverse transcriptase (RT) assays were used to detect viral replication. Spire et al. reported the first disinfection studies in 1984 using the RT assay (2). They reported that cell free virus was inactivated by 1:400 dilution of β-propiolactone, .01% glutaraldehyde (95% inactivation), 30 mM sodium hydroxide, and .2% sodium hypochlorite. Inactivation with ethanol and formalin was variable.

Martin and McDougal (4), using the ID-50 immunoassay and ELISA, reported that HIV was inactivated by .3% hydrogen peroxide, 50% ethanol, .5% paraformaldehyde, .5% Lysol® (a proprietary mixture of phenolics and surfactants), and .1% household bleach (52.5 ppm NaOCl). Over time, many laboratories have performed inactivation studies with various compounds (Table 3) (2,3,4,10,11,12,13-19). Sattar summarized the results of many of these experiments (10). The predicted susceptibility of HIV to a vary wide variety of chemical disinfectants was confirmed.

Inactivation with NaOCl has been investigated in many laboratories (Table 4) (4, 14-20). HIV inactivation has been studied for HIV in both the liquid and dried states. A range of dilutions of bleach and/or varying concentrations of serum or blood was not always tested in each laboratory. The concentrations of NaOCl reported to inactivate cell-free HIV ranged from a minimum of 52.5 ppm to 5000 ppm. The presence of blood or 50% serum increased the amount of available chlorine (Cl) required for complete inactivation.

Ingraham (8) wrote that the chlorine compounds are the most misunderstood and consequently the most abused disinfectants. Chlorine compounds can provide high degrees of disinfection. Chlorine works quickly as a bactericidal agent although its action is not fully understood. The toxicity can be due to a variety of factors including the pH, Cl ions, protein denaturation, nucleic acid inactivations, and oxidizing properties (8,21). Klein and Deforest reported that all of 25 viruses tested were inactivated in 10 minutes by a solution containing 0.02 % available chlorine (7). Available chlorine is a measurement of the total chlorine oxidizing potential in a given solution. Chlorine demand refers to the amount of Cl that is needed to react with impurities, both inorganic and organic. After this demand is met, any additional Cl is residual available Cl. Chlorine's disinfection ability is determined by the concentration of free and available chlorine in the solution. This is affected by the temperature, the presence of organic material, the pH, and the hardness of the water. Chlorine compounds usability may be limited by the corrosiveness and instability.

Serum proteins and other organic material in blood will react when mixed with chlorine compounds and reduce the chlorine available for microbial inactivation. For example, before using chlorine to clean up a blood spill, it is necessary to remove as much of the visible blood as possible with absorbent material. After this cleaning, material is appropriately discarded, the spill site may then be disinfected with bleach or other chlorine product. CDC recommends a 1:100 dilution of household bleach for cleaning blood-contaminated environmental surfaces that have been previously cleaned of visible material (22). The underlying principle is to remove as much of the organic material prior to using a Cl compound for disinfection.

The presence of infected cells in blood should also be considered when developing an inactivation protocol. Flynn (23) reported that whole blood is protective against disinfection of HIV. There was a step-wise increasing resistance to disinfection as the <u>in</u>

vivo situation was approached. That is, susceptibility to inactivation increased with cell-free HIV being the most sensitive, followed by cell associated, with cell-associated in blood being the most resistant. Dilute household bleach, 70% isopropyl alcohols and dilute liquid dish detergent were the most active of the tested disinfectants. Most experiments done with HIV-infected cells have focused on the testing of chemicals such as formaldehyde used to fix cells (both separated cells and in whole blood) for flow-cytometry and other laboratory procedures.

Moore (24) reported that HIV infected cells were inactivated in water, but this inactivation was not rapid. There was a 10-fold loss within 1 hour of tap-water exposure and a 100-fold loss after 8 hours. Attempts were also made to recover virus after the introduction of HIV-contaminated blood into tap water. Seropositive blood was diluted to a final total volume of 1 and 2 %. No virus was recovered after 1 minute in the 1% vol/vol experiment and after 5 minutes in the 2% vol/vol experiment.

Newmeyer (25) examined the transmission of HIV under simulated conditions of sharing of hypodermic equipment by intravenous drug users (IVDU). Hypodermic equipment was exposed to cell-free HIV in tissue culture medium and attempts were made to culture virus after different conditions of exposure. Viable HIV was cultured from the following conditions: contaminated needle and syringe left for an interval of 1 minute, exterior of needle exposed and left for 15 seconds, and decontamination twice with water. Viable HIV was not recovered from equipment under the following conditions: contaminated needle and syringe left for 60 minutes and decontamination once or twice with bleach. The researchers concluded that decontamination by bleach rinsing, but not water alone, appeared to be efficacious (25). Caution should be used in interpreting these experiments since whole blood was not tested.

As indicated, there are other disinfectants such as glutaraldehyde compounds, detergents, iodine, quaternary ammonium compounds, and alcohols which have been shown to inactivate HIV under certain conditions. Selection of another disinfectant, rather than NaOCl, to recommend for disinfection of needles and syringes designed for single use must take into consideration, ease of use, toxicity, effect on syringe and needle, disinfection capability in the presence of blood, and many other factors.

It is not surprising that the use of bleach for disinfection for syringes and needles contaminated with blood may not result in complete inactivation of cell-free HIV. The presence of organic material such as blood, liquid or dried, the absence of precleaning or rinsing with water, and the difficulty of cleaning a device not designed for reuse are all complicating factors. There is also the difficulty of documenting the effectiveness of disinfection strategies for IVDUs. Siegel (26) found that the greatest life-year savings were in areas of low HIV prevalence.

Clearly, the first course of action for drug users who are injecting drugs is to always use a sterile, never used needle and syringe obtained from a reliable source such as a pharmacy. This is the only safe recommendation for injecting drug users who cannot or will not stop injecting drugs. Disinfection procedures can reduce the amount of HIV or HIV-infected cells present in the injecting equipment, but can not guarantee complete inactivation every time.

ACKNOWLEDGMENT

The review by Walter Bond, CDC, is gratefully acknowledged.

REFERENCES

1. Barre-Sinoussi, F., Chermann, J.C., Rey, F. et al. 1983. Isolation of a T-lymphotropic retrovirus from a patient at risk for acquired immunodeficiency syndrome (AIDS). *Science* 220:868-71.

2. Spire B., Barre-Sinoussi, F., Montagnier, L., et al. 1984. Inactivation of lymphadenopathy associated virus by chemical disinfectants. *Lancet* ii:899-901.

3. McDougal, J.S., Cort, S.P., Kennedy, M.S., et al. 1985. Immunoassay for the Detection and Quantitation of Infectious Human Retrovirus, Lymphadenopathy-Associated Virus (LAV), *J Immun Meth* 76:171-83.

4. Martin, L.S., McDougal, J.S., Loskoski, S.L. 1985. Disinfection and Inactivation of the Human T Lymphadenopathy Virus Type III/Lymphadenopathy-Associated Virus, *J Infec Dis* 152:400-3.

5. Block, S.S. 1983. *Disinfection, Sterilization, and Preservation,* 3 ed., Philadelphia, PA. Lea & Febiger.

6. Favero, M.S., Bond, W.W. 1991. Chemical Disinfection of Medical and Surgical Materials, In Block, SS. *Disinfection, Sterilization, and preservation*, 4th ed., Philadelphia, PA, Lea & Febiger.

7. Klein, M, Deforest A. 1983. Principles of viral inactivation. In: Block, SS. *Disinfection, Sterilization, and Preservation.* 3rd ed. Philadelphia, PA: Lea & Febiger. 422-34.

8. Ingraham, A.S., 1992. The Chemistry of Disinfectants and Sterilants. *Cont Topics* 31:18-23.

9. Spaulding, E.H. 1972. Chemical disinfection and antisepsis in the hospital. *J Hosp Res* 9:5-31.

10. Sattar, S.A., Springthorpe, V.S. 1991. Survival and Disinfectant Inactivation of the Human Immunodeficiency Virus: A Critical Review. *Rev Infect Dis* 13:430-47.

11. Quinnan, G.V. Jr., Wells, M.A, Wittek, A.E., et al. 1986. Inactivation of Human T-cell Lymphotropic Virus, Type III by Heat, Chemicals, and Irradiation., *Transfusion* 26(5); 481-3.

12. Hanson, P.J.V, Gor, D., Jeffries, D.J., et al. 1989. Chemical Inactivation of HIV on Surfaces. *BMJ* 298:862-4.

13. Tjotaa, E., Hungnes, O., Grinde, B., 1991. Survival of HIV-1 Activity After Disinfection, Temperature and pH Changes, or Drying. *J Med Vir* 35:223-227.

14. Resnick, L., Veren K, Salahuddin, S. Z., et al. 1986. Stability and inactivation of HTLV-III/LAV under clinical and laboratory environments. *JAMA* 255:53-68.

15. Bloomfield, S.F., Smith-Burchnell, C.A., Dalgleish, A.G. 1990. Evaluation of Hypochlorite-Releasing Disinfectants Against the Human Immunodeficiency Virus (HIV), *J Hosp Inf* 15:273-8.

16. Aranda-Anzaldo, A., Viza, D., Busnel, R.G. 1992. Chemical Inactivation of Human Immunodeficiency Virus in Vitro. *J Viro Meth* 37:71-82.

17. Busnel, R.G., Aranda-Anzaldo, A., Viza, D., and Hutchinson, S. A. 1990 Parameters of HIV inactivation by disinfectants. *Int Conf AIDS* Abstract 1076.

18. Van Bueren, J., Salman, H., Simpson, R.A., et al. 1992. Survival of HIV and Inactivation by Heat and Chemical Disinfectants. *Int Conf AIDS*, Jul 19-24; 8(2):A69

19. Prince, D.L., Prince, R.N., Prince, H.N. 1990. Inactivation of Human Immunodeficiency Virus Type 1 and Herpes Simplex Virus Type 2 by Commercial Hospital Disinfectants. *Chem Times & Trends* January: 13-17.

20. Shapshak, P., McCoy, C. B., Rivers, J.E. et al. 1993. Inactivation of human immunodeficiency virus-1 at short time intervals using undiluted bleach. *J AIDS* 6:218-219.

21. Van Houton, J., Hayre, M. D. 1991. Disinfectants and sterilants: Their chemistry, use and evaluation. *AALAS Bulletin* 30:24-27.

22. Centers for Disease Control and Prevention 1993 *MMWR Morb Mortal Wkly Rep* 42:418-490.

23. Flynn, N., Jain, S., Keddie, E., et al. 1990. Bleach is not enough: giving IV drug users a choice of disinfectants when they share needles and syringes. *Int Conf AIDS* Abstract SC761.

24. Moore, B. E. 1993. Survival of human immunodeficiency virus (HIV), HIV-infected lymphocytes, and poliovirus in water. *Appl Env Micro* 59:1437-1443.

25. Newmeyer, J., Drew, L., Minor, R., 1989 HIV transmission in simulated conditions of sharing of hypodermic equipment. *Int Conf AIDS* Abstract D.707

26. Siegel, J.E., Weinstein, M.C., Fineberg, H.V., 1991. Bleach Programs for Preventing AIDS Among IV Drug Users: Modeling the Impact of HIV Prevalence. *AJPH* 81:1273-78.

TABLE 1

Descending Order of Resistance to Germicidal Chemicals*

BACTERIAL SPORES

Bacillus subtilis

⇓

MYCOBACTERIA

Mycobacterium tuberculosis var. bovis

⇓

NONLIPID OR SMALL VIRUSES

polio virus

⇓

FUNGI

Trichophyton spp.

⇓

VEGETATIVE BACTERIA

Pseudomonas aeruginosa

⇓

LIPID OR MEDIUM-SIZED VIRUSES

herpes simplex virus
hepatitis B virus
human immunodeficiency virus

---

*Adapted from Favero and Bond (6)

TABLE 2

Comparison of Environmental Protection Agency (EPA)Produce Table Terminology and Center for Disease Control and Prevention (CDC) Germicidal Process Terminology*

EPA Product Classification	CDC Process Classification
"Sterilant/Disinfectant" (e.g., glutaraldehyde, chlorine dioxide, hydrogen peroxide, or peracetic acid-based products)	"Sterilization" (sporicidal chemical prolonged contact time)
	"High-Level Disinfection" (sporicidal chemical, short contact time)
"Hospital Disinfectant" with label claim for tuberculocidal activity (e.g., phenolics, iodophors, or chlorine compounds)	"Intermediate-Level Disinfection"
"Hospital Disinfectant" with no label claim for tuberculocidal activity includes "Sanitizers" (e.g., quaternary ammonium compounds, some iodophors, and some phenolics)	"Low-Level Disinfection"

*Adapted from Favero and Bond (6)

TABLE 3

Summary of susceptibility of cell-free HIV to chemical inactivation.*

Chemical	Concentration or percent reported to inactivate cell-free HIV
Sodium hypochlorite	>52.5 ppm
Glutaraldehyde	0.0125%
Glutaraldehyde - alkaline	1-2%
Formaldehyde	0.04-2%
Formaldehyde + β-propiolactone	0.025-.25%
Paraformaldehyde	0.5%
β-propiolactone	0.025-25%
Acetone	50%
Ether	100 %
Hydrogen Peroxide	0.3%
Betadine II	0.125-.5%
Betadine surgical scrub	.005-.025 available I_2
Sodium hydroxide	0.12%
Phosphoric acid	2-8%

Other Chemicals reported to inactivate cell-free HIV (Concentrations Not Cited)

Ethanol
Isopropyl
Chlorhexidine solutions
Quaternary Ammonium compounds
Phenolics
Detergents
Triton X-100
Tri (n-butyl) phosphate + sodium cholate
Spermicides
  Nonoxynol - 9

*References (2,3,4,10,11,12,13-19)

TABLE 4

Inactivation of cell-free HIV with NaOCl: Summary of reported studies*

Cell-free HIV in liquid state

52.5 - 5,250 ppm NaOCl (4)**

262.5 ppm NaOCl (14)

2,500 ppm available CL in 10% plasma (15)

5,000 ppm NaOCl, equal volumes of virus and blood (complete killing after 2 minutes) (15)

525 ppm NaOCl (16)

262.5 ppm NaOCl inactivated 56ng of p24/ml (time must = 1 minute) (17)

Efficacy of NaOCl was reduced considerably in the presence of blood or serum (18)

HIV in dried state (19)

2625 ppm NaOCl (inactivation in presence of 2.5-50% serum)

1312 ppm NaOCl (inactivation in presence of 10% serum)

263 ppm NaOCl (HIV titer reduced in presence of 2.5-5% serum)

HIV in pelleted state (20)

52,500 ppm NaOCl = Undiluted household bleach

---

*Cell-free HIV was tested using laboratory cultured HIV. No viral replication was detected at concentrations/conditions indicated. Results are reported as given in references. A range of dilutions was not tested in every study.
**( ) = Reference

USE OF BLEACH BY INJECTION DRUG USERS

ALICE A. GLEGHORN, Department of Health Policy and Management,
The Johns Hopkins University, Baltimore, Maryland

INTRODUCTION

In 1986, distribution of household bleach to injection drug users (IDUs) began in San Francisco in an effort to stem the spread of HIV[1,2]. Prior to that time, reported cleaning efforts by IDUs who shared their works were limited to rinsing the syringe with water before use; only a small portion reported rinsing with alcohol or using boiling water to clean the injection equipment (19 and 16 percent, respectively)[3].

Instructions on "how to sterilise equipment"[2] were developed through a combined effort of several public service agencies in San Francisco, which formed the Mid-City Consortium to Combat AIDS. The initial instructions were based on a report by Resnick and colleagues on in vitro use of diluted bleach which held that "viral infectivity is undetectable and reduced more than 7 $\log_{10}TCID_{50}$ within one minute with 0.5% sodium hypochlorite"[4]. According to Newmeyer[5], "The MidCity strategists inferred from this data that a comparable reduction in virus activity could be accomplished by a few seconds' exposure to full-strength bleach." Froner[6] further suggested that during the cleaning procedure, bleach may be in the syringe for 20-30 seconds, "ample time to kill any virus present".

The procedure that was developed and recommended by the Mid-City Consortium was to fill the syringe full ("flush") twice with full strength bleach, followed by rinsing the syringe twice with clean water[7].

The use of these procedures for disinfection of syringes with bleach were widely and rapidly adopted throughout the United States and internationally[1,8,9,10,11]. However, concerns were raised about how IDUs would interpret the instructions, and whether the actual performance of cleaning strategies by IDUs in their environment would be adequate[5].

This concern resurfaced in Baltimore when Vlahov and colleagues found only a modest protective effect against HIV for reported use of chemical disinfection of injection equipment in an analysis of seroconverters and persistent seronegative IDUs[12]. These findings were supported in a follow-up of this cohort[13], and further analysis controlling for sexual risk factors did not alter this result[14]. Latkin et al. recently addressed concerns regarding the potential for a socially-desirable response bias by IDUs in this sample, and found that statistical adjustments for "self-deception" and "impression management" had an insignificant effect on the size of the relationship between risk behaviors and HIV serostatus[15].

Insufficient contact time of disinfectant with the syringe was one of several factors hypothesized to be related to the apparent modest protective effect of disinfection[12]. Several recent laboratory studies have noted that 30 seconds of continuous contact time with bleach is the minimum necessary to inactivate HIV[16,17]. Extended bleach contact time was also recommended in recently issued guidelines from a NIDA/CSAT/CDC Prevention Bulletin[18], although the guidelines do not make specific recommendations for a minimum number of seconds of bleach contact or a minimum number of flushes with bleach.

METHODS

To obtain a more objective assessment of IDU syringe cleaning techniques than have been typically obtained through questionnaires, we recently conducted a study which videotaped 161 active IDUs demonstrating the cleaning strategies used during their last injection episode. Videotaping allowed us to obtain bleach contact time, and quantify techniques intrinsic to the IDU environment. Since the taping was conducted prior to the publication of the new NIDA/CSAT/CDC guidelines, the videotape analysis allowed us to evaluate the concordance of cleaning strategies with the original Mid-City guidelines, and to determine the proportion of IDUs whose current practices approximate the new NIDA/CSAT/CDC guidelines. Each cleaning segment was viewed and scored by a trained coder according to a standard protocol of decision rules. Multi-lap stopwatches were used to measure time variables. Detailed interviews were conducted in conjunction with the videotaping. A complete description of this study and results has been reported previously[19].

RESULTS

Among the 161 study participants, 144 (89%) were male, 150 (93%) were black, and the median age was 38.5 years old (range: 25.2 to 64.1); 79 (49%) had less than 12 years of education, and 134 (83%) reported < $2500 of legal income in the prior six months (Table 1). By HIV status, 110 (68%) were seronegative, 33 (21%) were seropositive, and 33 (21%) were known seroconverters since 1988. In terms of drug use, the median duration of drug use was 17.5 years (range: 4 to 47). All had injected during the past six months; the proportion who injected less than weekly was 20%, weekly was 22% and at least once a day was 58%.

Of the 161, 15 (9%) denied needle cleaning procedures the last time they injected because their needles were new; these subjects were excluded from further analysis. Of the 146 who reported any needle cleaning, 61 (42%) did not use full strength bleach. Of the 61, 55 (90%) used water alone, 5 (8%) used isopropyl alcohol, and 1 (2%) used diluted household bleach.

Among the 146 drug users who reported needle cleaning attempts the last time they injected, 85 (58%) used full strength household bleach. For the bleach users, 82% demonstrated the sequence of cleaning steps recommended by the Mid-City Consortium which was to repeat twice the procedure of drawing bleach into the syringe and squirting it out (mean number of flushes 2.2, s.d.= .95), followed by several water rinses (mean 2.9, s.d.= 1.4) to clear the syringe of bleach; 18% of bleach users rinsed the syringe with water prior to flushing with bleach, the sequence recommended in the new NIDA/CSAT/CDC guidelines. A minority of bleach users (n=26, 30.6%) filled the syringe at least halfway. During the bleach cleaning step, 66% (n=56) agitated the syringe, while 71% (n=60) agitated the syringe at any point in the cleaning process. A small proportion (14%, n=12) of bleach users dismantled the syringe during the cleaning process. Of the bleach users, 30 (35%) reported that they clean the cooker, however, none of the subjects were observed to clean the cooker during videotaping.

For the 85 bleach users, we calculated the draw and contact time per each single flush and then for total flushes (to allow for multiple flushes with bleach) (Table 2). The median draw time was 6.6 seconds (range: 1.4 - 33.6 seconds), the median contact time was 9.4 seconds (range: 1.4 - 138.3 seconds), and the median time per flush was 16.1 (range: 3.6 - 152.4). When all flushes were combined, the median total draw time was 12.4 seconds (range: 4.1 -45 seconds), the median total contact time was 18.2 seconds (range: 4.3 - 138.2 seconds), and the median total flush time was 31.5 seconds (range: 8.8 - 152.4 seconds).

Based upon studies by Shapshak and colleagues (9), we used a flush time of 30 seconds to dichotomize the sample. Table 3 shows that 68 (80%) of the 85 bleach users had a total contact time of less than 30 seconds, and that 39 (46%) had a total flush time less than 30 seconds. Table 4 examines the characteristics that distinguish participants by bleach contact time. On univariate analyses, filling the syringe at least halfway full of bleach, (OR=3.22), having less than 12 years of education, (OR=3.65), and being older than 35 years of age, (OR=3.18), were positively associated with bleach exposure times of at least 30 seconds. In our sample, bleach contact was not statistically associated with HIV serostatus. Small sample size precluded meaningful multivariate analysis.

Because videotaping is unlikely to be feasible in most field situations, we compared selected actual and reported times for the bleach users. Correlations of self-report and videotape were performed separately for the bleach step of the cleaning process, and then for the duration of the entire cleaning process. We observed a consistent pattern that the median time of self-reports was about twice as long as the duration measured from the videotapes (e.g., median time of self-reports for bleach step = 60.0 versus 33.0 seconds observed from videotape, Pearson r = -0.04, median total cleaning time self-report = 120.0 versus 78.2 second observed, Pearson r = 0.06).

Discussion

The results of this study suggest that the majority of injection drug users we videotaped flush their works with some solution in an attempt to clean their syringe. However, a high proportion of these used only water to clean the works, a strategy unlikely to provide protection against HIV. Furthermore, of those who used full strength bleach, even fewer used bleach with a minimum exposure in the syringe of 30 seconds. The results of this study suggest that the majority of cleaning techniques commonly practiced by IDUs are probably insufficient to achieve adequate levels of disinfection.

The results also suggest that the majority of those who used bleach followed the general sequence of steps suggested by the early Mid-City guidelines, the same strategy which had been disseminated by local AIDS prevention organizations in Baltimore. However, only a small proportion of bleach users practiced the more specific recommendation of filling the syringe all the way full. This indicates that while IDUs in this sample may have adopted general guidelines for bleach use, some specific practices important for adequate disinfection were *not* demonstrated by the majority of IDUs in this sample.

Additional cleaning activities included in the revised disinfection guidelines[18] were observed here; the frequency of these practices has implications for the adoption and acceptance of the guidelines by IDUs. Since agitation of the syringe is a behavior intrinsic to drug use and it appears to have a mechanical "loosening" effect during cleaning, it is probably appropriate to include this activity as part of instructions to IDUs. Because agitation was practiced by a majority of bleach users in this sample, there should be a high level of compliance by IDUs with this recommendation. Other cleaning activities, such as dismantling equipment and a preliminary water rinse, occurred with less frequency in this sample, and may be adopted less readily. The discrepancy between the considerations recently disseminated in the NIDA/CSAT/CDC Prevention Bulletin[18] and the actual practices observed here indicate the need for further education of IDUs on effective HIV prevention strategies.

Whether drug users are amenable to using bleach and lengthening the contact time with the disinfectant requires further study. Another interesting finding was the discrepancy between observed versus self-reported contact time of disinfectant. Self-reported times on average were two times longer than observed times. Thus, simple instruction on counting to 30 seconds may still result in insufficient contact times. Instructing users to rely on external timing measures rather than on subjective impressions seems prudent unless few have clocks nearby. Doubling counts is another approach, although the correlation obtained for this sample suggests that the relationship between self-reported and observed times is more complex, and such advice might be incorrect for some IDUs. A third approach derives from the data showing that the median contact time per flush was about 10 seconds, suggesting that a minimum contact time of 30 seconds might be achieved if drug users perform at least *three* flushes where the syringe is filled completely with bleach. An additional method currently taught in Baltimore involves letting the syringe sit with bleach inside it while the IDU performs other tasks, such as cleaning the cooker and getting fresh rinse water.

REFERENCES

1. Watters JK, Newmeyer JA, Feldman HW, Biernacki P. Streetbased AIDS prevention for intravenous drug users in San Francisco: prospects, options, obstacles. In *Community Epidemiology Work Group Proceedings, Vol. 2.* Rockville, MD: National Institute of Drug Abuse. (1986), 2:137-143.

2. Chaisson RE, Osmond D, Moss AR, Feldmen HW, Biernacki P. HIV, bleach, and needle-sharing. *Lancet*, June 20, 1987:1430.

3. Chaisson RE, Moss AR, Onishi R, Osmond D, Carlson JR. Human immunodeficiency virus infection in heterosexual intravenous drug users in San Francisco. *AJPH*, 1987, 77:169-172.

4. Resnick L, Veren K Salahuddin SZ, et al: Stability and inactivation of HTLV/LAV under clinical and laboratory environments. *JAMA* 1986, 255:1887-1891.

5. Newmeyer JA. Why bleach? Development of a strategy to combat HIV contagion among San Francisco intravenous drug users. In *Needle Sharing Among Intravenous Drug Abusers: National and International Perspectives* (1988) (Eds. Battjes RJ and Pickens, RW) NIDA research monograph 80:151-159.

6. Froner, G. Disinfection of hypodermic syringes by IV drug users. *AIDS* 1987, 1:133-134.

7. Watters, JK. A street-based outreach model of AIDS prevention for intravenous drug users: preliminary evaluation. *Contemp Drug Prob* 1987, 14:411-23.

8. *MMWR*. Coordinated community programs for HIV prevention among intravenous-drug users- California, Massachusetts. June 2, 1989, 38, no. 21: 369-374.

9. Mckee MM, Caine VA & Bryson LM. Promoting safe injection technique and condom usage among injection drug users in Indianapolis, Indiana. *Int Conf AIDS*. 1992, Jul 19-24; 8 (2):D401 (abstract no. PoD 5085).

10. Loxley W, Marsh A & Hawks D. Differences in risk behaviour of injecting drug users between 1989 and 1990 in Perth, Australia. *Int Conf AIDS*, 1992, Jul 19-24; 8 (2):D447 (abstract no. PoD 5265).

11. Rodriguez Arenas MA, Donoghoe MC, Higueras I, Crosier A et.al. Differences in HIV prevalence and risk behaviour in injecting drug users in London and Madrid. *Int Conf AIDS*, 1992 Jul 19-24, 8 (3):184 (abstract no. PuC 8187).

12. Vlahov D, Muñoz A, Celentano DD, Cohn S, Anthony JC, Chilcoat H, Nelson KE. HIV seroconversion and disinfection of injection equipment among intravenous drug users, Baltimore, Maryland. *Epidemiol* 1991,2,6:444-446.

13. Vlahov D, Muñoz A, Celentano DD, Cohn S, Solomon L, Astemborski J, Nelson, KE. Field effectiveness of needle disinfection among injecting drug users. *J Acquir Immune Defic Syndr* 1994, 7(7):760-766.

14. Soloman L, Astemborski J, Warren D, Munoz A, Cohn S, Vlahov D, Nelson KE. Differences in risk factors for human immunodeficiency virus type 1 seroconversion among male and female intravenous drug users. *Am J Epi* 1993, 137:892-898.

15. Latkin CA, Vlahov D, Anthony JC. Socially desirable responding and self-reported HIV infection risk behaviors among intravenous drug users. *Addiction* 1993, 88: 517-526.

16. Shapshak P, McCoy CB, Rivers JE, Chitwood DD, Mash DC, Weatherby NL, Inciardi JA, Shah SM, Brown BS. Inactivation of human immunodeficiency virus-1 at short time intervals using undiluted bleach. *J Acquir Immune Defic Syndr* 1993;6:218-219.

17. Shapshak P, McCoy CB, Shah SM, et al. Preliminary studies of inactivation of HIV-1 in needles and syringes containing infected blood using undiluted household bleach. *J Acquir Immune Defic Syndr* 1994, 7(7):754-759.

18. Curran JW, Scheckel LW, Millstein RA. *HIV/AIDS Prevention Bulletin* April 19, 1993, DHHS, PHS, CDCP.

19. Gleghorn AA, Doherty MC, Vlahov D, Celentano DD & Jones TS. Inadequate bleach contact times during syringe cleaning among injection drug users. *J Acquir Immune Defic Syndr* 1994, 7(7):767-772.

TABLE 1

Demographic Characteristics of Injection Drug Users
Enrolled in Study of Bleach Contact Times, Baltimore Maryland, 1992

Characteristic	N (161)	Percent
Gender		
Male	144	89.4
Female	17	10.6
Race		
Black	150	93.2
Non-black	11	7.8
Age		
<35	58	36.0
≥35	103	64.0
Median	38.5 range	(25.2 - 64.1)
Education		
<12 years	79	49.1
≥12 years	82	50.9
Income		
≥$2500/6 month	22	13.7
<$2500/6 months	134	83.2
No Income	4	2.5
Unknown	1	0.6
HIV Status		
Negative	110	68.3
Positive	33	20.5
Seroconverters	18	11.2
Duration of drug use (years)		
Median	17.5 range	(4 - 47)
Frequency of Drug Use/6 Months		
Less than weekly	32	19.9
Weekly	33	21.7
At least once a day	94	58.4

TABLE 2

Median Draw, Contact, Flush and Total Times
in Seconds for Bleach Users (N=85)

Activity	Time in Seconds Median	Minimum	Maximum
Draw Time	6.6	1.4	33.6
Contact Time	9.4	1.4	138.3
Flush Time (Draw + Contact)	16.1	3.6	152.4
Total Draw Time	12.4	4.1	45.0
Total Contact Time	18.2	4.3	138.3
Total Flush Time	31.5	8.8	153.4

TABLE 3

Proportion of Bleach Users with Total Contact and
Total Flush Times Less Than 30 Seconds and Greater Than
or Equal to 30 Seconds

	N (85)	Percent
Total Contact Time		
< 30 seconds	68	80.0
> = 30 seconds	17	20.0
Total Flush Time (Draw + Contact)		
< 30 seconds	39	45.9
> = 30 seconds	46	54.1

TABLE 4

Odds Ratios and 95% Confidence Limits for total bleach flush time less than 30 seconds or greater than or equal to 30 seconds by selected variables

Characteristic		< 30 seconds (N=39)	≥ 30 seconds (N=46)		
		N (percent)	N (percent)	OR	95% CI*
Bleach level in Syringe	< 50 units+	32 (82.0)	27 (58.7)	1.00	
	≥ 50 units	7 (18.0)	19 (41.3)	3.22	[1.08,10.35]
Education	≥ 12 yrs	23 (58.9)	13 (28.3)	1.00	
	< 12 yrs	16 (41.0)	33 (71.7)	3.65	[1.49,8.92]
Age	< 35 yr	17 (43.6)	9 (19.6)	1.00	
	≥ 35 yr	22 (56.4)	37 (80.4)	3.18	[1.21,8.34]
HIV Status	Seronegative	27 (69.2)	31 (76.4)	1.00	
	Seroconverters and Positive Combined	12 (30.8)	15 (32.6)	1.09	[0.39,3.04]

* Cochran-Mantel-Haenszel confidence bounds

+ 100 unit "u100" diabetic syringe - 50 units = one half full

DISCUSSION: BLEACH DISTRIBUTION PROGRAMS

T. Stephen Jones

T. Stephen Jones observed that the presentations in this workshop session and other recent research make clear the limitations of promoting the disinfection of needles with bleach as a means of preventing HIV transmission. He characterized it as a second-rank intervention: imagine, he said, that you are in a health care facility and about to receive an injection. Given the option of having the injection with a new, sterile syringe or a well-bleached one that has been recently used by someone else, who might well be HIV positive, it would not be difficult to decide what the safer choice would be. However, when there is no safer option, that is, no sterile syringe, then one that has been cleaned well with bleach takes on a different aspect.

He noted that one of the points that is probably clear by now is that there is no body of scientific data to indicate what we ought to tell drug injectors about how to use bleach to disinfect needles and syringes. It is disconcerting to be in the situation of trying to tell people what they should do, but not having a solid scientific basis for what you say. Boiling a syringe for 15 minutes will probably sterilize it. But that is not a practical option in the real world of injection drug use.

Some general principles about how to disinfect syringes with bleach are known, however: reducing the bioburden--the amount of blood or other material that will interfere with the effectiveness of the bleach--is important; contact time is very important (longer is better); agitating the syringe is beneficial because it mixes things up and increases the contact time; and multiple repetitions are also beneficial. About compliance: the larger the number of steps involved, the greater the chance of only partial compliance, suggesting that bleach protocols must be simplified into something that is teachable and do-able in the field.

Finally, Jones said, to the extent that there is not a solid base of information regarding how it should be used in the field, bleach will remain a second-rank intervention for preventing the spread of HIV among drug injectors. It this regard, it should be kept in mind that the more readily available sterile needles are, the less need there will be for bleach as a disinfectant.

WORKSHOP AGENDA AND PARTICIPANTS

WORKSHOP ON NEEDLE EXCHANGE AND BLEACH DISTRIBUTION PROGRAMS

September 27-28, 1993, Baltimore, Maryland

LOCATION: LIBERTY BALLROOM A, MAIN LEVEL, Omni Inner Harbor Hotel
101 West Fayette St., Baltimore, MD 21201; *telephone*: 410/752-1100 and *fax*: 410/625-3805

AGENDA

September 27, 1993

8:30 a.m. *Light breakfast buffet in foyer outside meeting room*
9:00 a.m. *Welcome and introduction of participants*; *Description and purpose of the workshop*

PLENARY I: U.S. Needle Exchange Data

FOCUS: impact of needle exchange on HIV and drug use behaviors

9:15 a.m.	Data from Four Programs *New York City, New York* (DENISE PAONE) *Portland, Oregon* (KATHY OLIVER) *Tacoma, Washington* (HOLLY HAGAN) *San Francisco, California* (JOHN WATTERS)
10:15 a.m.	*Refreshment break in foyer*
10:30 a.m.	University of California Study: Description of Methods and Impact on HIV (PETER LURIE)
11:00 a.m.	University of California Study: Community Issues (BENJAMIN BOWSER)
11:30 a.m.	University of California Study: Cost-Effectiveness and Behavior Changes (JAMES KAHN)
12:00 p.m.	DISCUSSANT: ANDREW MOSS
1:00 p.m.	*Lunch buffet in foyer*

PLENARY II: International Evaluations of Needle Exchange Programs

FOCI: needle exchange programs in Canada, the Netherlands, and Australia; impact of such programs on the spread of HIV and drug use behavior

2:00 p.m.	Netherlands (ANNEKE VAN DEN HOEK)
3:00 p.m.	Canadian Data (CATHERINE HANKINS AND MARGARET MILLSON)
3:45 p.m.	*Snack and refreshment break in foyer*
4:00 p.m.	Australia (ALEX WODAK)
4:45 p.m.	GAO Study (ROSE MARTINEZ)
5:15 p.m.	DISCUSSANT: PETER SELWYN
6:15 p.m.	*Adjournment*

September 28, 1993

8:30 a.m.	*Light breakfast buffet in foyer outside meeting room*
9:00 a.m.	Summary of Day 1 (LINCOLN MOSES, PANEL CHAIR)

PLENARY III: Legal Issues and Drug Paraphernalia Laws

FOCUS: legal perspective of needle exchange programs

9:30 a.m.	Legal Climate: Prescription and Possession Laws (LARRY GOSTIN)
10:00 a.m.	Legislative Changes: The Connecticut Experience
	Pharmacies (LINDA VALLEROY)
	Survey of Injecting Drug Users (SAM GROSECLOSE)
10:45 a.m.	*Refreshment break in foyer*
11:00 a.m.	Canadian Pharmacist Survey (TED MYERS)
11:30 a.m.	DISCUSSANT: LANE PORTER
12:00 p.m.	*Lunch buffet in foyer*
	LUNCH SPEAKER: PETER LURIE

PLENARY IV: Evaluation Methods

FOCI: research methods and design; measurement issues associated with the evaluation of needle exchange and bleach programs

1:00 p.m.	Needle Exchange Evaluation Strategies (NOREEN HARRIS AND SHEIGLA MURPHY)
2:00 p.m.	Bleach Distribution Programs Evaluation Strategies (JOHN WATTERS)
2:30 p.m.	Math Modeling (EDWARD KAPLAN)
3:30 p.m.	DISCUSSANT: ROBERT BOOTH
4:00 p.m.	*Snack and refreshment break in foyer*

PLENARY V: Bleach Distribution Programs

FOCI: inactivation of HIV and use of bleach by IDUs

4:15 p.m.	Inactivation Issue and New Data (CLYDE MCCOY AND PAUL SHAPSHAK)
5:00 p.m.	Inactivation/Disinfection (LINDA MARTIN)
5:30 p.m.	IDU Use of Bleach (ALICE GLEGHORN)
6:00 p.m.	DISCUSSANT: T. STEPHEN JONES
6:30 p.m.	Adjournment

WORKSHOP ON NEEDLE EXCHANGE AND BLEACH DISTRIBUTION PROGRAMS
September 27-28, 1993
DISCUSSANTS, PRESENTERS, AND PARTICIPANTS

DISCUSSANTS

Robert BOOTH, Assistant Professor of Psychiatry
Project Safe
University of Colorado Health Sciences Center
1643 Boulder Street, Suite 101
Denver, CO 80211

T. Stephen JONES, Assistant Director for Substance Abuse and HIV Prevention
Office of HIV/AIDS (OHA)
Centers for Disease Control and Prevention (CDC)
Mail Stop D-21, 1600 Clifton Road, N.E.
Executive Park, Building 26
Atlanta, GA 30333

Andrew MOSS, Professor in Residence
Department of Epidemiology and Biostatistics
University of California, Box 1347
San Francisco, CA 94143-1347

Lane PORTER, Consultant
4007 Connecticut Avenue, N.W., Suite 403
Washington, DC 20008

Peter SELWYN, AIDS Program
Section of Infectious Diseases
Department of Internal Medicine
Yale University School of Medicine
135 College Street, Suite 323
New Haven, CT 06510

U.S. PRESENTERS

Benjamin BOWSER
Sociology Department
California State University
25800 Carlos Bee Boulevard
Hayward, CA 94542-3000

Alice GLEGHORN
School of Hygiene and Health
Department of Health Policy and Management
The Johns Hopkins University
733 Hampton House, 624 North Broadway
Baltimore, MD 21205

Larry GOSTIN, Visiting Professor of Law
Georgetown University Law Center
600 New Jersey Avenue, N.W.
Washington, DC 20001

Sam GROSECLOSE
Division of STD/HIV Prevention
Centers for Disease Control and Prevention (CDC)
Mail Stop E-63
1600 Clifton Road, N.E.
Atlanta, GA 30333

Holly HAGAN
Tacoma Pierce County Health Department
3701 Pacific Avenue
Tacoma, WA 98408

Noreen HARRIS (**deceased**)
Senior Epidemiologist and Principal Investigator HIV Epidemiology Unit
Seattle King County Department of Public Health
3rd Floor Yesler Building, 400 Yesler Way
Seattle, WA 98104
and
Clinical Assistant Professor
Department of Epidemiology, Mail Stop SC-26
University of Washington
Seattle, WA 98195

James G. KAHN, MD, MPH
Assistant Professor of Epidemiology and Health Policy
Institute for Health Policy Studies, Box 0856
University of California, San Francisco
San Francisco, CA 94143

Edward H. KAPLAN, Professor of Management Sciences and Professor of Medicine
Yale School of Management
Box 208200
New Haven, CT 06520-8200

Peter LURIE
University of California at San Francisco
74 New Montgomery, 6th Floor
San Francisco, CA 94105

Linda S. MARTIN, Director
National Institute for Occupational Safety and Health (NIOSH) HIV Activity
Centers for Disease Control and Prevention (CDC)
1600 Clifton Road, N.E., Mail Stop F-40
Atlanta, GA 30333

Rose MARTINEZ
NGB/Health Financing and Policy
441 G Street, N.W.
Washington, DC 20548

Clyde McCOY, Director
Comprehensive Drug Research Center (CDRC)
Dominion Tower, 2nd Floor
University of Miami School of Medicine
1400 Northwest 10th Avenue, Room 210 (D-93)
Miami, FL 33136

Sheigla MURPHY, Principal Investigator
Institute for Scientific Analysis
2595 Mission Street, Suite 300
San Francisco, CA 94110

Kathy OLIVER, Executive Director
OUTSIDE IN
1236 Southwest Salmon
Portland, OR 97205

Denise PAONE, Senior Research Associate
Chemical Dependency Institute
Beth Israel Medical Center
16th Street at First Avenue
New York, NY 10003

Paul SHAPSHAK
Department of Psychiatry - D-28
University of Miami School of Medicine
Elliott Building, Room 2006
1800 Northwest 10th Avenue
Miami, FL 33136

Linda VALLEROY, Epidemiologist/Anthropologist
NCID/DHA, Mail Stop E-46
Centers for Disease Control and Prevention (CDC)
1600 Clifton Road, N.E.
Atlanta, GA 30030

John K. WATTERS, Associate Professor
Urban Health Study
School of Medicine, Box 1304
University of California
San Francisco, CA 94143-1304

PRESENTERS FROM OUTSIDE OF THE UNITED STATES

Catherine HANKINS, Public Health Epidemiologist
Centre for AIDS Studies, Public Health Unit
Montréal General Hospital
1616 René Lévesque West, 4th Floor
Montréal, Québec, CANADA H3H 1P8

Margaret MILLSON, Assistant Professor
Department of Preventive Medicine and Biostatistics
Faculty of Medicine
University of Toronto, 12 Queen's Park
Crescent West, 4th Floor, McMurrich Building
Toronto, Ontario, CANADA M5S 1A8

Ted MYERS, Associate Professor
National Health Research Scholar - AIDS
Department of Health Administration
2nd Floor, McMurrich Building
12 Queens Park Crescent West
University of Toronto
Toronto, Ontario M5S1A8, CANADA

Anneke VAN DEN HOEK, Coordinator
AIDS Research Projects
Municipal Health Service Amsterdam
Department of Public Health and Environment
Nieuwe Achtergracht 100
1018 WT Amsterdam, NETHERLANDS

Alex WODAK, Director
Alcohol and Drug Service
St. Vincent's Hospital
366 Victoria Street, Darlinghurst NSW
2010 AUSTRALIA

PARTICIPANTS

Robert BATTJES, Deputy Director
Division of Clinical Research
National Institute on Drug Abuse (NIDA)
5600 Fishers Lane, Room 10A-38
Rockville, MD 20857

Peter BEILENSON, Health Commissioner
Baltimore City Department of Health
303 E. Fayette Street, 8th Floor
Baltimore, MD 21202

Michael BETHEA, Director of Outreach
Association for Drug Abuse Prevention
and Treatment (ADAPT)
552 Southern Boulevard
Bronx, NY 10455

Nancy H. CORBY, Co-Director
CSULB Community Research & Services
1407 E. Fourth Street
Long Beach, CA 90802
and
Principal Investigator
CDC AIDS Community Demonstration Project
Long Beach, CA

Susan COYLE, Health Scientist Administrator
DCR/CRB, National Institute on Drug Abuse (NIDA)
Parklawn Building, 5600 Fishers Lane
Rockville, MD 20857

Patsy FLEMING, Special Assistant to the Secretary
Department of Health and Human Services
200 Independence Avenue, N.W.
Washington, DC 20201

Ripley FORBES, Senior Staff Associate
Subcommittee on Health and Environment
House Annex 1, Room 512
Washington, DC 20515

Samuel R. FRIEDMAN
National Development and Research Institutes, Inc. (NDRI)
Beth Israel Medical Center
11 Beach Street
New York, NY 10013

Sander GENSER, Branch Chief of Clinical Medicine Branch
National Institute on Drug Abuse (NIDA)
Parklawn Building, Room 11A-33
5600 Fishers Lane
Rockville, MD 20857

Peter HARTSOCK
Division of Epidemiology and Prevention Research
National Institute on Drug Abuse (NIDA)
Parklawn Building, Room 9A53
5600 Fishers Lane
Rockville, MD 20857

Bernard MERRILL, Special Assistant to the Coordinator
Office of the National AIDS Policy Coordinator
Executive Office of the President
750 17th Street, N.W., Suite 1060
Washington, DC 20503

Richard NEEDLE, Chief of Community Research Branch
National Institute on Drug Abuse (NIDA)
Parklawn Building, 5600 Fishers Lane
Rockville, MD 20857

Beny J. PRIMM, Executive Director
Addiction Research and Treatment Corporation
22 Chapel Street
Brooklyn, NY 11201

Lourdes QUINONES, Registered Nurse
Substance Abuse Program
Saint Luke's Roosevelt Hospital, Simms Building
428 West 59th Street
New York, NY 10019

Margaret R. REINFELD, Director
Education and International Program
American Foundation for AIDS Research (AMFAR)
733 3rd Avenue, 12th Floor
New York, NY 10017-3204

Harvey SIEGAL, Professor and Director
Substance Abuse Intervention Programs
School of Medicine
Wright State University
Dayton, OH 45435

Ronald O. VALDISERRI, Deputy Director
Division of STD/HIV Prevention
Centers for Disease Control and Prevention (CDC)
1600 Clifton Road, N.E., Mail Stop E-02
Atlanta, GA 30333

Timothy WESTMORELAND, Counsel
Subcommittee on Health and the Environment
2415 Rayburn House Office Building
Washington, DC 20515

Linda WRIGHT-DeAGUERO
Division of STD/HIV Prevention
Centers for Disease Control and Prevention (CDC)
Mail Stop E-44, 1600 Clifton Road, N.E.
Atlanta, GA 30333

EDITOR

Jean SHIRHALL
Center for Substance Abuse Research (CESAR)
University of Maryland
4321 Hartwick Road, Suite 501
College Park, MD 20740

TRANSCRIPTIONIST

Romelle MILLION
Million Reporting
P.O. Box 2419
Alexandria, VA 22301

PANEL ON NEEDLE EXCHANGE AND BLEACH DISTRIBUTION PROGRAMS

Lincoln E. MOSES (CHAIR), Professor
Department of Statistics
Stanford University, Sequoia Hall
Stanford, CA 94305

Ronald S. BROOKMEYER, Professor
Department of Biostatistics
School of Hygiene & Public Health
The Johns Hopkins University
615 North Wolfe Street
Baltimore, MD 21205-3179

Lawrence S. BROWN, Jr. **[unable to attend]**
Assistant Clinical Professor of Medicine
Department of Medicine, Harlem Hospital
College of Physicians and Surgeons, Columbia University
New York, NY 10035
and
Senior Vice President
Division of Medical Services Evaluation and Research
Addiction Research and Treatment Corporation
22 Chapel Street
Brooklyn, NY 11201

Richard F. CATALANO, Jr., Associate Director
Social Development Research Group
University of Washington
146 North Canal Street, Suite 211
Seattle, WA 98103

David S. CORDRAY **[unable to attend]**
Vanderbilt Institute for Public Policy Studies (VIPPS)
1207 18th Avenue South
Nashville, TN 37212
and
Chair, Department of Human Resources
Peabody College, Room 110 Jesup Building
Vanderbilt University, 18th Avenue South
Nashville, TN 37203

Don C. DES JARLAIS, Director of Research
Chemical Dependency Institute
National Development & Research Institutes, Inc.
Beth Israel Medical Center, 11 Beach Street
New York, NY 10013

Caswell A. EVANS, Jr., Director
Public Health Programs & Services
Assistant Director of Health Services
County of Los Angeles Department of Health Services
313 North Figueroa Street, Suite 909
Los Angeles, CA 90012

Mark B. FEINBERG, Assistant Investigator
Gladstone Institute of Virology & Immunology
P.O. Box 419100
San Francisco, CA 94141-9100

Herbert D. KLEBER, Professor
Department of Psychiatry
College of Physicians and Surgeons
Columbia University
and
Executive Vice President & Medical Director
Center on Addiction and Substance Abuse
Columbia University
722 West 168th Street
New York, NY 10032

Patrick M. O'MALLEY, Research Scientist
Institute for Social Research
University of Michigan, Box 1248
426 Thompson Street
Ann Arbor, MI 48106-1248

Nancy S. PADIAN, Assistant Adjunct Professor
Department of Obstetrics, Gynecology, and Reproductive Sciences, University of California
San Francisco General Hospital
1001 Potrero Avenue, Ward 6D, Room 14
San Francisco, CA 94110

Marian Gray SECUNDY, Professor
College of Medicine
Department of Community Health & Family Practice
Howard University
520 W Street, Room 2400
Washington, DC 20060

David VLAHOV, Associate Professor of Epidemiology
School of Hygiene and Public Health
The Johns Hopkins University
Hampton House, Room 894
624 North Broadway
Baltimore, MD 21205

W. Wayne WIEBEL, Principal Investigator
AIDS Outreach Intervention Project (M/C 925)
and
Professor, School of Public Health
University of Illinois at Chicago
Epidemiology-Biostatistics Program
2121 West Taylor Street, Room 556
Chicago, IL 60612-7260

David R. WILLIAMS, Associate Research Scientist and Associate Professor of Sociology
Institute for Social Research
University of Michigan
426 Thompson Street
Ann Arbor, MI 48106

NRC PANEL STAFF

COMMISSION ON BEHAVIORAL AND SOCIAL SCIENCES AND EDUCATION

Jacques L. NORMAND, Study Director
National Academy of Sciences
2101 Constitution Avenue, HA 178
Washington, DC 20418

Susanne A. STOIBER, Director
Division on Social and Economic Studies
National Academy of Sciences
2101 Constitution Avenue, HA 172
Washington, DC 20418

Sahr J. KPUNDEH, Staff Officer
National Academy of Sciences
2101 Constitution Avenue, HA 166E
Washington, DC 20418

M. Elaine McGARRAUGH, Research Associate
National Academy of Sciences
2101 Constitution Avenue, HA 156M
Washington, DC 20418

Susan R. McCutchen, Senior Project Assistant
National Academy of Sciences
2101 Constitution Avenue, HA 178
Washington, DC 20418

INSTITUTE OF MEDICINE

Michael STOTO, Director
Division of Health Promotion and Disease Prevention
National Academy of Sciences
2101 Constitution Avenue, FO 3026
Washington, DC 20418

Leslie HARDY, Program Officer
National Academy of Sciences
2101 Constitution Avenue, FO 3032
Washington, DC 20418